WOMEN'S CANCERS

---　❖　---

"WOMEN'S CANCERS is fully comprehensive, helpful to patients and healthcare workers alike. Recommended."
—*LIBRARY JOURNAL*

"Discussions of exactly what happens during surgery or while getting chemotherapy are excellent—both authors are oncologic nurses—and so are explanations of how different cancers develop. The authors suggest reasonable explanations for why people get cancer—the mix of cancer-causing factors in each woman's life will be unique—thereby downplaying fear-mongering news reports that say the cause of cancer is this chemical or that bad habit.
WOMEN'S CANCERS will benefit women and their families, and should help some beat their disease."
—*NATURAL HEALTH*

"Readers will find all the answers to questions either patients are afraid to ask their doctors or that doctors don't know how to answer themselves."
—*THE RICHMOND REVIEW*

"Between them [McGinn and Haylock] have crafted an easy-to-understand book that explains difficult medical terms and issues in a layperson's language."
—*MENLO PARK'S ALMANAC*

"This book is a helpful addition to the information resources that both women and men need. It provides the reader an opportunity to be well-grounded in important basic information about cancer."
—**Neal D. Barnard, M.D.,** President, Physicians Committee for Responsible Medicine

This book is dedicated to the many women who have taught us the meaning of courage and hope.

WOMEN'S CANCERS

How to Prevent Them, How to Treat Them, How to Beat Them

Kerry A. McGinn,
R.N., B.S.N., M.A.

&

Pamela J. Haylock,
R.N., M.A., E.T.

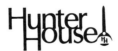

Acknowledgement is made for permission to reprint illustrations on pp. 41, 48, 54, 55, 193, 195, 197, 198, 199, by Ken Miller from Kerry A. McGinn, *The Informed Woman's Guide to Breast Health*, CA: Bull Publishing, rev. 1992; illustrations on pp. 335–337 from Judy Sandella, *Oncology Nursing Forum* 14(6): 71–73, Oncology Nursing Press, Inc., 1987; illustrations on pp. 174, 248 courtesy the National Cancer Institute; illustrations on pp. 53, 212, 213, 222, 236, 238 courtesy Susan Schoen.

Library of Congress Cataloging-in-Publication Data

McGinn, Kerry Anne
Women's cancers: How to prevent them, how to treat them, how to beat them /
Kerry A. McGinn and Pamela J. Haylock.
p.cm.
Includes bibliographical references and index.
ISBN 0-89793-102-5 (soft cover): $14.95 — ISBN 0-89793-103-3 (hard cover): $24.95
1. Cancer—Popular works. 2. Women—Diseases. 3. Breast—Cancer. 4. Generative organs, Female—Cancer. I. Haylock, Pamela J. II. Title
RC281.W65M36   1993
616.99'4'0082—dc20   92-41408

Cover design and illustration by Teresa Smith   Book design by *Qalagraphia*
Project Editor: Lisa E. Lee   Copyeditors: Anne Ingram, Lisa Lee, Kiran Rana
Production Manager: Paul J. Frindt
Marketing: Corrine M. Sahli   Promotion: Robin Donovan
Customer Service: Liana S. Day
Publisher: Kiran S. Rana

Typeset by 847 Communications, Alameda, CA
Printed and bound by Griffin Printing, Sacramento, CA
Manufactured in the United States of America

101120

9 8 7 6 5 4 3 2   First edition

Contents

❖

Acknowledgments

No book—especially one as extensive as this—happens without plenty of help. There are many people who helped in pulling it together, and our special thanks go to:

—the following health and social work professionals for the interviews they graciously gave: Susan Diamond, L.C.S.W., psychotherapist, group therapist, Stanford University; Lyssa Friedman, R.N., O.C.N., oncology nurse, Pacific Hematology-Oncology, San Francisco; Jerold Green, M.D., radiation oncologist, California Pacific Medical Center (CPMC); I. Craig Henderson, M.D., chief, Oncology Center, University of California, San Francisco; Peter Richards, M.D., oncologic surgeon, CPMC; Diane Scott, R.N., Ph.D., nurse-psychotherapist for women with cancer, San Francisco; Helene Smith, Ph.D., researcher/director, Geraldine Brush Cancer Research Institute, San Francisco; Ange Stephens, M.F.C.C., clinical director, Cancer Support Community, San Francisco; and Kelly Van Bokkelen, M.S.W., social worker, radiation oncology, CPMC;

—members of several cancer support groups from the Cancer Support Community who generously shared their stories and expertise;

—Theresa Koetters, R.N., M.S.N., oncology specialist, who efficiently and helpfully reviewed the manuscript; and Saskia Thiadens, R.N., founder of the National Lymphedema Network, and Bryant A. Toth, M.D., reconstructive surgeon, CPMC, for reviewing specific sections;

—artist Susan Schoen, who drew the original illustrations;

—our publisher Kiran Rana, who believed in the project, and Lisa Lee, our editor, who kept pushing gently.

We also thank each other for mutual support and, last—but definitely not least—we thank our families who put up with all the tribulations of being around authors on deadline.

Important Notice

The material in this book is intended to provide a review of information regarding the cancers that affect women. Every effort has been made to provide accurate and dependable information, including an overview of what is new and often speculative, and a review of unconventional and unproven therapies. The contents of this book have been compiled by professional research and in consultation with medical professionals. However, healthcare professionals have differing opinions and advances in medical and scientific research are made very quickly, so that some of the information may become outdated.

Therefore, the publisher, authors, editors, and professionals quoted in the book cannot be held responsible for any error, omission, or dated material. The treatments described should be undertaken *only* under the guidance of a licensed healthcare practitioner. The authors and publisher assume no responsibility for any outcome of the use of any of these treatments in a program of self-care or under the care of a licensed practitioner. If you have questions concerning your care or treatment, or about the application of the treatments described in this book, consult your healthcare professional.

Foreword

❖

Cancer touches each of our lives in some way. It directly affects one in four families, and the incidence of women's cancer, especially breast and lung cancer, is on the rise. To change this, women must feel empowered to make a difference in their personal health care. Early detection and prevention can work if women consistently use resources like regular checkups, and self-care methods like breast self-examination.

Cancer is one of the most feared diseases in the United States. A diagnosis of cancer is a major blow and thoughts of therapy raise doubt and concern. Cancer care was once limited in scope, with few choices and questionable chances of success. Today, combinations of new therapies improve survival rates for some types of cancer, but making the "right" treatment choices is still difficult. Never before has the need to understand options and gather accurate information been so great.

Current healthcare systems are also often confusing and sometimes impossible to understand. At one time, a single physician cared for individuals and families throughout their lifetime. They knew each other well and usually formed a strong personal bond. Now, many specialists care for different aspects of our health, and insurance carriers, instead of us, often choose these healthcare providers. Ultimately, we are left feeling cold and distanced from our health care, instead of feeling taken care of. A Massachusetts mother describes the situation well when she says, "My daughter was under the care of an oncologist, a neurologist, an endocrinologist, a surgeon, an internist, and a radiation oncologist, but no one was addressing her pain." Understanding how to make the system work effectively for each individual is indeed a challenge.

It is no surprise that cancer changes a person's life forever. Women who are diagnosed with it often feel uncertainty, fear, and a profound sense of loss. Without time to deal with these emotions, a person must consider different treatment options and make quick decisions under a great deal of pressure. Further, it is rare to be faced with only a single right decision. Instead, a series of choices confronts the already confused and overwhelmed person dealing with cancer. Only by approaching cancer and its treatment options with accurate information and an understanding of your personal lifestyle and life goals can you reduce anxiety and fear, and make positive changes in your health and your life.

Women's Cancers is the place to start. Authors Haylock and McGinn use their expertise as experienced oncology nurses and nursing leaders to give updated and comprehensive information about the cancers that affect them most, and the conventional and complementary therapies used to treat them. A particular strength of this book is that it encourages women to be assertive about their personal needs and to insist that they are considered in healthcare plans. It offers specific suggestions for how readers can become actively involved in their healthcare decisions and avoid common pitfalls. Once empowered with accurate information and options, women can tailor their care to their individual beliefs and values.

This book also speaks to the personal experience of cancer. McGinn and Haylock generously and sensitively share their own experiences with cancer and cancer therapy. They describe the frustration and turmoil as well as many obstacles in our healthcare system, and they give practical hints for coping with common cancer issues.

Women's Cancers is not just a book for women with cancer. Health professionals and women of all ages can learn from this easy-to-read guide and share the important information with others. In today's healthcare system, this book is an important resource for women to become knowledgeable and involved in choices that have a lasting impact on their lives.

Carol P. Curtiss, R.N., M.S.N., O.C.N.
Franklin Medical Center, Greenfield, MA
President, 1992–93, Oncology Nursing Society

Introduction

❖

Empowerment. It is a strong word—and a concept we like. We want *Women's Cancers* to be a book that empowers women and encourages them to be knowledgeable and assertive healthcare consumers. We want it to be a book that may even help them save their own lives.

What is this book about? It is about the cancers that occur only or primarily in women: cancers of the breast, cervix, ovary, uterus, vagina, and vulva. Women's cancers are not necessarily the most deadly cancers for women—lung cancer kills more women now than any women's cancer does—but they present a special group of challenges. Because these cancers attack the female organs, they seem to threaten a woman's "femaleness" as well, which is why we are looking at all of them together.

This book is for every woman who has ever been diagnosed with a women's cancer. It is meant to be both an instructive guide and a supportive friend, giving not only up-to-date information but also practical help from women who have "been there." It deals with the disease and with what it means to be a *woman* with this disease.

This is also a book for every woman at risk for one of these cancers—and that means *every* woman. In addition, it is for anyone who cares, either personally or professionally, for someone with a women's cancer: family, friends, health professionals.

We realize that no book can erase the fear that goes with cancer. But we also believe that knowing what to expect—the "how, why, when, who, and what" that goes with any cancer diagnosis—makes the path easier to travel.

Both of us are cancer nurses who have cared for many women with cancer. We have also both met cancer close-up: Kerry as a breast cancer survivor and the daughter of a cancer patient, Pam as the daughter of a cancer patient. As Kerry says,

"This book says what I wish I had known!"

In writing *Women's Cancers*, we divided up the chapters so that each of us wrote about the subjects she knew best. Thus, although we share the same goal, we write with two separate voices from two distinct sets of experiences. We hope this will give the book a richer perspective. Pam discusses the cancers of the reproductive tract, the issues of cancer cause and prevention, unorthodox therapies, and cancer as a political issue. Kerry writes about breast cancer and the other general cancer topics. While we both draw from our personal experiences, Pam is more likely to search the literature, Kerry to interview healthcare providers and women with cancer. For clarity, the name of the primary author appears at the end of each chapter.

Part I of the book discusses women's cancers in general, including such topics as prevention, diagnosis, treatment, and emotions. Part II focuses on breast cancer. Part III looks at the cancers of the female reproductive tract: cervical, ovarian, uterine, vaginal, and vulvar. Part IV talks about "afterwards" issues, such as surviving (and thriving) after treatment ends, and dealing with the politics of women's cancers.

For the woman who has been diagnosed with a cancer, we discuss what the disease and treatments do to her body, and what she might be feeling, along with plenty of practical tips for self-care. For women who have questions and concerns about cancer, we talk about prevention and early detection. We hope to erase needless fears, stimulate interest in developing healthy habits, and help women make informed choices.

As women ourselves, we have great confidence in the strength, determination, and resilience of women. We know that women are more likely than men to seek out the health information they need for themselves and for their families. However, we are also convinced that women have received the short end of the stick when it comes to healthcare research and funding. This makes us hope for politically aware and active women who will push for a more equitable share of both—so that maybe, some day soon, there will be no need for a book called *Women's Cancers*.

To our health!

PART ONE

❖

"YOU HAVE CANCER..."

"I felt like Alice down the rabbit hole . . . . "

" . . . as if this had to be a horrible dream, and if I just tried hard enough, maybe I would wake up."

" . . . as if my emotional circuit breaker was overloaded and had tripped."

It was a reunion potluck of my cancer support group sisters, and we were comparing notes on how we felt when we first heard that we had cancer. As we munched appetizers and caught up on everyone's news, we paused for a moment to look back.

"You have cancer." Such a short statement—but it marks an absolute division between *before* and *after*. We could recall the doctor's words with painful clarity, eerily etched in our memories, like hearing those first words from Dallas that President Kennedy had been shot.

What the doctor said next we remember less well. There is a blank there, or a recollection of a sense of unreality and doom, of thoughts and feelings tumbling over themselves too fast to be caught.

Take it back. It can't be true. The report must be wrong. You can't be serious! Why me? Why don't we wait a few months and check it again? Am I going to die? What am I going to do? What is going to happen to me? Even years later, the memory is still painful.

For me, the news was not a complete surprise. The breast lump just felt "different" from the many nonserious lumps I'd had over the years. I had one of those gut feelings about it, and spent sleepless nights fretting. I persuaded my surgeon to withdraw a few cells through a needle to find out what the lump was—and learned that I had cancer. To this day I have not figured out how I carried on a seemingly intelligent conversation with the surgeon and then drove myself home.

However "prepared" I was for the news, it was not enough. No one among my family and close friends had been diagnosed with breast cancer. I felt I wanted to protect my family and not upset them any more than necessary. But my wayward feelings bewildered me, and so did all the immediate decisions I had to make. I roller-coastered from moment to moment, between being in perfect control and collapsing in fear, anger, and uncer-

tainty. Some mornings I woke up feeling fine—until I remem-
bered. There I was: a registered nurse, who had even written
health books (including, ironically, one about breast changes
that were not cancer). But what I knew could not save me from
feeling very frightened. Cancer was just too overwhelming an
experience to go through without help.

There was also a vague but growing inner sense that something good ought to come about as a result of this experience.
Cancer is a crisis. Like other crises, it is also an opportunity for
us to look at what we are and what we really want. It is a
pressure-cooker that forces us to change. If I had to change, I
wanted it to be for the better.

Plainly, I needed help, and it was my good fortune to find
it. My healthcare professionals, my family and friends and co-
workers, a breast cancer support group, a nurse-psychotherapist
and others all pitched in. Sometimes I felt as if there was an
immense network of joined hands buoying me up in deep waters
during the times when I was too exhausted to swim. (Of course,
there were moments when I wanted them all to just leave me
alone!) At other times, I became part of that network, offering
a hand to someone else.

Cancer is scary for any human being. Even the word itself,
cancer—the crab—makes us think of sharp claws, pincers, and
pain. And each of us experiences cancer in an individual way,
based not only on the specific disease we get but also on who
we are, where we have been in life, and what our environment
is like. My particular combination of temperament, available
support, and past coping techniques, for instance, helps to create my own experience.

But there are common threads. Despite infinite variations
among women, most of us tend to bring some "woman-ness"
with us as we face cancer: how we talk about the experience,
how we cope, what we value. Being a woman does not necessarily make cancer easier or harder to bear, just different. On
occasion, we may complain about some aspect of being a
woman, but we *are* women. Having a "women's cancer" seems
to strike at the heart of this woman-ness, to threaten a crucial
part of what makes us who we are.

Next week, my cancer support group plans to gather again for another reunion dinner. We will laugh and cheer each other on and enjoy each other's company, as we have done together for years now. We will also mourn our losses, because that is part of the picture. We will remember yesterday—which makes today all the sweeter—and we will look toward tomorrow.

We cannot change the fact that we have had cancer. But, as I look around the room at my support group "sisters," I know that I will be awed and amazed yet again by how we have *risen* to that challenge.

Kerry McGinn

Chapter 1

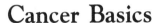

Cancer Basics

What is cancer, anyway?

It is an abnormal growth of cells in the body that do not obey the rules. To be considered "cancer," the cells must

— look different from normal cells

— divide rapidly enough to upset the body's status quo

— have the potential both to "invade" adjoining cells and tissue and to spread to other parts of the body

Cancer is not one disease but more than 200 different diseases. Each has its own personality, from slow-growing, sleepy "lapdogs" of cancers to those that move quickly and aggressively, but which may be better targets for some of our current anticancer therapies.

THE WRONG KIND OF CELLS

A normal body cell viewed under a microscope looks rather round, oblong, or cube-like and has certain predictable parts. Cells that have similar functions in the body look alike because a particular kind of cell does a specific job best. Thus normal breast duct cells look like each other, but very different from normal red blood cells.

Sometimes, in all the trillions upon trillions of cells in the body, a glitch occurs in the quality control producing a cell that looks different or abnormal or **atypical** under the microscope. The shape may be irregular, the components (such as the cell membrane and the nucleus) broken or disrupted and there may be extra parts or missing ones.

Some of these cells are slightly different, others are wildly atypical. A group of cells that is slightly abnormal is still considered **benign** (not cancer); the very deviant ones are called **malignant** (cancer) cells.

Even among malignant cells, though, there is a wide variation in just *how* abnormal the cells are. Many cancer cells still somewhat resemble the normal cells from the same organ or tissue; at the other extreme are cells that look utterly bizarre. How abnormal these cancer cells appear under a microscope provides clues to how they are likely to behave.

Cancer cells are not "super" cells. In fact, they are poor-quality cells: weaker, less resilient, and less functional than normal cells. They are not invincible and they can be killed.

TOO MANY CELLS

The life cycle of every normal cell in the body follows a particular timetable. Each breast duct cell, for instance, divides about as often and lasts about as long as each other breast duct cell, but has a totally different pattern from that of a red blood cell. When a normal cell reproduces, on schedule, it divides into two daughter cells just like itself. The daughter cells mature to do whatever they are supposed to do, wherever they are supposed to do it, and then reproduce in turn. Because normal cells also wear out and die on schedule, the adult body maintains a "zero population growth" cell balance.

If, for any reason, the status quo is upset and there are too many cells, the resulting overgrowth is called **neoplasia**, or new growth. These cells can clump together as a **tumor**, one kind of neoplasm. Tumors and neoplasms can be either benign or malignant.

Benign neoplasms include those in which older (but normal) cells pile up because they are living longer than they

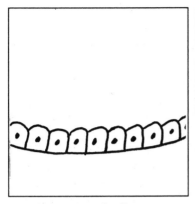

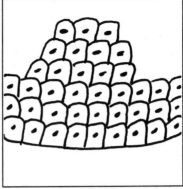

Normal cells

Proliferative change without atypia (hyperplasia)

should and/or the body is not disposing of dead cells quickly enough. As long as the buildup in cells is not caused by the cells reproducing more often than they should, this is called **nonproliferative change**. If some cells begin dividing more often than normal, but the cells themselves are normal, the result is **proliferative change without atypia** (also called **hyperplasia** for "too much" growth). A freckle, a wart, an ovarian cyst, and most benign breast tumors are examples of one of these two kinds of benign neoplasms.

If those cells which are dividing too often include some which are abnormal—but not too abnormal—the condition is still benign and is called **proliferative change with atypia** or **dysplasia** (pronounced dis-play-ze-ah—"bad" or abnormal growth). This kind of change may reverse itself during the normal turnover of cells, may stay the way it is, or may grow worse. A change like this is *not* in any way cancer, but it is a warning that a quality control problem exists which can be temporary and minor or more serious. It can somewhat increase the chance that a cancer will develop in that organ later.

If the cells look quite atypical, but are confined to one area such as the duct of the breast or the top layer of the cervix, the changes are called **carcinoma in situ** or **noninvasive carcinoma,** among other names. The labels—carcinoma means can-

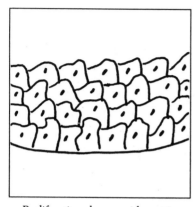

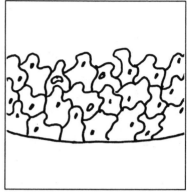

Proliferative change with atypia (dysplasia)

Carcinoma in situ

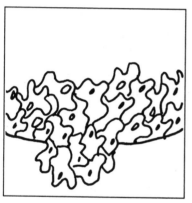

Invasive cancer

cer—are a holdover from earlier years when doctors considered this the very earliest stage of cancer. While some doctors still believe this, others believe that the cells have not shown that they are abnormal enough to behave like cancer cells (that is, invade neighboring tissues); they may never become that atypical. In any case, while the area needs to be removed or destroyed, it is not in itself life-threatening. However, carcinoma in situ does significantly increase the risk of an invasive cancer developing in that organ later.

An **invasive** (or **infiltrating**) **cancer** means that the cells that are dividing too often are sufficiently abnormal to behave in ways that can threaten the body. The doctor can see under the microscope that the cells have invaded adjoining tissues. A cell that can invade another has the potential to spread elsewhere in the body.

How Cancer Cells Behave

At best, the cancer cell is a parasite, taking up space, devouring nourishment and crowding out the normal cells. Because it is abnormal, the cancer cell lacks the capacity to function as a full team member. Depending on how abnormal it is, the cancer cell may still do some of the things that normal cells are supposed to, but it usually contributes little or nothing to the body community. It works less efficiently than a normal cell and thus needs larger amounts of cell nutrients to keep going. The cancer cell exists primarily to eat and reproduce.

What is more dangerous is that the cancer cell pays little heed to the body's territorial rules. Normal cells with intact cell parts keep to themselves, and stay at a distance from other kinds of cells. Even when benign cells overgrow and jostle or push against neighboring tissue, which is what is happening when benign tumors cause discomfort, they still respect the boundaries of other cells.

Not so the cancer cell when it gets pushed into adjoining body tissue. Lacking a normal "wall" and needing to survive in this new terrain, it penetrates and takes over the cells there for its own use. This is invasive cancer.

These maverick cancer cells can break away, hitch a ride through the circulatory systems, and wander elsewhere (**metastasize**) in the body. Extremely abnormal cells are able to plant themselves and grow elsewhere in the body, away from the organ where they originated. This spread is called **metastatic cancer.**

How Cancer Comes About

We do not know yet what causes cancer, but we are learning more about how it happens. For cancer to develop, there must be an abnormal cell, a mechanism for it to divide rapidly and establish a colony, and a body immune system that does not destroy it.

Inside the nucleus or command chamber of each body cell are 23 pairs of chromosomes along the double helix ("twisted ladder") molecule of DNA. DNA contains the general information for any living cell. The pairs of chromosomes with the DNA contain millions of genes; each gene carries the code for a specific characteristic. This genetic code, which is passed from the parent cell to its offspring, tells the daughter cell which parts of the DNA message it should read and follow: what kind of cell it is, what it is supposed to do, when to divide, and how to repair itself.

When the cell divides, the DNA "ladder," along with its chromosomes, splits down the middle through the rungs. Each half of the ladder is completed again with material brought to it by the cell's supply source (RNA) and becomes the DNA for one of the two daughter cells.

A mistake in one of the millions of genetic messages in a cell produces a change or **mutation**. The change may be for the better and make the cell function more effectively, or it may be so catastrophic that the cell dies immediately. It may also be a flawed message that can get passed down from generation to generation of daughter cells without noticeable effect. But a cell with a flawed genetic message—the atypical cell—is more vulnerable than the normal cell to additional mutations, and may eventually become a cancer cell. The more atypical the individual cell is, and the more atypical cells there are, the greater the chance for a cancer to develop.

Many cancer researchers now believe that cancer occurs, not because of a single major event that turns a normal cell cancerous, but as a result of *multiple* hits to the genes. Thus, damage accumulates until it reaches a kind of critical mass, at which point the cancer "switch" turns on. The result of a combination of hits may be far greater than the sum of the individual effects. So, whether or not cancer occurs seems to depend not only on how many hits there are, but also on what kinds they are, how often they come, how strong they are, and how much chance the body has to recover between them.

Some hits are called initiators because they can cause direct damage to the genes. Substances that produce these hits are called **carcinogens** or **mutagens** because they can produce cancer or cell mutations. Tobacco is a known initiator for lung cancer, for example, as is the hormone DES for one kind of vaginal cancer. Other hits, like alcohol, are promoters—they encourage atypical cells to grow. Then there are miscellaneous hits such as heredity, a family history of a certain cancer, for instance.

The likelihood of developing most cancers increases with age. The longer a person lives, and the more genetic messages that get passed on, the more opportunities there are for a message to get scrambled.

The total number of cells in the body is normally controlled by a balance of growth genes that urge a cell to divide and suppressor genes that tell it to wait. If the suppressor genes are not functioning for some reason, the cells just keep dividing; if the cells themselves are abnormal mutants, the result is cancer.

Cells in the body normally reproduce very rapidly while a person is growing (from a single cell to a baby in nine months is impressive!) or repairing a broken bone, or is pregnant or breastfeeding. Except at these times, cells divide on a strict schedule; they only replace those that die and thus maintain the body's status quo.

Cancer researchers believe that some of the "rapid growth" genes that program the cells to divide so frequently during the first nine months of life are "switched off" after birth (suppressed by other genes). They may lie dormant in the body, but potentially could get switched on again later in life if there is a mutation and they are no longer suppressed adequately. These **oncogenes** ("onco" is a prefix meaning "tumor") could then cause the rapid multiplication of cancer cells. But what switches on the oncogenes? How can they be switched off again? We do not know yet.

Researchers are also studying a particular gene, p53, which controls cell division and ordinarily protects against the abnormal cell division found in cancer. However, when p53 is damaged—by tobacco smoke, for example—it can mutate and begin pushing the cell to reproduce itself too often.

Scientists looking for a common mechanism in the development of different cancers have found that p53 appears to be damaged in about 90% of all human cancers. The mutation may occur decades before cancer appears and is only one of several genetic changes that move the cell along the path toward cancer—but it appears to be a necessary step. If this step could be prevented or reversed . . . .

Scientists researching p53 are looking for the "fingerprints" of factors that may have led to the original mutation. For instance, recent discovery of the fingerprint of an unknown carcinogen in the p53 of breast cancer patients suggests that some environmental chemical may play a role in the development of the disease.

Our bodies defend us against atypical cells all the time. The cell itself may repair some small mutations. Some abnormal cells may lose the ability to reproduce. Normal cell turnover disposes of abnormal cells as well as normal ones.

Throughout our lives, the body's immune system recognizes atypical cells (including cancer cells) as "enemy" and destroys them. Unfortunately, some cancer cells seem able to slip through the body's surveillance: they pass for normal or disguise themselves. Others may divide so rapidly or are so aggressive that they overwhelm even the strongest body defenses.

Or, the immune system may be exhausted or operating at partial power. People with AIDS or people on certain medications that suppress the body's immune system (to keep it from rejecting a transplanted organ, for instance) are especially vulnerable to cancer. When the immune system is stressed severely and continuously by *anything*, such as poor diet, personal losses, or relationship difficulties, it may become less effective, less able to search out rogue cancer cells and destroy them.

SEARCHING FOR CANCER CAUSES

With our current knowledge we cannot say, "Thus-and-so caused this cancer." If we were to try to indicate the causes for an individual cancer on a pie-shaped graph, we would have to draw a piece for the person's inherited vulnerability, a piece for age, a piece for possible initiators (many of which we do not know yet), a piece for a weakened immune system, and so on. Each person's graph would be different and, knowing what we do now, we could only guess at how big each section of the pie would be.

But more information about possible causes of cancer comes in all the time, much of it from researchers working at the molecule and gene level. Statisticians and epidemiologists (the scientists who look at patterns of disease in large populations of people) continue searching for common factors among women diagnosed with a particular women's cancer. The challenge for all these researchers lies in clarifying which factors actually contribute to the disease, which are effects of the disease, and which are innocent bystanders.

Every day medical stories report this or that astonishing research finding, often contradicting what was believed yesterday. Research is the way scientists verify their proposed answers to questions, but not every research study is equally valuable. The woman trying to make sense of all the conflicting medical research needs to ask:

- ◆ Was the research conducted on animals or on humans? (Humans often react quite differently from animals.)

- ◆ How many individuals were studied? (The results of larger studies are less influenced by chance or coincidence.)

- ◆ How large or significant was the effect? (Did women with a particular factor develop cancer slightly more often, for instance, or five times as often?)

- ◆ How common is the condition being studied? (It is generally not worth worrying about a factor that significantly increases the risk for a specific cancer that almost no one gets.)

- ◆ Was the study a reasonable way of exploring the question? (Did it study the right population and change one factor—and only one—that might be expected to make a difference?)

- ◆ Are there other possible explanations for the findings?

- ◆ Has the study been repeated to confirm the findings?

How Cancer Grows

If something goes wrong in the genes of a normal cell (malignant transformation), and that cell then divides, the result is two cancer cells, a doubling. If those two daughter cells survive, they in turn divide so that there are four cells. Eventually, unless something happens to stop the process, there will be a trillion cells doubling at the same inexorable rate. The time it takes for the number of cells in a tumor to double is called the **doubling time**.

Each cancer has its own doubling time, coded in its genetic message. The doubling time for one cancer may be one week; for another, six months. Barring another change in the genetic message, this doubling time will remain constant. For instance, a cancer with a doubling time of four months will take four months to double from two cells to four, but also four months to double from two billion cells to four billion.

It takes 10 doublings to reach about 1,000 cells, 20 doublings to reach about one million cells. It takes about a billion cancer cells to form a lump that can be felt. That represents about 30 doublings, which means that a long silent period—often several years—may have passed since the first cancer cell began dividing.

Every cancer has the potential to invade adjoining tissues and metastasize to other organs, but each follows its own timetable. Some tend to stay in their own local area where they can grow quite large, while others begin metastasizing very early.

When cancer penetrates adjoining tissues within the organ where it started, this is called **local invasion**. The logical way to treat a local problem is with local therapies: removing the cancer cells surgically or destroying them in that area with controlled high-energy nuclear beams of **radiation therapy**.

If the cancer cells continue to invade neighboring tissues, they may reach a new organ (ovarian cancer cells may begin invading the nearby bladder, for instance). This is called **regional extension**, and it can sometimes be treated at the same time and/or with the same therapies as a local invasion.

CANCER METASTASIS

Much more serious is **distant metastasis,** which occurs when cancer cells break off from the parent tumor, transplant themselves to another organ, and continue doubling there. This continues to be the same kind of cancer, though. For example, if breast cancer spreads to the lung, it still looks, behaves like, and *is*, breast cancer; it does not behave like a cancer which started in the lung.

How do cancer cells get to distant organs? Either one of the body's two parallel circulatory systems can be a possible route for metastasis: the **artery-vein system** and the **lymphatic system.**

To feed their voracious appetites, cancer tumors develop their own connections with the body's artery-vein blood supply and may even develop new blood vessels of their own, a process called **angiogenesis.** Some cancer cells may then invade the blood vessel walls, break off, and travel through the veins, arteries, and smaller blood vessels until they reach receptive tissue. Most either die a natural cell death, are hunted down and killed by specific kinds of defender blood cells, or never find an appropriate place to settle.

Currently, unless doctors know that there is a distant metastasis, they cannot be certain whether cells from an invasive cancer have made their way into the bloodstream. When they look at slides of the tumor under a microscope, however, they may be able to make a knowledgeable guess based on the blood supply near the cancer.

In the lymphatic system, a fluid called lymph flows through a network of small vessels, scavenging and draining substances that the body recognizes as used up, foreign, or dangerous. A series of lymph-nodes, way-stations along the lymph system, filter the lymph. They trap, and often destroy escaping cancer cells. Circulating white blood cells in the lymphatic system also kill cancer cells. The lymph eventually empties into a large vein near the heart and thus joins the artery-vein system.

The lymph nodes are a fall-back defense system for the body. When a lymph node is positive for cancer (has cancer cells in it as seen under a microscope), that may mean that it has trapped cancer cells that have strayed from the original organ.

Unless there is clear evidence of distant metastasis it is impossible to know whether any cancer cells have evaded this filter system. The more positive lymph nodes there are, however, and the more cancer cells there are in each one, the greater the chance that some cancer cells have escaped, although it may be years before a metastasis shows itself.

If medical **oncologists** (cancer doctors) either know that there is distant metastasis or suspect that there might be cancer cells in transit that could eventually establish a distant colony, they may prescribe systemic treatment, which treats the whole body and backs up the body's own defenses. **Chemotherapy** uses powerful medicines to kill rapidly-dividing cells (such as cancer cells) anywhere in the body. **Hormone therapy** changes the hormone balance in the body to create a hostile environment for cancer cells. **Biological therapy** bolsters the body's own defenses so they are better able to destroy cancer.

Obviously, the best strategy for beating cancer is to prevent it. Until we learn how to prevent it, we must try to detect and treat it early, before any cancer cells have a chance to metastasize. If some cancer cells escape from the organ where they originate, we try to destroy them before they can settle and grow in a vital organ, an organ necessary for life. (Women's cancers—breast and gynecological cancers—do not arise in vital organs.) Cure is possible up until this point. Even in the case of distant metastasis, treatment can often buy a woman time, comfort, and a good quality of life. And sometimes more . . . .

Some of our weapons against cancer have been around for centuries. Some are as new as today. Having them all available and being open to whatever new ones tomorrow brings gives a woman a real chance of surviving cancer.

"Died in her sleep . . . natural causes . . . age 102?"
Why not?

Kerry McGinn

Chapter 2

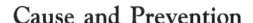

Cause and Prevention

In each section of this book, we will describe risk factors that are linked to specific women's cancers. But there are many other cancers which women are susceptible to that will affect them in some way. Women, as family members, are also likely to be affected by the cancer of loved ones—friends, husbands, children, sisters, and relatives. So, in this chapter, we have included a basic, general overview of known risk factors related to the development of cancer, and information on what you can do to help prevent cancer.

Sometimes it seems like everything causes cancer. Cigarette smoke almost certainly causes cancers, despite the tobacco industry's claims that it does not. This is pretty frightening for those of us who have inhaled second-hand smoke over many years. We know that toxic chemicals cause cancer, and that there are several carcinogenic pollutants in rivers, lakes, drinking water, and the air. Too late to do anything about it, I discovered I had been exposed to asbestos dust throughout my childhood. It is entirely possible that the fresh country air in Iowa where I grew up was loaded with toxins from farm supplies—fertilizers, pesticides, and weed killers. Just when I thought I had found an acceptable diet soda, I learned that saccharine may cause cancer. More recently, and more critical to my current tastes, I read that wine can be related to the development of breast cancer. The good news is that red wine might prevent some forms of heart disease.

Is there anything any of us can do to decrease our risk of

getting cancer? Sure there is. But, again, keep in mind that cancer results from a combination of factors: heredity, exposure to toxic chemicals and environmental hazards, and most important of all, personal and social habits, such as cigarette smoking, alcohol consumption, and a high-fat diet. Just as there is no one cause of cancer, there is not likely to be one cure.

When we talk about cancer prevention, we mean taking action to get rid of or limit exposure to risk factors, to avoid the additive effects that might lead to cancer. Many people are both skeptical and fatalistic. A common response is, "Why should I go to great lengths to change if I am going to get cancer anyway?" Others say things like, "I've got to die from something—it might as well be cancer." (This response often comes from people who are reluctant, for whatever reasons, to give up smoking.) It is true that we usually cannot prove beyond a shadow of a doubt that some thing or event causes cancer. Much of the evidence we have is based on the effects of substances on animals, and transferring those results to humans is difficult and not completely accurate.

Many studies suggest that 80–90% of all cancers are due to lifestyle and occupational exposures. Most people agree on the need to regulate exposure to environmental carcinogens, but disagree on who should impose the regulations and how and what to regulate. Lifestyle exposures are determined by individual choice, circumstance, or both. Decisions about what risks are acceptable are personal and, hopefully, can be made with good, solid facts and information. Each person needs to consider the relative risks that go with certain choices, certain exposures.

For example, the decision to smoke cigarettes must be considered in light of the risks associated with smoking: the chance of nicotine addiction, the certainty of lung damage, and the possibilities of heart disease, lung cancer, cervical cancer, mouth, nose, and throat cancers, and bladder cancer. In other words, the "relative risk" associated with cigarette smoking is pretty high. On the other hand, the relative risk that goes with using the artificial sweetener saccharin is probably quite low. Rat studies used to define the cancer-causing potential of saccharin involved massive doses over a short timespan—much more than a human would consume in a lifetime.

The occurrence of different types of cancer varies in different countries. Different ethnic and cultural groups have their own social, dietary and environmental risk factors. Migrant populations develop types of cancer that are characteristic of where they live, rather than those of their ethnic group. For example, native Japanese have a higher incidence of stomach cancer but lower rates of colon cancer compared to Americans. After one or two generations in America, Japanese-Americans have the same, lower incidence of cancer of the stomach and higher incidence of colon cancer affecting other American populations.

TOBACCO

Making the decision *not* to smoke cigarettes is the major thing any woman can do to decrease her chance of developing cancer. Although we do not know what causes *all* cancers, we do know that tobacco is the major carcinogen in industrialized nations. The risk of lung cancer is ten times greater by middle age for smokers versus lifelong nonsmokers. Cigarette smoking is also linked to cancers of the mouth, larynx (voicebox), pharynx, esophagus, bladder, pancreas, kidney, stomach, and liver. Smokeless tobacco (chewing tobacco and snuff) is related to cancers of the mouth. *At least 85% of lung cancer deaths and 30% of all cancer deaths are caused by smoking tobacco.*

This means that of the 170,000 people in the U.S. diagnosed with lung cancer every year, 136,000 cases were preventable. Each year, 66,000 women are diagnosed with lung cancer, and 53,000 women die from it. It is a shame to think that somewhere around 53,000 women *every year* would not die from lung cancer if they only did not smoke. Some molecular biology studies suggest that women might be more susceptible to the carcinogens in tobacco smoke than men—making smoking even more dangerous for women. Tobacco and alcohol used in combination create a higher risk for cancer than when either substance is used alone. In other words, a woman who smokes and drinks alcohol is more likely to develop a cancer than another woman who drinks alcohol but does not smoke.

So what about those people we all know who smoke and never get cancer? Everyone has a story about a relative or friend who smoked a couple of packs a day, lived to a ripe old age, and died of "natural causes." We also know of people who have never smoked who get lung cancer, but most of these are linked to industrial exposures like asbestos. These individuals do throw a wrench into the theory, but they are exceptions to the rule.

Ironically, thousands of women are up in arms about claims that the government has not funded studies on breast cancer and other diseases that affect women—yet, almost 30% of American women continue to smoke (probably a larger percentage in European countries) and continue to be exploited by the tobacco industry. Although thousands of women are affected by breast cancer, most can be treated. Many *more* women die from lung cancer. Lung cancers are not usually found early, and most cannot be effectively treated. Most lung cancers and at least 30% of other cancers could be prevented by women changing only *one* thing—stopping smoking.

People who quit smoking, regardless of age, live longer than people who continue to smoke. Smokers who quit before they are fifty have half the risk of dying in the next 15 years compared with those who continue to smoke. Quitting smoking decreases risks of cancers of the lung, larynx, mouth, pancreas, bladder, and cervix. Keep in mind, too, that stopping smoking can also help prevent other serious diseases: heart disease and strokes, emphysema and bronchitis, and peripheral vascular disease (poor circulation in the legs).

DIET

Both undernutrition and overnutrition have been linked to various types of cancer. Low-fiber diets have been blamed for cancers, but the way fiber actually prevents cancer is not really defined. Researchers think that fiber speeds up the time it takes food products to move through the colon, which in turn limits the time the inside of the colon is in contact with carcinogens contained in foods.

High-fat diets are also linked to cancer. As fats are digested, some chemicals are produced that are thought to be carcinogenic. Additives used in food processing in the United States and other industrialized countries may also be related to the development of cancer.

It is estimated that in the United States, about one-third of all cancers can be linked to dietary factors. The National Research Council recommends that fat intake not exceed 25% of total daily calories (the average American diet is made up of more than 40% fat) and the number of fruits, vegetables, and whole grain cereals in our diet be increased. The American Cancer Society offers seven guidelines for a common-sense approach to dietary cancer prevention:

1. Maintain a desirable weight.

2. Eat a moderate and varied diet.

3. Include a variety of vegetables and fruits in the daily diet:

   — include foods rich in vitamin A (for example spinach, carrots, sweet potatoes, peaches, and apricots)

   — include foods rich in vitamin C (for example oranges, grapefruit, strawberries, red and green peppers)

   — include cruciferous vegetables (for example cabbage, broccoli, brussel sprouts, kohlrabi, and cauliflower).

4. Increase fiber intake to 20–30 grams per day by eating whole grain cereals, fresh fruits, and vegetables.

5. Reduce total fat intake to less than 25% of caloric intake by substituting low-fat for high-fat foods.

6. Reduce consumption of alcohol.

7. Limit consumption of salt-cured, smoked, and nitrite-cured foods (for example, sausage, bacon, lunch meats, hot dogs, fried meat, and fried fish).

ENVIRONMENT

Our environment includes where we live and work, and most cancers in the United States seem to be linked in some way to our physical surroundings. Certain occupations have known cancer risks: chemicals and other substances used in some industries are known to cause cancer. For example, arsenic compounds are linked to lung and skin cancer. Aromatic amines, manmade chemicals used in dye and drug manufacturing, increase the risk of bladder cancer. Asbestos is a factor in several cancers, including lung cancer—especially mesothelioma. The additive effects of asbestos and tobacco smoke are especially deadly. Dioxin from chemical plant emissions or inadequate chemical waste disposal and pesticide residues in food products are environmental exposures that may or may not be contributors to the overall human cancer problem. These exposures are manmade and therefore should be controllable through regulatory safeguards.

Radiation

Radiation exposure increases the risk of leukemia and cancers of the breast and lung. Sources of radiation occur in the natural environment in minerals like radon, uranium, and radium. As these sources decay naturally some radiation is released into the air and water. We can be exposed to radiation through foods or water contaminated by a radioactive substance. Other types of radiation can be breathed in through the respiratory system—as people in Nevada discovered after early nuclear bomb testing.

Minor exposure to radiation occurs through diagnostic X-rays and use of radioactive substances in treatment, but the risk of developing cancer from a diagnostic test is estimated to be one out of a million tests per year. Even though the risk is low, there is concern about the risk of radiation exposure. Medical centers take care to select people who truly need diagnostic X-rays and limit routine procedures where the risks outweigh the benefits.

Radon, a gas that occurs in nature as a decay product of radium and uranium, has been recognized as a possible cause of lung cancer. It is present in nearly all soil and rock, and may be linked to lung cancer in people who mine uranium and other underground minerals. Radon is carried indoors with air that passes from the soil into a building. Many houses built on certain geologic formations, such as the Reading Prong in Pennsylvania, have been found to have high radon levels. In seven states surveyed by the Environmental Protection Agency (EPA), nearly one of three houses had high radon levels. Advisory warnings were issued from the U.S. Public Health Service in 1988 that urged housing testing for radon. You can contact the EPA for the pamphlet "A Citizen's Guide to Radon," which provides guidelines for monitoring and sets a national standard for the annual average radon concentration in the living space of homes. Copies of the pamphlet are available directly from EPA offices. Radon detection services can be located through county building departments and through listings in local telephone directories and yellow pages.

Cancers related to exposure to radiation include cancers of the breast, thyroid, and blood-forming tissues. Certain leukemias have been related to radiation, and most of them occur two to four years after the exposure. The occurrence of certain tumors and blood-system cancers increased after the use of the atomic bomb in Japan near the end of World War II. A similar increase in the rate of radiation-related cancers is already being observed as a result of the 1986 nuclear accident in Chernobyl, in the former Soviet Union.

Ultraviolet radiation sources include the sun and industrial equipment like welding arcs and germicidal lights. It is thought that this radiation causes damage to DNA and eventually leads to skin cancer.

Exposure to sun

Most of the 600,000 cases of skin cancers diagnosed each year are thought be related to exposure to sun and there is some speculation that the diminishing size of the ozone layer will increase skin cancer rates. Most of these cancers (the majority of which are basal cell or squamous cell cancers) are both preventable and curable. Melanoma is a serious skin cancer that is not as amenable to treatment as other forms. Risk factors for all skin cancers include excessive exposure to the sun, fair skin, and occupational exposure to coal tar, pitch, creosote, arsenic compounds, or radium. Skin cancer incidence is very low among blacks and more common in people with light skin who live near the equator. There is a link between severe sunburns during childhood and the development of melanoma later in life.

Preventing skin cancer starts with limiting exposure to the sun's ultraviolet rays. The sun's rays are strongest from 10 A.M.– 3 P.M. and exposure at these times should be avoided. Sunscreens should be used and reapplied frequently. It is especially important to protect children from sunburn, not forgetting that they need sunglasses to protect their eyes, too.

Skin cancer presents an interesting cultural dilemma. It has become very fashionable—particularly among Caucasians— to have what is marketed as a "deep, dark tan." Teenage women seem particularly susceptible to the marketing of this idea. In one study, people 30 and younger were surveyed about their use of sunscreens and knowledge of sun protection factors and sun exposure risks. The study showed that knowing the risks did not improve their use of sunscreens. Yet the incidence of melanoma has continued to increase at the rate of 4% each year since 1973.

Electromagnetic fields

Electromagnetic fields are created by the flow of alternating electric current (AC). People are exposed to electric frequencies ranging from "extremely low frequency" (ELF) to radio, television, radar and microwave frequencies, ultraviolet rays, and X-rays, to the high end of the range, the high-energy ionizing radiation that both causes and cures cancers! Electric fields are easily shielded by all kinds of materials, including buildings and human bodies. Magnetic fields pass through most of these substances. Studies of the health effects of electromagnetic fields focus on the magnetic field, which is assumed most likely to have biologic effects.

The first scientific study of a link between electromagnetic fields and cancer was published in 1979. Many studies since then suggest a strong association between exposure to electro-magnetic fields and the development of cancer, but none are conclusive. The strongest association seems to be with the development of brain cancer—especially in electrical workers and children living near electrical structures such as high voltage wires, subways, or transformers. Other cancers being studied for possible links to electromagnetic field exposure include melanoma and leukemia. One study produced weak evidence linking leukemia and brain cancer when mothers used electric blankets during pregnancy, and linking leukemia to children who used electric blankets.

So far, studies have not offered proof of a direct cause-and-effect relationship between exposure to low electromagnetic frequency radiation and cancer. The risks have not been clearly identified. The studies are confusing because there are so many other variables that could color study results. Measures of exposure vary from one study to another, and in some cases, vary even within one study. The actual frequency of each exposure has not been (or cannot be) controlled. Also, the effects of electromagnetic frequencies that occur naturally cannot be eliminated or controlled either. It is not known if there is a cumulative effect to exposures over time.

So what is a person to do? Clearly, no one can totally avoid electromagnetic exposure. It is most important to be aware of the potential risks and make informed decisions about where to live and occupational and environmental exposures.

VIRUS

The capacity of viruses to cause cancer is evident through the relationship of the hepatitis B virus to liver cancer, the Epstein-Barr virus to Burkitt's lymphoma, human T-cell lymphotrophic virus to adult T-cell leukemia and lymphoma, and human papillomavirus (HPV) or "venereal warts" to cervical cancer (see

Chapter 17). Overall, few viruses that actually *cause* cancer have been identified. As with other carcinogens, the actual agent or event is difficult to pinpoint. Current theory is that the virus becomes part of the DNA of the cells, which results in cell mutation.

Avoiding exposure to viruses is easier said than done. Still, women can decrease their chances of exposure to HPV by limiting sexual partners. Using condoms during sexual relations—even if intercourse is not a part of that activity—is an important protective action; exposing the genitals and the inside of the mouth to the virus can result in infection.

IMMUNE SYSTEM

The immune system protects the body from things it recognizes as "foreign," such as bacteria, viruses, and cancer cells. People who have deficient or damaged immune systems are more likely to develop cancer. Nearly 70% of people with AIDS develop certain cancers, such as Kaposi's sarcoma. Children younger than 2 years and adults older than 60 have immune systems that function at a less than optimal level, and have above-average cancer rates. People who take immunosuppressive drugs to reduce the chance of organ rejection have a higher chance of developing cancer too.

AGE

Many women believe that their risks for the "female cancers" decline after the childbearing years. This could not be farther from the truth. Age is the single most important risk factor for cancer. Over half of all cancer occurs in people over 65. Studies indicate that cancer in this older population, as in most other population subgroups, is related to exposure to carcinogens and other known risk factors.

Knowing that increasing age is related to cancer risk cannot help anyone prevent cancer, but it can help us be more watchful for *signs* of cancer. Spotting cancer early is the second-best defense against it—which is why early detection is also sometimes referred to as "secondary prevention."

Fewer women over 65 have Pap smears, and as a result, older women with cervical cancers are diagnosed at a much later stage of disease than younger women. When women over 65 are screened, they tend to have more abnormal Pap smears—mostly because they have not been screened often or have never been screened at all. Cervical cancer screening may not occur as regularly after a woman passes the childbearing years. Non-gynecologic doctors may think of cervical cancer screening as the territory of the gynecologist. Some general practitioners may not have good skills or any interest in gyne-cologic care. More than a few older women cannot do the gymnastics required during the gynecologic exam (bending at the waist, flexing at the ankles and knees, and flexing and rotating the hips). Doctors may also need to use special exami-nation techniques because of these normal changes in aging women.

Breast cancer is the most common kind of cancer found in women over 65, lung and colon cancers the second and third. The American Cancer Society recommends that women over 65 be examined yearly. The exam should cover general health counseling and a cancer checkup that includes examination of the thyroid, ovaries, lymph nodes, mouth and skin, breast exam and mammogram, Pap test and pelvic exam, digital rectal exam, and a test for blood in the stool.

HEREDITARY FACTORS

Some cancers occur with greater frequency among relatives. Breast cancer occurs at rates higher than expected in daughters and sisters of women who have been diagnosed with breast cancer before menopause. Colon cancer is more likely to be found in relatives of people who have had colon cancer. Some families are known to have higher rates of different types of cancer than would normally be expected. The role of environment, diet, and other factors in the development of cancer in these families is difficult to define.

A few cancers occur because a defective gene is inherited from one parent—cancer might develop at a later time when that gene is exposed to a carcinogen. Such cancers include retino-blastoma, a tumor starting in cells of the retina of the eye, and Wilms' tumor, a tumor in the kidney that mostly affects children.

Other inherited conditions are linked to the development of cancer. For example, children with Down's syndrome have a higher than normal risk of developing leukemia. Familial polyposis, a condition in which polyps develop in the colon, is strongly linked to colon cancer.

Some abnormal chromosome patterns also appear to increase a person's risk. In people who develop chronic myelocytic leukemia, more than 95% have an inherited chromosomal change called the Philadelphia chromosome. Other chromosome alterations have been noted in people with other forms of leukemia, lymphomas, and solid tumors.

RACE

Cancer rates vary among races. American Cancer Society data shows that African Americans have more new cancer diagnoses and higher death rates than Caucasians. The cancer rate is at least two times higher for blacks compared to whites for cancers of the esophagus, cervix, liver, and stomach. Some of the differences could relate to differences in lifestyle and behaviors that add to the risk of cancer—smoking is a risk factor for all of these cancers except liver. Even though the major cancer sites are the same among all races, the ranked order is slightly different. Of new cancers found among blacks, lung cancer was the most common, followed by breast cancer in women, prostate cancer, and cancers of the colon and rectum. Cancer rates for Hispanics and other ethnic minorities are lower than for the white and black populations. This is attributed to cultural, socioeconomic, and life expectancy factors.

When we think about the risk for developing cancer, race and genetics cannot be considered alone. Behavior that is related to a culture or ethnic group, diet, economic and social factors all have to be taken into account. Cancer rates and survival are very often related to economic factors, like access to healthcare services.

It is impossible to separate geographic and racial factors from other factors that define a person or a group of people. People in this century have become very mobile—moving from town to town or from one continent to another. For example, the Chinese population in San Francisco, California, has a high incidence of nasopharyngeal cancer. The incidence drops in later generations in the United States. It is unclear if the high rate of this form of cancer is related to social or environmental factors (the nitrite content of prepared foods is suspect) or to the Epstein-Barr virus, which is also found very often in people with nasopharyngeal cancer.

THE CANCER PERSONALITY

Speculation about personality traits, emotional reactions and development of disease is not new. Some people believe that cancer develops, at least partly, as a result of several serious life changes, continued demands for readjustment, and the potential for wear and tear on the body's protective systems. As early as 1956, Hans Selye showed that body structure and function could change in response to stress. Work by several researchers demonstrated that negative events or negative stressors are related to onset of some illness. Some have even demonstrated a relationship between loss experiences and onset of cancer. Onset of illness in these studies usually follows experiences of greater than normal life change within a year.

Some people infer that a cancer personality exists in which the person perceives the world as generally dissatisfying and negative. Louise Hay first wrote about her thoughts on this in 1976 in her book *What Hurts*. In the 1991 edition of *Heal Your Body* Hay calls illness "dis-ease," which reflects her belief that illness is caused by an inability to be at ease with one's self. She reveals in the introduction that she had vaginal cancer, and describes her background of being raped and battered as a five-year-old child. She says "it was no wonder I had manifested cancer in the vaginal area." Hay believes that "cancer comes from a pattern of deep resentment that is held for a long time, until it literally eats away at the body. . . . " Hay advocates the power of self-healing. She is a metaphysical counselor, known for her workshops and books using affirmations, visualizations, meditation, and forgiveness.

Dr. Bernie Siegel, author of *Love, Medicine, and Miracles*, has said that the most powerful stimulant for the immune system is love, and that love heals. Many methods of natural healing derive from ideas about self-care, self-love, getting rid of old resentments and hurts, and achieving a state of balance in the body. The question that follows is, what wears the immune system down and makes us sick—ourselves? All of these ideas imply the existence of a cancer personality.

On the other hand it can be pretty hard for someone to think she is responsible for causing her own cancer. Some interpret Louise Hay's teachings to mean that a person with cancer should forego traditional medicine and instead invest her time in working out deep resentments and go through body detoxification. I am a proponent of a balance between traditional and complementary medicine. Complementary treatment has a role, but I would hate to see anyone give up their medical options while exploring methods of natural healing and metaphysical renewal.

CANCER RISK ANALYSIS

Cancer risk means an estimate of the chances of development of cancer and the seriousness of the effects the cancer would have. Many cancer centers offer cancer risk analysis. This service may be performed by a medical doctor, a medical geneticist, or a nurse. Cancer risk analysis is controversial: many doctors do not believe it is worthwhile; some think it causes people to worry more. Others believe that knowledge of cancer risks can relieve unnecessary fears by providing useful information for a healthcare program.

Risk is the possibility of an unwanted result of an event. Risk involves both the probability of the event happening and the seriousness of the event's effects. There is no such thing as zero risk—some gambles cannot be avoided, and tradeoffs are sometimes needed between quality of life and the quantity of life. For most of us, a gamble involves trading some risk for some type of gain—the "risk-to-benefit" ratio of cancer treatment, for example.

Factors that cause cancer can be divided into two basic groups: those that are under a person's control and those that are not. Risk factors can also be divided according to whether they affect only one person or are shared by a whole group.

The major risk factors that are thought to be responsible for 70–79% of cancers in people in Western industrial societies can be placed in these categories:

A. Environmental
    1. Nonoccupational
        a. Habits
            — smoking
            — alcohol consumption
            — sunbathing
            — diet
        b. Customs
        c. Air and water pollution
    2. Occupational
        a. Chemical (for example, asbestos)
        b. Physical (for example, radiation)
B. Sex differences (hormonal, anatomical)
C. Virus
D. Race
E. Habitat: rural versus urban
F. Genetics
G. Marital status
H. Psychological

1. Personality profile theory
2. Stressful life events
I. Socioeconomic class
J. Medical therapy—related cancers

(Cohen & Frank-Stromberg, 1990)

Thinking about cancer risk factors in these categories helps to develop a personal cancer-risk profile. Some risk factors can be altered to decrease the chance of developing cancer. If you have risk factors that cannot be altered, you can come up with a life plan for health measures that will help you find cancers early, in the most curable stages. Cancer risk analysis may also identify options to help people make realistic decisions about their own health care. Healthcare plans can be tailored to the person's risk and ability to live with that risk. A key point to remember is that the risk of developing cancer is not the same as the risk of dying.

A comprehensive cancer risk analysis should include:

— identification of risks

— estimation of the likelihood of the risk occurring

— some measure of the acceptability of that risk

— suggestions for risk management or control

For example, a cancer risk analysis might indicate that a woman is at a higher risk of developing breast cancer. So, she might wish to increase her knowledge and practice of breast self-examination skills. She would also probably want to have more frequent mammograms or at least clinical breast examinations by a nurse or doctor who specializes in breast care. Similarly, a woman who has a positive history of infection with the human papillomavirus will want to have Pap smears at least yearly—with testing done by a doctor or nurse who is aware of her risk for cervical cancer.

A woman with a major family history of ovarian cancer might have a screening program that includes not only pelvic examinations every six months, but also regular use of a special tumor-marker blood test for ovarian cancer, ultrasound (soundwave) studies of the pelvic region, and perhaps experimental tests of blood flow in the area of the ovaries.

We are exposed to cancer risks all the time—in our food, environment, and lifestyle. The key to cancer prevention lies in making informed decisions. By balancing acceptable risks in our lifestyle choices, we can control the risk factors around us.

Pamela Haylock

Chapter 3

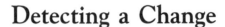

Detecting a Change

For me, it was finding a tiny lump in my breast. Something was different. What did it mean?

Finding the answer to that question is what the diagnostic process is all about. It has three phases:

1. **Detection**, in which a woman or her healthcare professional finds a change from normal. The doctor gathers enough information about it to decide if it is necessary to proceed further.

2. **Diagnosis**, in which cells or tissues from the "different" area are removed from the body and examined under a microscope to see what the change means.

3. If the diagnosis is cancer, doctors find out as much about it as they can, including how extensive it is (**staging**) and how it looks and behaves (**grading**), so that they can treat it most effectively.

This chapter is about detection. The next chapter is about diagnosis, and staging and grading.

As it grows, cancer eventually becomes large enough to produce a symptom: it can be felt as a lump, causes pain as it presses on nearby tissues, leads to bleeding as it grows into blood vessels, or in some other way changes the way the body works. On the other hand, many things that have no connection at all with cancer can cause identical symptoms.

However a change is detected, the doctor assesses it by

taking a "history"—listening to the woman and asking her questions—and performing a physical examination. Additional information can come from **imaging procedures** (such as mammograms or other X-rays) that picture the area and from laboratory tests such as blood counts.

EARLY DETECTION

Since we do not know how to prevent many cancers, we try to detect them as early as possible. If a cancer is discovered during its silent period, we will be dealing with a smaller tumor that has had less time to cause damage. How early a cancer is diagnosed and treated is not the only factor in cancer **prognosis** (the statistically likely outcome), but it is an important one.

Early detection includes screening measures that check for cancer in the woman who is asymptomatic (without signs or symptoms of disease). A sensible screening program balances the woman's risk of developing a particular disease with the ability of current tests to detect the disease at a stage where it makes a consistent difference in survival and ease of treatment—as well as with the safety, cost, convenience, and availability of these tests.

Thus, a woman considered at high risk for ovarian cancer because of family history might undergo various screening tests every year. These may be appropriate for her—but have not yet met the cost/benefit criteria for mass screening. On the other hand, it makes sense for a woman at average risk for the disease to be screened with regular pelvic examinations.

The Pap smear

The Pap smear of the cervix is an appropriate screening test for large groups of women. This simple test, in which a health professional scrapes some loose cells from the surface of the cervix and stains and examines them under a microscope for any sign of abnormal cells, has saved countless lives.

The best time for a Pap smear is at the midpoint of a

woman's menstrual cycle, when the cervical canal is more open, so that better samples can be taken. For example, if a woman menstruates every 28 days, the best time for a Pap smear is at or around 14 days after the first day of her last period. Women should *not* douche before having a Pap test because the douche might remove cells or fluid that are crucial to the accuracy of the test.

To do the Pap test, a doctor or nurse uses a small, plastic brush (called the "cytobrush") to get a sample of the fluid from the cervical canal and to scrape the outside of the cervix. Both samples can be tested using one glass microscope slide, which saves handling costs. Pap tests should *not* cause pain, but women often feel some pressure during the exam, which is usually done during a full pelvic examination. Pap tests can also detect some other gynecologic cancers by picking up cells sloughed or shed from the cancer.

A major concern about Pap tests is the high rate of "false negative" tests. A woman can help ensure the most reliable test results by asking that the pathologist who examines her Pap test slides be someone who has had training in cytopathology—the study of cells in disease—and that the laboratory doing her tests is staffed with trained cytotechnologists.

Many women develop cervical changes that may progress to cancer if they are not treated. Finding and treating these changes early makes a major difference in the survival rate as well as in the ease of treatment. The vast majority of women with dysplasia, carcinoma in situ, or cancer that has not spread beyond the cervix survive, often with minimal therapy. But only a very small percentage of those diagnosed with advanced cervical cancer survive for five years or more. The Pap smear finds these changes reliably and conveniently, with minimal cost and risk.

The Pap smear does not diagnose a specific cancer; it simply says that something is abnormal somewhere in the reproductive tract and alerts the doctor to the need to look further. Researchers are currently working to develop a similar screening method for breast cancer using a drop of breast fluid suctioned from the nipple.

LABORATORY TESTS

Standard blood tests can show nonspecific suspicious changes. Along with a regular physical examination, doctors often routinely order a complete blood count to show the numbers of red cells, white cells, and platelets in the blood and perhaps a blood chemistry panel, which measures several components of blood against a normal range of values.

If test results are too high or low, the doctor focuses on certain body systems to see what is wrong. A high "alkaline phosphatase" value on a standard blood chemistry panel, for instance, is a clue to possible bone or liver disease. Bone or liver metastasis from a cancer could cause this change—as could many other conditions that have nothing to do with cancer.

Other blood tests are more cancer-specific because they measure amounts of certain chemicals called **tumor markers**. These are proteins found in the blood after they are produced (or produced in greater than normal amounts) by particular cancers. Ovarian cancer may give off a protein called CA-125, for instance; the blood of the woman with breast cancer may show higher than normal amounts of carcinoembryonic antigen (CEA) and/or of CA 15-3.

Unfortunately, the blood tests we have now cannot trace these proteins early enough and reliably enough for them to be appropriate screening techniques for large groups of women. If the blood level becomes elevated at all, it may not do so until the cancer is beyond the early detection stage.

However, the tumor marker counts still have very important uses. They can provide additional information when a doctor suspects cancer. Often, repeated tumor marker assays can "follow" a cancer during treatment to check how effective the therapy is. For example, a CEA that is high when a breast cancer is diagnosed and then drops to normal after chemotherapy indicates that the treatment is working. In addition, tumor marker assays every few months after the end of therapy can give early warning if cancer recurs so that it can be treated as soon as possible.

IMAGING TECHNIQUES

Imaging studies provide a picture of the inside of the body. The doctor can visualize body organs without having to cut through the skin. Imaging studies, however, detect changes rather than diagnosing cancers. No matter how abnormal an imaging study may look, cells and/or tissues from the suspect area are still necessary for firm diagnosis.

Imaging studies can be used to screen asymptomatic women, to give more information when cancer is suspected or has been diagnosed, to help check the effectiveness of treatment (is a tumor gone, or is it smaller?), and to follow up over the years after a cancer diagnosis to check for any changes.

Used wisely, imaging studies can save a woman's life, protect her from unnecessary surgery, or define the scope of her treatment. They can also be overused. Before any imaging study, a woman can ask, "Will the results of this examination influence what treatment I receive?" and "If I do need an imaging study, is this the most appropriate one for my situation?"

Standard X-rays and mammograms

The most common imaging studies are **X-rays**, which show bones and certain tissues well. With the addition of a "contrast medium" (which is injected into a vein, swallowed, or given as an enema), X-rays can outline some additional organs. While they do not image the organs in the pelvis well, X-rays can indicate whether a cancer has spread to other organs which do show up well on the films (the lungs, for instance).

Before major abdominal/pelvic cancer surgery, X-rays using a contrast medium can provide the surgeon with a road map of where organs in the abdomen and pelvis are located. Thus, an intravenous pyelogram (IVP) uses dye injected through an arm vein to outline the urinary tract. A woman may swallow barium before upper gastrointestinal X-rays (UGI series), or she may have a barium enema to show the lower end of the digestive tract.

Mammograms are special X-rays of the breasts. They can

image lumps or thickened areas in the breast tissue as well as places where the normal "architecture" of lacy fibers in the breast may be distorted by a tumor. The particular magic of mammograms, however, is their ability to show the tiny white specks of calcified tissue called **calcifications** or **microcalcifications.** These accompany many completely innocent breast changes, but clusters of calcifications with certain shapes may be the only sign of carcinoma in situ or may signal the presence of an early invasive cancer before there is a lump to feel.

The mammograms done today usually look like large black-and-white film negatives. Previously, they often looked like blueprints on paper and were called xeromammograms after the Xerox corporation that developed them. To obtain mammograms, the technologist uses a plastic "paddle" to compress each breast in turn against the platform of the machine. Breast and machine are repositioned to provide pictures of each breast from the side and from top to bottom. If the doctor has questions about a specific area, magnified views provide enlarged pictures to show more detail. The procedure can be uncomfortable because the breast is compressed, but should not be very painful. Mammograms use minimal amounts of X-ray energy and are considered quite safe.

A radiologist, a doctor who specializes in "reading" imaging studies views the mammograms after they are taken, compares them to any earlier ones, and checks for abnormalities.

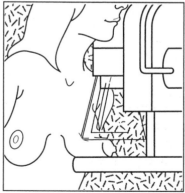

Mammography
(*courtesy of* The Informed Woman's Guide to Breast Health)

Mammography is used not only to give more information when a woman has a symptom, but also as a screening technique for large groups of women. Because mammograms can show relatively early changes—which is when cancer is most curable and requires the least amount of treatment—the American Cancer Society recommends one set of baseline mammograms for all women by age 40, mammograms every one to two years for women 40–50, and every year for women over 50.

Women who are pregnant or breastfeeding should not have screening mammograms, and it is wise to wait three months or more afterward for the breasts to get back to their prepregnancy state. However, if there is a lump to evaluate, mammography can be used safely as long as the uterus is well shielded. Women whose breasts have been augmented with implants can get clear mammograms from a technologist who takes extra views and uses a special technique to bring the breast tissue forward, in front of the implant.

Mammography is currently the "gold standard" of breast imaging techniques, but it is not perfect. How much it can be trusted depends on the equipment itself, the experience and skill of both technologist and radiologist, and the breasts of the individual woman.

It makes sense to insist on "dedicated" equipment (used only for mammography) which is relatively new (preferably less than five years old), so that it gives maximum clarity in its films with minimum radiation exposure. Generally, the greater the number of mammograms done at an institution, the better: getting the best films and reading them correctly takes constant experience. More and more mammography departments are choosing to apply for the voluntary accreditation offered by the American Society for Radiology, which says that the specific institution has met strict standards for state-of-the-art equipment and staff.

Even in the best of hands, however, mammography may produce **false positives**, in which a change which looks like cancer turns out to be benign. Much more dangerous are the **false negatives**, in which a change that is cancer does not show up. Under optimal conditions, the overall rate of false negative mammograms is about 10%. However, since most of these occur in younger, premenopausal women, the rate of false negatives in this age group is actually considerably higher. Young women normally have large amounts of glandular tissue in their breasts. In some women this may image clearly, but in others this normal breast tissue is so dense that the mammograms look as if they were filmed through a heavy cloud. A cancer or a cluster of microcalcifications may show up, or it may not. After menopause, the glandular tissue is usually replaced with fatty tissue, which mammograms show much more clearly.

Mammograms can detect some breast cancers years before they can be felt. But, because the technique is not fail-proof, the wise woman combines mammography with monthly breast self-examination (see Chapter 12) and regular, thorough breast examinations by a health professional.

Other imaging techniques

Ultrasound, or **sonography,** projects high-frequency sound waves into the body. These sound waves bounce off different kinds of tissue in different, characteristic ways. A computer reads the pattern of echoes and generates a picture from them (rather like radar). Ultrasound images the ovaries and uterus well, and is useful for telling whether a breast lump that can be felt is solid or fluid-filled. It is considered safe to use during pregnancy.

For conventional ultrasound tests, a technologist or radiologist applies a slippery gel or cream to the skin over the organ to be imaged and then glides a hand-held instrument over the skin to produce the sound waves and pick up the echoes. Transvaginal sonography involves inserting an ultrasound probe into the vagina. This can give a more precise image of the ovaries than conventional ultrasound.

Doppler studies use sound waves to image blood flow to an area. These may be able to detect increases in blood vessels around a "hungry" cancer, and researchers are trying this special ultrasound technique to detect ovarian cancer.

Computerized tomography (CT, CAT, computed tomography) and **magnetic resonance imaging (MRI)** both give clear cross-sectional images of body parts that cannot be seen well with standard X-rays, including some pelvic and abdominal structures. Neither test shows moving parts of the body well (such as the intestine), but they can provide distinct pictures of "quieter" organs.

The woman undergoing CT lies still while a CT scanner (inside what looks rather like a giant flat doughnut) rotates rapidly around the table and takes X-ray images of narrow "slices" of the body (tomograms) from different angles. A computer then assembles these images into pictures. Sometimes a contrast material is swallowed or injected into an arm vein before the test.

Magnetic resonance imaging uses a magnetic field to align radio waves and provide its pictures. The woman, lying on a stretcher, is wheeled headfirst into a narrow tube. She lies without moving for an hour or so and hears loud clicking noises while the computer collects its data. Contrast material may be given. Anyone who is somewhat claustrophobic can ask for a sedative before the test.

CT and MRI have revolutionized cancer detection and treatment because they can clearly show organs that could not be seen well before without surgery. Research goes on to find ways to make them even more useful. For instance, researchers are studying breast MRIs taken after an injection of a substance called Gadolinium into an arm vein. This may be able to give more information about breast anatomy in women with very dense breasts after a cancer has been diagnosed. However, both CT and MRI are too expensive to use for mass screening. In addition, CT employs fairly high doses of radiation, which makes it inappropriate for repeated use.

Doctors may order **nuclear scans** after diagnosis of a woman's cancer to see if the disease has spread to a particular organ. Many doctors use them for routine followup as well (a yearly bone scan after breast cancer treatment, perhaps). For a bone, liver, or brain scan, a tiny amount of radioactive substance is injected into a vein, travels through the body, and is absorbed by the target organ. A scanner then moves back and forth, looking for "hot spots" in the target organ where cancerous areas have absorbed more radioactivity. A computer assembles the information into a black and white film negative.

The injection is given well before the scan. Depending on the organ being scanned and how long it takes the radioactive substance to reach it, the woman may leave the nuclear medicine department for a time. She should drink lots of water or other fluids and urinate frequently during this period (about three hours for a bone scan) to dilute the radioactive substance, move it safely through the body and out through the urinary tract. The dose of radioactivity is minuscule, and it is safe to be around other people during this time. She then returns to the nuclear medicine department and lies as directed on a table while the scanner moves back and forth over her (or under the table) for about an hour.

Researchers continue to look for the perfect imaging technique, trying to capitalize on differences between normal and cancerous tissue. **Diaphanography**, or transillumination, relies on an intense light shining through the organ (typically the breast) to show a tumor. **Thermography** uses some kind of heat-sensing material to try to detect warmer areas from increased blood flow to a cancer. Other researchers are exploring differences in electrical conductivity between normal and cancerous tissues. In their current states of development these tests may be used in specific situations, but they have not proven their worth for mass screening.

Kerry McGinn

Chapter 4

Diagnosis and Beyond

After a change has been detected, diagnosis requires obtaining a specimen of cells or tissue from the suspect area and examining it under a microscope to see if cancer is present. The surgeon, gynecologist, or another doctor collects the cells or tissues, but it is the pathologist, the physician specializing in microscopy, who looks at the specimen and makes the diagnosis. Even if a doctor is 99.99% sure that a cancer exists because of the history, physical examination, imaging and laboratory studies, there can be no firm diagnosis without a pathologist's analysis of a specimen of cells or tissue.

The challenge with any diagnostic procedure is obtaining the right tissue or cells. If cancer cells in a suspicious area are clustered in one small spot, a diagnostic procedure that samples the wrong spot will miss the cancer entirely. Plainly, any diagnostic procedure must be performed as carefully and completely as possible.

How is the specimen obtained?

Sometimes the doctor can see an obviously suspicious area and reach it easily to get a specimen. During a routine pelvic examination, for example, the gynecologist may notice an abnormal-appearing spot outside the vagina or, after spreading the vaginal walls with a speculum, may see something worrisome inside. The doctor then takes a biopsy, snipping or scraping out a small piece of tissue for the pathologist to look at under the microscope.

Depending on the organ and the situation, if the area is

not obvious and accessible, the doctor may

- ◆ use a needle through the skin to withdraw cells or tissue (needle aspiration or wide needle biopsy)

- ◆ take a biopsy with the aid of some kind of "scope" to see better than or beyond what could ordinarily be seen (colposcope, endoscope, or laparoscope, for instance)

- ◆ scrape out the lining of the uterus and remove it through the cervix (dilation and curettage) so that the pathologist can examine it

- ◆ cut out a cone-shaped piece of the cervix through the vagina (conization, also called cone biopsy)

- ◆ perform an "open" biopsy of some kind, surgically cutting through skin to reach and remove the suspicious area

Sometimes there is not a separate biopsy at all. For instance, the doctor may perform a hysterectomy when a large tumor in the uterus must be removed in any case because it is causing symptoms. Afterward, the pathologist examines the removed uterus to see whether the tumor is benign or cancerous.

INFORMED CONSENT

Before surgery or any other "invasive" procedure and before a patient participates in any experimental study, doctors must explain what they are doing, what they expect to achieve, and what the risks and options are. Thus informed, the patient agrees in writing to the procedure; this is called informed consent. Some states have other requirements, such as California's law that all women diagnosed with breast cancer must receive certain information about treatment options.

No doctor can predict how a particular procedure or therapy will affect an individual woman. There are no guarantees. What the doctor is responsible for is telling her the statistically common outcomes and risks.

FINE NEEDLE ASPIRATIONS AND NEEDLE BIOPSIES

With some breast lumps, the doctor can simply aspirate (with-draw) some cells through a thin needle to obtain a pathology specimen. This **fine needle aspiration (FNA)** is especially ap-propriate for on-the-spot diagnosis of a lump that feels as if it might be a cyst, a benign fluid-filled lump that is common in the breast. The doctor scrubs the skin with an antiseptic, stabi-lizes the lump with the fingers of one hand, inserts the needle of a regular hypodermic syringe through the skin into the lump, and then tries to withdraw whatever is inside. This may smart a bit and may leave a temporary bruise. Some doctors inject a little local anesthetic under the skin first.

If the lump is a cyst, it will collapse as the fluid is sucked out, an instant diagnosis. If the lump is solid, the aspiration may obtain some cells for the pathologist. An alternative is a **needle biopsy**, using a larger needle called a **tru-cut needle** to obtain a larger specimen. This "cutting" needle may be inserted several times in different places to sample a solid lump. Most women prefer local anesthetic for this procedure.

Fluid that is clearly from a cyst often does not need to be sent to pathology at all. The final pathology report on cells from a solid lump may take 24 hours or longer.

New technology may make it possible to perform a fine

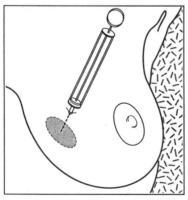

Needle aspiration into cyst

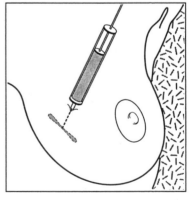

Needle aspiration with fluid
(*courtesy of* The Informed Woman's
Guide to Breast Health)

needle aspiration (or a "core" biopsy with a larger needle) for breast abnormalities that can only be seen on a mammogram, so that there is nothing for the surgeon to feel. With a **stereotactic guided needle biopsy**, a computer system uses mammogram views to place the needle in the abnormal-appearing area. The woman lies face down on a special table with the breast hanging down through an opening while several samples of tissue are withdrawn with a biopsy "gun." This procedure is relatively expensive and probably will not be as spur-of-the-moment as a standard FNA.

Women prefer FNAs because they avoid surgery and the anxious waiting for an operating room date, are much cheaper than surgical biopsies, and do not leave a scar or internal scar tissue. The drawback with a needle aspiration or needle biopsy of a solid lump is that it may not sample the right spot. If a needle biopsy is positive for cancer, the result can be trusted. However, a negative needle biopsy of a solid lump or a mammographic abnormality—a biopsy that does not show cancer—may need to be followed up with a surgical "open" biopsy in which the abnormal tissue is removed.

BIOPSIES WITH A SCOPE

Abnormal Pap smears of the cervix are graded by how abnormal the cells look. If they appear quite abnormal, the gynecologist knows that a source somewhere in the cervix, vagina, or uterus is sloughing off "different" cells, and this area needs to be found and perhaps treated. But if, even after washing the vaginal canal with a stain to show up abnormalities better, the gynecologist still cannot find anything obviously strange, what then?

To see the area better the gynecologist may spread the vaginal wall with a speculum, and use a **colposcope**, a piece of equipment which looks like a glorified pair of binoculars mounted on a stand with wheels. The colposcope provides both a powerful light and a set of magnifying lenses that can enlarge the area up to twenty times. It can be wheeled into place and raised and lowered to give the best view.

Looking through the colposcope, the gynecologist can take pinhead-sized specimens of tissue for biopsy using a instrument somewhat like a paper punch: a **punch biopsy.** This can be done without anesthesia in the doctor's procedure room. If the woman is prompted to cough at the moment of the biopsy, she often avoids the brief sharp pain of the procedure. The whole process takes only a few minutes. The woman may have slight bleeding afterward or some cramping "period" pain. Gynecologists also use the colposcope to view the area while treating local abnormal areas (see Chapter 7).

Another kind of scope is the **endoscope,** an instrument inserted through a body opening to see an internal area. Different types of endoscopes, named after the Greek word for the part of the body viewed, let a doctor see and reach into the body without having to cut through the skin.

To look into the uterus, for example, the gynecologist may be able to insert an **hysteroscope,** a narrow, lighted magnifying probe, through the cervix to see into the uterus. This can be done in the doctor's office, and a specimen of abnormal-appearing endometrium, the tissue lining the uterus, can be scraped out in an endometrial biopsy.

A doctor who wants to check the bowel wall for signs of cancer can look at it directly through a **proctosigmoidoscope,** a long, lighted tube, often flexible, that is threaded up through the anus into the sigmoid colon. A **colonoscope** is a longer tube through which the doctor can see the whole large intestine. To see into the bladder, the doctor can insert a **cystoscope** through the opening of the bladder. Through these and other scopes, the doctor can snip out a piece of tissue for biopsy.

Still another kind of scope, the **laparoscope,** requires a tiny slit in the skin around the navel (this is sometimes called "bandaid" surgery). Through this the doctor can examine and remove tiny specimens from the pelvis or abdomen. A **culdoscope** is similar to a laparoscope except that it is inserted through a small slit in the vagina rather than through the skin and it allows the doctor to see the area in the cul-de-sac between the uterus and the rectum.

Many scopic exams can be performed in the doctor's office

or a special-procedure room. Depending on the exam, the woman may need no medication or may receive a sedative. For a laparoscopy, she may be hospitalized briefly and given a general anesthetic.

DILATION AND CURETTAGE (D&C)

When the doctor needs a pathology specimen from the uterus or inside the cervix, a dilation and curettage (D&C) can provide it without any incision into the skin. In this procedure, the gynecologist dilates (widens) the cervical canal and then inserts a curette, an instrument with a sharp spoon-shaped tip, to scrape off the surface layer of the uterus. This whole layer is then sent to the pathologist to be checked for cancer cells (or other changes, since D&Cs are used to diagnose and sometimes treat a wide array of noncancer-related gynecologic problems).

A D&C is ordinarily performed in the doctor's office—almost never in the hospital. The woman has the D&C and can return home in a few hours. She lies on an operating table with her feet in stirrups in the standard pelvic exam position while the vaginal area is thoroughly cleaned with a solution to kill any germs. She is usually put to sleep for the fifteen minutes or so that the procedure takes with a short-acting general anesthetic injected through an arm vein; sometimes, a local anesthetic is used instead to numb the cervical area, perhaps along with a sedative.

When the woman is asleep and her muscles are completely relaxed, the doctor performs a careful bimanual (two-handed) **examination** of the pelvic organs, using the fingers of one hand in the vagina and the other hand on the outside of the pelvis. Then the doctor inserts a speculum, grasps the cervix with a special clamp to hold it steady and, if a local anesthetic is being used, injects this into the cervix and the area around it.

A "dip-stick" rod is threaded through the cervix to measure the depth and position of the uterus. Then the doctor inserts a tapered rod into the cervix to begin stretching the opening and uses progressively larger rods until the opening is dilated to about half an inch. Finally, the curette is inserted and the endometrium and possibly part of the lining of the cervical canal is gently scraped out. After the curette and other instruments are removed, the woman is kept in a recovery room until she is fully awake. The final pathology report is usually available within a week.

The cervix may take a week or two to close to normal. In the meantime, many women experience some bleeding and cramping. Most doctors recommend that a woman not use tampons or douches during the period when the cervix is still open. While some doctors allow sexual intercourse with a condom if the woman is not actively bleeding, many others ask her to abstain for ten days or so to prevent infection. The woman who still menstruates may have heavy or irregular periods for a few months after a D&C.

CONIZATION (CONE BIOPSY)

In a cone biopsy, the gynecologist surgically removes a cone of tissue from the center of the cervix—rather like coring an apple. This used to be standard procedure after an abnormal Pap smear; with the advent of colposcopes that can pinpoint small abnormal areas for punch biopsies it has become much less common. However, it still has value, especially when the doctors cannot tell whether an area is carcinoma in situ or an early invasive cancer, conditions that require different treatment.

Conization is done in an operating room at the hospital under local, spinal, or general anesthesia. The woman is placed in the pelvic exam position, a speculum is placed in the vagina, the cervical area is washed thoroughly, and anesthesia is given.

The gynecologist steadies the cervix by putting stitches on each side, cuts a shallow circle around the opening that includes all the affected area, and then continues to cut deeper and toward the center of the cervix until a cone of tissue has been loosened. The doctor removes the cone and sends it to the pathologist, and then stitches the cut edges of the cervix with sutures that the body will absorb after a few days.

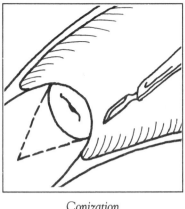
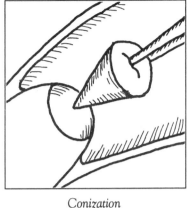

Conization

Conization
(courtesy of Susan Schoen)

Heavy bleeding is common, either right after surgery or about ten days later when the sutures are absorbed. Sometimes, a woman finds it more difficult to become or stay pregnant after conization because of scar tissue buildup.

OPEN BIOPSY

In an open biopsy to sample an area of the body which cannot be reached any other way, the doctor cuts through the skin over the suspect area and removes some tissue so that it can be examined by the pathologist. An **incisional biopsy** cuts into a tumor and takes out a piece, perhaps a wedge from a large tumor. An **excisional biopsy** cuts out or excises *all* of the suspect area, along with a margin of nonsuspicious tissue all around.

All open biopsies are performed in an operating room. Often the woman is admitted to the hospital as a "same day surgery" patient.

In the operating room, the skin is swabbed repeatedly with germ-killing solutions and then draped so that only the area to be cut shows. The surgeon may mark the area where the incision will be.

Depending on the circumstances and her preference, the woman may receive either a local or a general anesthetic. For a biopsy under "local," the surgeon will inject an anesthetic similar to novocaine under the skin; this can sting briefly. If the woman needs general anesthesia, a short-acting anesthetic is given through the vein. If the surgery will be longer than a few minutes, a tube is passed through the woman's mouth into her windpipe after she is asleep and a mixture of anesthetic gases and oxygen is administered. The tube is removed before she wakes up but it may leave her with a temporarily irritated throat and the feeling that she is coming down with a cold.

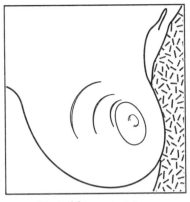

Typical biopsy incisions
(these illustrations—on pages 54 and
55—courtesy of The Informed
Woman's Guide to Breast Health)

The woman lying awake on the operating table during a biopsy probably will not be able to watch, even if she is so inclined, because a screen is placed between her face and the surgical area. As long as the area is sufficiently numbed she will not feel pain but may feel sensations of pressure and tugging; if there is any pain, it is time to ask for more local anesthetic. She will hear unfamiliar noises, like the faint hiss of the electric cauterizing wand that stops bleeding from tiny blood vessels. Some surgeons explain what is happening during the procedure.

The surgeon cuts through the skin and other layers of tissue to find the suspicious area, removes all or part of it, and sends it to the pathologist. For an immediate **frozen section** the pathologist quick-freezes a piece of the specimen, slices it thinly, stains it, and then looks at it under the microscope. This report is about 98% accurate and can tell the surgeon immediately if more tissue needs to be removed. (The surgeon who excises a lump that shows cancer will want to remove a "clear margin" of tissue around it.) For the final report, available in a few days, the pathologist painstakingly prepares a **permanent section** from the specimen, a process that takes about 24 hours.

The surgeon may stitch the underlying tissues together with sutures that do not need to be removed, and closes the skin with special tape strips or stitches. The tape strips fall off in about two weeks; skin sutures are removed by the surgeon after a week or so. The surgeon bandages the area with a protective bulky gauze dressing. If the biopsy was performed under general anesthetic, the woman usually wakes up in the post-anesthesia recovery room.

The amount of post-biopsy pain, bruising, and scarring depends on the individual surgery and the woman who undergoes it. Pain from a simple biopsy usually subsides within a day or so, and can be relieved with pain pills. Complications from a biopsy are rare, but include the possibility of infection, a collection of fluid at the site (seroma), or bleeding into the surrounding area (hematoma).

WIRE LOCALIZATION BIOPSY

What if the biopsy is for a breast abnormality such as a cluster of microcalcification that appears only on a mammogram? Since there is nothing to see or feel, the surgeon must turn to the radiologist for help in localizing the spot. This can be done either with a stereotactic guided biopsy or with a special procedure called a wire or needle localization biopsy.

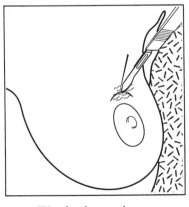

For a wire localization, the woman goes to the X-ray department before she goes to the biopsy room. There the radiologist uses mammograms to decide on the proper spot for inserting one or more wires or needles; these may have tiny hooks to keep them from moving. After their placement is determined, a little dye may be inserted to mark the spot; the dye often stings at first.

Wire localization biopsy

Wires and dye in place, the woman is taken to the operating room, where the surgeon follows the track of the wire with the scalpel and removes the marked area as in a regular biopsy. Since the abnormality can only be seen on a mammogram, the biopsy specimen is x-rayed (specimen radiographed) so that the pathologist can see if the abnormal area—and all of it—has been removed.

FEELINGS ABOUT A BIOPSY

It is scary to have a biopsy or other diagnostic procedure. Whatever the outcome, most of us feel upset, frightened, and helpless at the prospect. No matter how well we understand intellectually that this is simply a necessary step to find out what is happening, and that most biopsies reveal only benign changes, our feelings may not match our thoughts.

Many women admit to being surprised and horrified by their emotional reactions. One minute they are convinced that all will be well; the next moment they are rehearsing deathbed scenarios. There is anxiety about what the biopsy may show, of course, and every day of waiting makes it worse. To face a biopsy is to confront the possibility of serious illness and our own mortality—but it is also to inhabit an unreal, in-between time of *not knowing*. And we may feel apprehensive about the procedure itself: will it hurt? What about scars?

It is common to become angry at health professionals, family members, and friends, because they may seem insensitive or blasé about what is, for us, a very difficult experience. Professionals sometimes forget that what is everyday for them is not so for us, or they may protect themselves emotionally by pulling away from patients. Family and friends are often so scared that they retreat into themselves or behave in unpredictable ways. Our own strong feelings may also distort what we perceive.

Sometimes, though, our anger is a smokescreen for feelings that are even more painful to accept in ourselves. Thus, "I can't believe what a jerk that doctor is!" or "Why do I have to be cut open to find out that I'm perfectly healthy?" masks "Do I have cancer? Will I die?"

These feelings are strong stuff, but they are normal. It is human to feel scared, sad, and/or angry before a biopsy. Our emotions may make us uncomfortable, sometimes acutely so, but if we can look at them clearly and talk about them freely, we can also draw on all that energy to help us recover quickly. It is the emotions we do not acknowledge that corrode our souls.

It helps to know that we are normal. It also helps if we get information about what the procedure will be like so we know what to expect. If we admit we need someone to talk to, doctor, nurse, spouse, or friend may be able to help.

Biopsies and other diagnostic procedures are not fun. They are both physically and emotionally uncomfortable. But the news is often good and, even if the diagnosis is cancer, a biopsy lets us know where we stand so that we can begin to take action.

TIMELY DIAGNOSIS

Nobody wants an unnecessary diagnostic procedure. On the other hand, failing to detect a curable cancer at an early stage because either the doctor or the patient refuses a biopsy is tragic.

One all too common scenario is a woman with a "dominant" breast lump and a doctor who says, "You're too young to have breast cancer, so this must be benign. I'll see you in a year." No matter how young the woman, no matter whether or not the lump hurts, if there is a persistent dominant breast lump—or a symptom of any other kind of cancer—it *must* be diagnosed.

Waiting a month to see if the lump goes away with the next menstrual cycle is reasonable, and may well save a biopsy. Performing a fine needle aspiration in the doctor's office is also reasonable. Waiting a year to check it again is not.

If a woman has a suspicious symptom, she has a right to timely diagnosis or to referral to another doctor who can diagnose the condition. If she is not content with what is being done, she has both the right and the responsibility to herself to ask for an explanation; if the explanation is not satisfactory, she can ask for a second opinion or change doctors.

STAGING A CANCER

A cancer can behave like a lapdog or a school of piranhas. If the diagnosis after the biopsy is cancer, the doctors still want to learn much more about it in order to treat it most effectively. This involves learning how extensive it is (its **stage**) and how aggressive it is likely to be (its **grade**).

Cancer is named by the type of body tissue involved. Most women's cancers are **carcinomas**, cancers that develop in the epithelial tissues (the surface or lining tissues of internal organs or passageways). A few are **sarcomas**, cancers that grow in the supporting or connective tissue of the body: muscles, bones, tendons, blood vessels, or nerves. The kind of tumor makes a difference in how to treat it.

Staging a tumor is based on three aspects: how large the **tumor** itself is (**T**); how much, if any, the tumor has spread to the lymph **nodes** (**N**); and whether there is any known **metastasis** or spread to distant organs (**M**).

A number after each letter answers the question "how much," so a T1 cancer of an organ is smaller than a T3 of the same organ. On the other hand, what falls into each "how much" group varies with each organ. Thus a breast cancer classified as T2 N1 M0, for instance, would be between about 1 and 2 inches (2–5 cm) in diameter, would have one or more lymph nodes from the armpit that show some cancer but not so much that they cannot move freely, and would have no known distant metastasis. A cancer of the same size which appeared in the ovary, however, might have a very different T number.

How do doctors discover a cancer's node and metastasis status? They may be able to feel some enlarged lymph nodes even before surgery, but many nodes are not close enough to the skin surface to be palpated. Removing the nodes closest to the cancer and having them examined by a pathologist is the only way to find nodes in which there are tiny islands of cancer cells (**microscopic nodal invasion**).

Because common places for women's cancers to metastasize are the bone, lung, liver, and brain, these areas are checked especially. Does the woman report any bone pain, shortness of breath, or other complaint that could possibly mean a metastasis? Is there anything the doctor can see or feel, such as a swollen liver? Usually, the woman undergoes a staging workup, including laboratory tests and imaging studies. The doctor also searches for any sign of regional spread, such as bladder signs or symptoms with ovarian cancer, or spread to the opposite breast of breast cancer. Biopsies may be performed.

Cancer stages range from 0 or I to IV, with subgroups, and define where the cancer diagnosed fits in the TNM framework. Stage 0 means an in situ carcinoma, a tumor which has not invaded any neighboring tissues and thus cannot have spread to any lymph nodes or distant sites. Not all cancers have an in situ stage, but breast, cervical, vaginal, and vulvar cancers do. The TNM status for this would be T0 N0 M0. Stage I is a relatively small invasive cancer without node involvement or known metastasis. Depending on the organ, Stage I may be subdivided into A and B or more subgroups. Stages II, III, and IV are progressively more extensive cancers, but may represent different TNM combinations. A Stage II breast cancer, for example, has no evidence of distant metastasis, but could be quite small with some spread to nearby lymph nodes, or considerably larger with no known node involvement.

The TNM classification gives doctors a common language to use. However, there are other classification systems and gynecologic cancers are frequently classified using the FIGO (International Federation for Gynecologic Oncology) system.

GRADING THE CANCER

A pathologist looking at slides of a cancer under the microscope can tell several things about how it might behave. And every year new tests appear that offer more information.

The pathologist sees how different the individual cells are from a normal cell in that organ. The cells that still look quite a bit like a normal cell—the **well-differentiated** cancers—tend to behave more like normal cells and to be less aggressive. The

poorly-differentiated cancers are at the other extreme, and **moderately-differentiated** cancers fall somewhere in the middle.

How fast is the cancer growing? The pathologist counts how many cells in the slides are in the process of dividing (mitosis) for an estimate of the cancer's growth pattern. Cancers with a shorter doubling time grow more quickly and have more cells dividing at any one time; for instance, it is likely that the pathologist will catch more cells in the process of dividing in a cancer whose cells are programmed to divide every two weeks than in one with a doubling time of four months.

The pathologist looks at the particular types of cells, the presence of any necrotic (dead) areas, how the cells fit together, what the nucleus and other cell parts look like, how many tiny blood vessels are in the area of the tumor, and so on. How have other cancers with this profile behaved?

Tumor material can be subjected to assorted tests, some of which are very new. These can provide valuable clues about treatment options. For instance, breast cancer cells are tested with hormone receptor assays to see if and how much the cancer cells respond to the female hormones estrogen and/or progesterone. Cancers that thrive in the presence of estrogen, for instance, may be treated by depriving them of the hormone, an additional therapy option.

Flow cytometry measures the DNA material in cancer cells: those with a normal amount (**diploid**) tend to have a better prognosis than the **aneuploid** ones. Tests can analyze the cancer cells' life cycle to see what its synthesis phase (S-phase) is. The S-phase is when the cell prepares to divide; checking what percentage of cells are in this phase is a more precise method than the pathologist's estimate to tell how fast the cells are dividing. Other tests detect abnormal tumor proteins, oncogenes, and increased amounts of growth factors that may be related to more aggressive tumors.

The idea behind all these tests is to find out what kind of treatment is most likely to help a woman live longer and better after a diagnosis of cancer. The most aggressive cancers, those with a high **nuclear grade**, require an "elephant gun" approach, while a lazier cancer may be destroyed with a gentler treatment.

If, no matter how aggressive the cancer is or is not, there is only one possible treatment, then it is a waste of time, effort, and money to find out how aggressive it is. On the other hand, for a cancer with multiple variations and many treatment options—such as breast cancer—it makes sense to learn everything we reasonably can before deciding on therapy.

PROGNOSIS

"What are my chances?"

After receiving a cancer diagnosis, many women ask (or wonder silently) about **prognosis**, the statistical odds of what will happen to a woman with this condition. The prognosis depends on the kind of cancer, how extensive and aggressive this individual case is, how successful the current treatments for it are, and whether there are other personal or medical factors that are likely to make a difference.

Postmenopausal women with very early stage breast cancer, for instance, are likely to have an excellent prognosis, a very good chance of being cured. The woman with widespread ovarian cancer faces a poorer prognosis.

But—prognosis says nothing about what will happen to this individual woman. She may face higher odds with a poor prognosis, but that is all. Years later, many a woman with a terrible prognosis is still around, enjoying life, thumbing her nose at the prognosticators.

In addition, all it takes is one effective new therapy to turn a bad prognosis into an excellent one. Many years ago, my sister-in-law was diagnosed in her 20s with Hodgkins's disease, a cancer of the lymph system that was then considered almost invariably fatal. Horrified, we searched for information, and learned that a doctor at Stanford University Medical Center was getting exciting results with Hodgkin's with a new program of radiation therapy.

So Chris and the family moved in with us for four months so that she could commute to Stanford. With four adults and six young children in a three-bedroom, one-bath San Francisco flat, it was close quarters, but worth it. Twenty years later, Chris is still vibrantly healthy, a pioneer in one of the treatments that have turned Hodgkin's from a virtual death sentence to a cancer that most people survive.

Kerry McGinn

Chapter 5

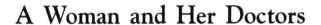

A Woman and Her Doctors

For most of us, cancer is too big a battle to fight alone. It takes a team effort.

On my team, I wanted

- ◆ myself at the center of the team—after all, it was my body, and I insisted on having a voice and making choices about what happened to it

- ◆ the best doctors I could find: smart, knowledgeable, and the kind of people I could work with

- ◆ lots of other very important people: healthcare workers other than doctors (including practitioners of any complementary therapies, such as acupuncture, that I chose to use); people who had "been there" as mentors and perhaps a support group; my family, friends, and co-workers; information resources, and so on

I felt shell-shocked after my diagnosis—vulnerable and overwhelmed by the choices that needed to be made promptly. As I gathered my "get well team," however, I regathered my own strength and sense of control as well. We were not perfect, any of us. We all made mistakes sometimes, failed to communicate, had bad days, or stepped on each other's toes. But at the same time, each person contributed something valuable—the will to get through this, specific chemotherapy drugs, or a care package of paperback mysteries sent with love. Woven together, these strands became far stronger than each alone. A rope? A safety net? A tapestry?

A *team.*

JOINING THE TREATMENT TEAM

Some women want to hear as little as possible about their cancer and prefer to leave all the control and decision-making in their doctors' hands. They have always trusted their doctors to make the right medical choices for them and see no reason to change that pattern now. This is a legitimate way of coping, and the woman might tell her doctor something like, "I will follow whatever treatment you advise. I really do not want to hear any more about this than I have to."

But "Yes, Doctor," "No, Doctor" is simply not enough for a growing number of women. Instead, they expect to be functioning members of their own treatment teams, and they do not wish to leave all the decisions to their doctors. As much as they trust their physicians, these women are profoundly aware that the doctors are not the ones who will have to live day after day with the choices that have been made.

These women expect their physicians to present treatment *options*—including no treatment. The doctor may argue strongly for a particular option, but must explain the pros and cons of each choice so that they can understand them. They ask questions, read, tell the doctor what they observe and how they feel—and they seek second opinions when appropriate.

To participate in her own treatment, a woman does not have to become a medical expert, she just needs to trust her intelligence and good sense. She is capable of learning about cancer and its treatment, and of making rational decisions. And she can contribute what no doctor can. Since she lives in her body every day, she is in the best position to notice and monitor subtle changes. She knows her own needs and desires better —and cares more about her health—than any doctor does.

Thinking of herself and her doctors as *partners* in a team effort does not mean she has to make all the decisions or always be in control. Part of being on a team is contributing what she can; the other part is welcoming the strengths of her teammates. Before getting cancer, I had grand notions about my role as a member of my healthcare team. I envisioned myself briskly making intelligent decisions and participating fully as its center. It worked like that sometimes, and I made some good decisions and some crucial observations. In truth, however, there were other times during diagnosis and treatment when I was barely slogging along, or was being carried by my teammates. That is what the team approach is all about.

CANCER DOCTORS

Usually a gynecologist or a surgeon obtains the biopsy tissue. Then a pathologist examines the biopsy specimen under the microscope to tell whether cancer is present. If cancer is diagnosed, some kind of treatment is often necessary, and many doctors might become involved in recommending cancer therapy and carrying out treatment.

A surgeon or gynecologist may perform more surgery (or other local treatment such as freezing or laser therapy) to remove a larger area after the biopsy. This doctor may be a general surgeon or gynecologist, or perhaps a doctor who specializes in cancer treatment: a **surgical** or **gynecologic oncologist.** For some women, this is all the treatment they need. If there is a reasonable possibility that there are stray cancer cells in the vicinity that the surgery has not removed, a **radiation oncologist** (or **radiation therapist**) may join the treatment team. This is a specialist who has received years of training in how to destroy local areas of cancer with high-beam X-ray energy. Although the titles sound similar, a radiation oncologist has a very different job from a radiologist, who reads imaging studies and thus helps detect cancer, but does not treat the disease.

But cancer is frequently both a local and a systemic (whole body) problem—and no single therapy currently available treats both parts of the problem adequately. Often, doctors cannot tell whether any cancer cells have escaped from the local area and prefer to play it safe. This means that a woman with cancer may have to deal with a combination of therapies: one or more local treatments (surgery, freezing or burning, and radiation), and one or more systemic treatments (chemotherapy, hormone therapy, and biological therapy).

Many women choose a **medical oncologist** to help fit the pieces together. This doctor not only coordinates care but also specializes in the systemic therapies for cancer. After completing training to become a doctor of internal medicine (internist), the medical oncologist has pursued advanced training in cancer therapy. When people refer to "my oncologist," they usually mean a medical oncologist.

Depending on the situation, any of these specialists, or the woman's family doctor or internist, may assume the role of the primary cancer doctor. The primary cancer doctor prescribes and/or coordinates treatment and sees the woman frequently during treatment, and at regular intervals afterward for the rest of her life. If she has more than one cancer doctor, a woman often continues to check in with each of them regularly after treatment finishes, perhaps alternating the appointments so that she sees each doctor at least once a year.

FINDING A DOCTOR

The gynecologist, internist, or family doctor may suggest a particular doctor to treat the cancer. Recommendations may also come from a nearby medical school, the local medical society or American Cancer Society chapter, a nurse on the oncology ward at the hospital, or from friends. They may provide further information: Is the doctor aggressive in treatment or more conservative? What about communication skills and bedside manner? Is she or he involved in clinical research? A call to the Cancer Information Service of the National Cancer Institute (NCI) at 1-800-4-CANCER will bring a list of cancer specialists.

Choosing the best doctor from among several candidates may be a problem for the woman with adequate health insurance living in or near a city, but many women do not have easy access to any doctor with expertise in cancer therapy. If there is only one doctor within 300 miles, for instance, and if this doctor rarely treats cancer patients, the woman with cancer may need to travel or have her records sent to a cancer center for assessment, development of a treatment plan, and perhaps therapy.

CHOOSING THE RIGHT DOCTOR

If all doctors made the best possible use of cancer therapies available today, more women would survive cancer. This is too serious a disease and the long-term relationship with the primary cancer doctor too crucial to settle for the wrong doctor. But how does a woman find the right one?

No doctor is perfect and no doctor can be expected to combine all the qualities a woman wants all the time. Most women have to choose a cancer doctor under less-than-optimal conditions: their anxiety levels are sky-high and they are under pressure to start treatment soon. Most women also do not have the time and money to interview several doctors, although they may be able to talk to more than one (by phone if not in person) and can also weigh what they have heard from other people.

With the stakes as high as they are in cancer treatment, however, it makes sense for a woman to think hard about what really matters to her in a doctor: what is essential, what is important but negotiable, and what she would like but could do without in a pinch. In fact, most women seem to find a cancer doctor they both like and trust. As one woman said, "My oncologist is the perfect combination of hope and reality. He does not soft-pedal the bad news, but he can always be counted on to be there and to cheer me on."

Basic credentials are essential. *The Directory of Medical Specialists* or the *American Medical Directory*, available in many libraries, lists such factors as a doctor's education and specialty preparation. For instance, is the doctor board-certified in the specialty? The doctor or office staff should be willing to supply this information as well. Many women insist that their doctors be members of relevant professional organizations such as the American Society of Clinical Oncology for medical oncologists.

Non-negotiable requirements often have to include that doctors be covered by the woman's insurance plan and that they have admitting privileges at a hospital included in that plan. The woman with Medicare or Medicaid (Medi-Cal in California) coverage needs a doctor who accepts this form of payment.

Competence and experience come next. The doctor must have the basic skills to take care of a patient with this type of cancer. If there is an unusual condition, the woman may need to see a "super-specialist" who has dealt with similar situations before. If one surgeon is the acknowledged national master of the rare kind of surgery I need, I may bemoan the fact that he or she has the communication skills of a turnip, but I will have that surgeon do my surgery anyway.

Beyond these essentials, the right doctor for one woman may not fit another woman's needs at all. One woman may place a premium on bedside manner, while another happily sacrifices empathy for access to clinical trials. If a woman has a choice between two or more well-qualified doctors, she should weigh what matters most to her. How clearly and honestly does the doctor communicate the whats, whys, and wherefores of diagnosis and treatment? Are the treatment recommendations backed up with convincing reasons? Is this a doctor who will not gloss over the risks of therapy while being a cheerleader for the benefits? Some doctors rely on their staff (oncology nurses, perhaps) to pass along some of the necessary information, and this can be a satisfactory arrangement.

How carefully does the doctor listen to the woman? Does he or she obviously respect the woman's input and look upon therapy as a shared venture? This is a key consideration for the woman who wants to work *with* her doctor, rather than simply to follow directions. It does not mean that the doctor will always agree with her, however, or say just what she wants to hear.

Is this physician involved in research and/or clinical trials? Some women prefer a doctor who is on the cutting edge of treatment, while others prefer a more conservative approach.

What is the doctor's treatment philosophy? To work well, cancer treatment often must be quite aggressive, but there is still a range of reasonable treatment styles. One oncologist builds a reputation for no holds barred treatment, *never* gives up, and always has another possible therapy to try. Another oncologist ordinarily suggests comfort care when cure is unlikely, and is much more ready to say "enough." All oncologists are bound by the individual woman's wishes, but most women will feel more comfortable with a doctor whose treatment philosophy meshes with their own desires.

What about the doctor's bedside manner? Cancer doctors have to present painful news and difficult choices all the time. To protect themselves emotionally—and perhaps save their energies for the long run—some fine doctors distance themselves from patients and may seem or become reserved, detached, or clinical. Others fear that a personal relationship will jeopardize their objectivity.

Many oncologists, however, recognize how therapeutic, how vital a part of effective treatment their manner can be. While a cancer doctor is not a mother, a father, or a buddy, basic friendliness and moral support are important. "Detached" may be adequate; "cold machine" is not. It makes sense for a woman to insist on doctors she can both respect and like enough to follow the treatment plan they decide on.

Susan couldn't stand her oncologist. She spent her whole treatment period quietly rebelling by flushing her chemotherapy pills down the toilet and missing appointments. Her early-stage cancer spread soon afterwards and she died quickly. Those of us who loved her will always wonder if things might have been different with a better doctor-patient relationship. Of course, because cancer doctors are often the bearers of bad news and unpopular treatments, they may become the innocent targets of a woman's anger. But if it is more than that, and if the anger seriously interferes with the treatment process, it is crucial to either renegotiate the patient-doctor relationship or find another doctor.

Health care is a product and patients are its consumers. While a woman cannot expect perfection, she has a right to competent, considerate care. This includes reasonably helpful office staff, appointments scheduled so that she does not routinely have to wait, and adequate telephone access in case of a problem.

THE PATIENT-DOCTOR RELATIONSHIP

Like other relationships, the patient-doctor relationship carries with it both rights and responsibilities. What does this mean for a woman?

She listens. Ideally, a few days after diagnosis, when she is past the initial shock, she should bring a family member or friend with her, a small tape recorder or a pen and notebook with questions written beforehand, and sit down with her doctor for a comprehensive treatment-planning session. Doctors know that anxiety blocks a person's capacity to listen and are accustomed to repeating what they have to say more than once; that is just the nature of communication during a period of high stress, and does not indicate any deficiencies on the woman's part. However, bringing someone along for any serious appointment, as a backup listener, saves missed information and misunderstanding; a tape recorder also lets the woman replay the conversation later for herself and her family.

Many women complain that they do not understand what the doctor and other health professionals say, that the vocabulary is unfamiliar and the explanations too technical. But medical concepts can all be explained in ordinary words; medical terminology cannot be allowed to become a barrier between doctor and patient.

The right to clear explanations in words she understands must be a woman's non-negotiable demand. It is always appropriate to ask, "Would you please explain that again in simpler terms?" or "Could you rephrase that?" or "This is what I think you said—is that right?" Many nurses have become proficient at explaining medical concepts, while medical book illustrations, drawings by the health professional, and books and booklets can all be helpful. It also makes sense for a woman to ask where she can get more information if she is interested.

The woman needs to think about what she wants and communicate it as clearly as possible. No matter how sensitive they may be, doctors cannot read minds. Unless the woman answers questions honestly and brings up issues that concern her, the doctor cannot know what is happening. (I have been guilty of that myself, thinking "He must know that—and if he doesn't, he should.") Cancer treatment is no place for guessing games. In particular, the woman accepts responsibility for either following the treatment plan she and her doctor have devised or communicating any problems so that they can be resolved.

Sometimes women may be too embarrassed to tell their doctor about some sensitive area in their lives. Most doctors are virtually unshockable, however, and find their jobs much easier if they can deal with a candid patient. If appropriate, the woman can request that certain items not go into her medical record.

Many women do not know what to ask or are reluctant to ask "silly" questions. Focusing on what is important to her is the key to asking sensible questions, and she can ask family or friends for input. Cancer books or booklets often include questions to ask the doctor. Many women find it helpful to keep a notebook handy so that they can jot down questions when they arise. Before an appointment, a woman can review her list and bring it with her. And if she does not know something and wants information, no question she asks is silly.

Many women have problems being assertive with doctors. They do not want to cause trouble or take too much of the doctor's time, and they shy away from anything that might lead to a confrontation. But the woman is fighting for her *life* and it is absolutely necessary that she say what she has to say with enough "oomph" to make her point. This does not mean being rude, but it can mean being very definite. She has the right to insist on appropriate concern for her problems and thoughtful answers to her questions, not only because she is the healthcare consumer paying for this service but also because she is a person of intrinsic worth. If a problem arises, remembering that this is a *partnership*—to which the doctor brings medical expertise and the woman brings the equally valuable contributions of her intelligence, personality, ability to observe, and coping skills—

makes it easier for some women to ask for the care they deserve. Many women also find it helpful to rehearse with a mentor or in a support group more effective ways to communicate with doctors and other health professionals.

The woman needs to take time to make treatment decisions. While it is important to begin any therapy reasonably soon, it ordinarily does not make any difference to her long-term survival if a woman takes a few extra days—or even two or three weeks—after a cancer diagnosis to get information and mull over what she wants before making any serious decisions. Often, in fact, it is not the doctor who is pressing for a prompt decision but the woman's own urgent sense that something needs to be done.

Most women do not want to be just "that breast cancer in Exam Room Four." They want to be real people to their health-care providers, and that means opening up enough to them so that their personality shows through. Interests, goals, fears, and stresses are important information to share.

If she expects her doctor to treat her courteously, the woman must return that consideration. That includes taking time before her appointment to collect her thoughts and questions, so that the doctor can meet her needs without having to change the whole day's appointment schedule. It also means such basics as keeping appointments or informing the office if she cannot, using advice phone calls reasonably, and not taking out her anger at the cancer itself on the medical staff.

Both the woman and her doctor are human, and only human. Accepting each other as human beings, sharing their strengths, and acknowledging their mutual fallibility are all part of forging a strong but flexible bond between them.

SECOND OPINIONS

Cancer therapy changes all the time. What was state-of-the-art just last year may be outdated now. In many cases, doctors do not know yet the best way to treat particular cancers. That means that good doctors may legitimately disagree about what therapy to recommend. It often makes sense for a woman to find out about what different doctors think about the therapy options for her cancer.

For instance, she may see a medical and/or a radiation oncologist after a biopsy but before any more surgery. If there are several possible acceptable ways to treat a particular cancer (as with breast cancer), the surgeon or gynecologist is more likely to look at surgical solutions, the radiation oncologist to recommend radiation, and the medical oncologist to propose systemic therapy.

This process tells a woman she has choices and helps her clarify what each might mean to her. In the long run it may save her from having to repent at leisure a decision hastily made. In the short run, however, hearing all these different points of view may be confusing and distressing. If we have choices, it means we have to make choices. There were times when I longed for someone to take that responsibility out of my hands. However, after floundering for days weighing imperfect options, I woke with a start at about 3 A.M. one morning knowing clearly what my choice had to be—and I have never regretted it. Had I followed my initial instincts, I doubt that I would have been happy with them six months later.

A woman can seek a second opinion from another doctor in the same specialty who is not connected with the original doctor, such as another surgeon who practices at a different hospital. This does not mean that she does not trust her original doctor. Most doctors consider second opinions routine and welcome; they are a safety mechanism that protects both patient and doctor. Of course, it is possible to go overboard getting second opinions. Visiting two surgeons makes sense; seeing six is usually too much.

Second opinions are common before surgery or other cancer treatments. Many women do not think about getting a review of the biopsy microscope slides from a second pathologist with special expertise in her type of cancer, but slides and other medical records can be safely and quickly mailed for a prompt second look.

A woman can get several second opinions at one time if

her case is reviewed by a tumor board, a group of health professionals from different cancer specialties who meet periodically at a regional hospital. They listen to a presentation of the case and view any visual evidence, such as imaging films or biopsy slides, and then pool their expertise to recommend a course of treatment. Any woman can travel to one of the hospitals designated as a Cancer Center by NCI (there were 57 in 1992), where new methods of cancer diagnosis and treatment are investigated. About half of these qualify as "comprehensive" centers, meeting several specific criteria for large-scale research set by NCI. A list is available from NCI's Cancer Information Service (see Resources).

Traveling to a cancer center or having her case reviewed there before treatment starts makes special sense for the woman who has limited access to specialized cancer care in her community, an uncommon cancer, or a cancer with either no standard treatment protocols or many therapy options. Some women may be candidates for, and choose to participate in, a clinical trial (a study to evaluate a new therapy). These are administered by cancer centers, or sometimes by oncologists in the community, and the treatment is without cost (see Chapter 8, Clinical Trials).

A woman's local doctor benefits from any second opinion information. Also, her doctor can access computer programs such as the on-line data base *Physicians Data Query* (PDQ) of NCI for up-to-date research and treatment protocols. The better informed *everyone* is, the better care a woman will get.

Kerry McGinn

Chapter 6

❖

The Rest of the Team

And then there are all the other members of the team. Whether they are professionals, like other healthcare workers, or contribute in other ways, they can become an indispensable part of a woman's cancer journey.

Depending on the treatments she receives, a woman with cancer can come into contact with a bewildering array of healthcare workers besides her cancer doctors.

Nurses, whether in the hospital or at the doctor's office, include general nurses, specialist nurses such as oncology certified nurses (O.C.N.s), and clinical nurse specialists (with a Master's degree in a specialty). Nurses frequently administer chemotherapy drugs in the oncologist's office or the hospital. Because of their education and focus, nurses may be especially interested in teaching patients and in quality of life issues.

The woman may need the services of several kinds of technicians and/or technologists, including personnel who draw blood samples, perform imaging tests such as mammograms or bone scans, or administer radiation treatments. A physical therapist can help the woman regain her strength and a full range of movement if she has undergone treatment that has affected these. In the hospital or as an outpatient, depending on her needs and wants, the woman may see a dietician, respiratory therapist, social worker, volunteers, admission clerk, office staff, and the hospital chaplain, among others.

Many women value the time spent with a psychotherapist or other mental health professional. Seeking help in coping emotionally with a cancer diagnosis does not mean a woman is maladjusted or crazy; it simply means she is making good use of resources to make her life better in a very difficult situation. Counseling can also come from a social worker or other licensed counselor.

The woman who includes complementary therapies in her treatment package may see such helpers as a relaxation training teacher, an acupuncturist, an herbal medicine specialist, and so on. Sometimes it seems like a blur of different people, with no time to get to know any of them. Many of them may be unsung members of her team—but they are an essential part of it.

MENTORS AND SUPPORT GROUPS

Even with the best medical care in the world, many women long to compare notes with someone who has been there: "Did you feel like this?" "What did you do about that?"

A woman may find someone who has been through the experience to act as a mentor for her. The woman who has undergone breast cancer surgery, for instance, can visit with an American Cancer Society *Reach to Recovery* volunteer who has recovered from a similar surgery. Instead of medical advice, the volunteer offers moral support, practical information, a simple temporary prosthesis (breast form) if the woman has had a breast removed—and the living, breathing proof that a woman can live well after breast cancer. This is ordinarily a short-term relationship: a visit and a phone call or two. Some doctors or hospitals automatically refer their breast cancer patients to *Reach to Recovery*. Otherwise, a woman can call the local ACS unit and refer herself for this free service.

Some women find a mentor by asking their doctors to recommend a woman who is doing well after treatment for a similar cancer. Referrals from friends provide more mentors, too: "Yeah, I know this woman who was diagnosed with cervical cancer years ago. I bet she'd be happy to talk with you."

Before cancer, I never thought of myself as the support group type and sometimes even looked down on people who "needed" the help of a group to get through life's troubles. Cancer changed that.

My cancer support group sisters understood what I was feeling without my having to spell out each detail. The group provided information (especially practical tips on dealing with treatment side-effects) a safe and accepting place for fears and tears, laughter and celebration, and a strong sense of a shared effort in getting well.

Separately, we were all reasonably strong and interesting women; together, we were that—and more. And where else could we go on at length about treatments for vaginal dryness after some kinds of chemotherapy, or fantasize about redecorating the oncologist's gloomy waiting room?

Being in a group gave me a sense of perspective and progress. At first, others who were further along in treatment were cheering me on; later, I could lend a hand to those just beginning and could appreciate how far I had come. I saw firsthand the positive changes other women were making in their lives after a cancer diagnosis. I was also forewarned of common emotional potholes so I could avoid some completely and get through others more easily.

By spending a couple of hours each week concentrating intensely on the experience, we began integrating it into our lives, but also got to put it out of mind some of the rest of the time. Our group was a place where we could find out how common and normal our feelings were, talk about them without burdening family and friends endlessly, and discover coping strategies that worked for others. The group gave us all a chance to rehearse more effective ways of communicating with health professionals, family, and friends. And it provided a chance to help others, to know that we were still contributors to life rather than just takers.

When psychiatrist David Spiegel of Stanford began investigating support groups for women with cancer, he fully expected that the groups would make women feel better but would not affect their survival. To his astonishment, he found that in his research sample of women with advanced metastatic breast cancer, the average survival rate after diagnosis was almost *double* for women who were in a support group as compared to those who were not. A larger-scale study by Dr. Spiegel is getting underway to prove or disprove these findings.

Why would support groups make a difference? Theories include increased access to information about cancer therapies, support and practical tips so that women persist in difficult treatments, and/or actual changes in the immune system from the psychosocial benefits of group work.

Groups may be short-term (six to eight weeks, for instance, or a weekend retreat) or much longer; homogeneous (women currently undergoing treatment for breast cancer, perhaps) or more mixed; oriented primarily toward information or toward mutual support; limited to cancer patients or open to family and/or friends; open, with new participants continuing to join, or closed. There are also groups strictly for family members or friends. Some support groups have a particular focus, such as holistic treatment. Every group has a different personality, depending on its goals, members, and group leader.

It helps to have a facilitator who may or may not have had cancer, but has experience in guiding groups. That way, members can explore painful feelings safely and freely, because they know there is a hand available to pull them out of any emotional quagmire.

Any type of group can be helpful and effective—or not. A few are actively detrimental. I would promptly leave a group that induced strong guilt feelings in its members for having cancer, or advised members to use alternative therapies *instead* of standard treatments for potentially curable cancers.

The local ACS chapter usually has information about different cancer support groups in the area. Women may hear about them from the oncologist, a nurse, or from friends. ACS itself sponsors *I Can Cope*, a series of eight education/support seminars for cancer patients and their families. One among several other possibilities is *The Wellness Community*, listed in Resources.

Support groups, even when readily available and very good, are not for every woman. Some women take on every other woman's burdens and suffer for everyone; others feel extremely uncomfortable in a group setting. A potential difficulty for every woman is the possibility that she will have to cope with the premature death of one or more "sisters." For many women, however, a cancer support group is well worth checking out—or even starting.

FAMILY AND FRIENDS

Health professionals call them "significant others": spouses, family members, lovers, best friends. However strange the term is, it does reflect the fact that a special person makes a difference. Often, not-quite-so-significant others—friends, acquaintances, coworkers—can play major roles in a woman's cancer journey as well.

A diagnosis of cancer is difficult and distressing not only for the woman herself, but for everyone around her. Serious illness changes roles and rules in relationships. Family members may have to face new responsibilities, often with little help or instruction; family and friends may have to cope with their own feelings of fear, sadness, anger and, perhaps, guilt.

Some people respond to cancer in someone close to them by being consistently loving, supportive, and helpful. They are there for her, accept her low days, show her that she is still loved and accepted, and bring her news and encouragement from the outside world.

However, cancer treatments often take a long time and it is common for family and friends to react differently at different times. People may be supportive part of the time and run out of steam at other times. No matter how much they love a woman, family members and friends are not immune to fatigue, other responsibilities, and strong and difficult feelings of their own.

I have been both patient and a close family member, and I contend that being the patient is sometimes easier. As a patient, no matter how miserable I was, I knew my limits and trusted my strengths; as a family member, often all I could do was look on helplessly.

While it is not her job to make everyone around her feel comfortable, a woman with cancer can encourage a helpful response from others by being frank about what is happening and what she wants and needs. By talking freely about the cancer, she can give cues to other people that they do not need to tiptoe around the subject. At the same time, if she can talk about other subjects as well and avoid concentrating exclusively on her illness, she reminds them—and herself—that she is a person who just happens to have cancer, rather than a cancer that just happens to have a person attached. Of course there are some times, such as right after diagnosis, when the ability to think or talk about anything but cancer may be too much to expect.

The woman may justifiably feel sad or angry, but she will scare off family and friends if she continually makes them the targets of her anger, or if she mopes for months and expects them to bear the weight of her depression. A mentor, a support group, or, better yet, a psychotherapist or counselor may help her move out of this emotional tunnel.

Some people just cannot handle being around a person with a cancer diagnosis. This is their problem and is in no way the fault or responsibility of the woman with cancer. Even if they do not believe cancer is contagious (a myth that some people still hold), they may feel scared and vulnerable. They avoid facing the possibility that they might be in the same situation someday by avoiding the woman. Or they may be so afraid that they will not know what to say or will start crying that they just stay away.

On the other hand, a woman may wish that some people *would* stay away, and may have to communicate this forcefully, if necessary. Some friends become so gloomy, pessimistic, or overly concerned that they make the situation worse. Others hover endlessly or overstay their welcome. My own least-favorites are the armchair psychologists who try to convince the woman that her feelings have caused the cancer and that she needs to "deal with her feelings" so that she can heal herself.

The woman may not have the stamina during this time to deal with exhausting emotional issues with others, including family members. This can wait until she feels better. And many women find themselves caught between opposing groups—close friends and family, perhaps, who have different ideas of what she should do. She may need to say "You people resolve this between yourselves. I don't want any part of it." A helpful booklet, *Taking Time: Support for People with Cancer and the People Who Care About Them*, is available free from NCI's Cancer Information Service (see Resources). It discusses many relationship issues, including coping within the family, sharing the diagnosis and the feelings involved, and maintaining and building relationships.

What about children? I remember driving home from the doctor's office and blurting out the news of my diagnosis to my husband. Together we planned for several days how best to break the news to our grown children and other family. It is crucial that children still at home be told very clearly (and repeatedly, if necessary) that they will be taken care of—and that they are *in no way to blame* for the cancer. Most children are sensitive to undercurrents of emotion. They react better to a simple, reasonably hopeful explanation than to a wall of silence that leaves them imagining the worst. Of course, the explanation needs to be tailored to the situation and the age of the child. A mother beginning chemotherapy who has a young child, for instance, might say something like, "I got sick. I have to take medicine for a while so I will get well. The medicine makes me feel very tired so I can't take you to the park today— but I still love you as much as always . . . . "

A useful booklet for older children, *When Someone in Your Family Has Cancer*, is available free from the Cancer Information Service.

INFORMATION SOURCES

Beside the specific information about her case that she gets from health professionals and any second opinion sources, a woman can learn a great deal about her type of cancer and cancer in general from other sources. The American Cancer Society has chapters in most areas and provides booklets. The phone number in the local phone book.

Trained personnel at the Cancer Information Service answer general questions and will send free packets of information on almost any cancer topic. Physician's Data Query (PDQ) of NCI offers up-to-the-minute treatment guidelines for anyone with access to a FAX machine (301-402-5874).

Phone lines such as the Y-ME Breast Cancer Support Program (800-221-2141) or DES Action for women with cancers related to the drug DES (510-465-4011) are just two of several cancer hotlines that answer questions and provide emotional support.

Bookstores and libraries (including hospital, medical school, and health consumer libraries) offer an array of reading material. As always, it makes sense for a woman to examine the author's credentials and the reasonableness of the material presented. A number of good books are listed in the back of this book under Resources.

A woman may be able to perform a medical literature search if she has access to a computer modem, or use of a medical center library system. If that is not feasible, she can have a search done for her for a fee, perhaps by a health information resource center such as Planetree (415-923-3680).

THE HOSPITAL EXPERIENCE

Many women have never been patients in a hospital, or have been there only for childbirth. It is a foreign territory—and they would just as soon keep it that way. Many women with cancer never need hospitalization at all, or stay in a Same Day Care Unit for only a few hours after a biopsy, for instance. Others enter the hospital for more extensive surgery, certain kinds of chemotherapy or radiation therapy, or for some complication.

What can a woman expect if she is hospitalized? For insurance reasons, most patients now stay in the hospital the shortest possible time. This means that anything that can be done before admission—blood work, imaging studies, physical examinations—may be done on an outpatient basis. It also means that hospitalized patients may be discharged from the hospital before they are fully recovered, and may need more help at home than would be required after a longer hospital stay. Because patients are not hospitalized now unless they truly need acute care, and because the number of hospital staff often does not reflect the high level of care needed, hospital personnel are often stretched—and stressed.

It makes sense to read and follow carefully any preadmission instructions from the hospital. Valuables, except for a few dollars, perhaps, and a wedding ring or watch, are best left home; if they are brought, the hospital staff will lock them up. It helps if people bring a list of any medications they are taking at home, including the name of the drug, the dosage, and frequency, but not the pills themselves. Hospitals must follow strict fire safety regulations and may have special rules for small electrical appliances such as hair driers.

Hospitals provide nightgowns, and often slippers and robes. Women can bring their own, but may choose to wear hospital gowns part of the time because they are opaque, often easier to put on and take off, and can save the woman's nightwear from stains and soil after surgery. On the other hand, wearing one's own sleepwear helps preserve a bit of personal turf in unfamiliar territory. Likewise, many women bring a family photograph or something similar to put by their bedside to mark this as *their* spot and remind them of life beyond the hospital. This also tells healthcare workers that this is a *person* here and can serve as a conversation starter.

If she has surgery or other treatment in a teaching hospital, a woman may tell her story to, be examined by, and receive much of her everyday treatment from "house staff": residents and interns who have finished medical school and are licensed physicians but are honing their clinical skills under the supervision of more experienced doctors. (Interns are not the same as internists, doctors who have received specialty training in internal medicine.) A woman will probably have "her" intern who has primary house staff responsibility for her case. The house staff makes rounds once or twice a day, in a group, to examine her. When "her" intern is not available, another on-call intern will have information about her. The interns rotate or move to another service every month or so.

The surgeon or other cancer doctor acts as an attending doctor, supervising the house staff. The attending doctor usually sees each patient once or twice a day or has a covering doctor see her (on weekends, perhaps). If a problem requiring medical attention arises at another time the nurse usually notifies the intern in a teaching hospital; if the intern or resident cannot resolve the problem, the attending doctor is notified.

Hospitals have their own vocabulary, and it is always okay to ask what something means. Some common items include: "p.r.n.," the Latin words for "as needed," referring to medicines or treatments given only at the patient's request; "NPO" for "nothing by mouth," meaning the patient is not supposed to eat or drink anything; and "void" for urinate. Many pain medications are ordered p.r.n.; if the woman does not specifically request it, it will not be given.

The woman in the hospital deserves considerate and respectful care, information about her diagnosis and treatment in words she can understand, and concern for her privacy. Her rights are further spelled out in the Patient's Bill of Rights, formulated by the American Hospital Association and often given to patients at admission or on request.

On the other hand, consideration works both ways. That means, for example, using the nurse call bell when one needs help, but also asking oneself first: is this a necessary request, something for which I need a nurse? Could I consolidate two or more requests?

A few hospitals encourage interested patients to read and contribute information to their own medical charts. This is a small but growing movement, and reinforces the concept of patient and healthcare workers as members of a team working together for the woman's health.

Kerry McGinn

Chapter 7

❖

Local Treatments for Cancer

Cancer is a thoroughly nasty disease—and the conventional medical treatments for it will not win any popularity prizes either. It is a tradeoff: if we choose to undergo the discomfort of a cancer treatment now, it is because we think there is a good chance we will be better off in the long run. The therapies we have now for cancer are tolerable, and may be worth enduring if they cure the disease or make it better.

There are three goals in cancer therapy. Treatment can **cure** the cancer outright, dousing the fire completely so that the woman lives cancer-free for the rest of her days.

If cure is not possible, the backup goal is **control**, often for very long periods of time. While there may be cancer cells around, they do not cause the woman any complaints. Therapy may be able to keep cancer in this suspended mode for years and give a woman an extended disease-free interval. Another control scenario is the cancer that smolders most of the time, flaring up occasionally. Therapy puts out each small fire as it occurs, and the woman is symptom-free the rest of the time.

If neither cure nor control is possible, **palliation** almost always is. Palliation means relieving or reducing symptoms, making the person with advanced cancer comfortable, keeping the fire at bay. All three goals—cure, control, and palliation—are worthwhile ones.

WHAT LOCAL THERAPIES DO

The women's cancers are all solid tumors that begin in one location. Local therapies are those that work for eradicating local disease: surgery and radiation. These are no help at all, however, in tracking down any cancer cells that have left the immediate vicinity.

When the doctor says, "I recommend such-and-such therapy," a woman may wonder, "If I choose to do that, what am I letting myself in for?" This chapter provides an overview of the answers. Closer looks at specific treatments appear in the chapters about individual cancers.

SURGERY

Cancer surgery is considered elective rather than emergency surgery, which means that it usually does not have to be performed immediately. The woman waits anxiously, torn between "I don't want to do this," and "Let's get this over with—the cancer cells could be spreading right this minute!"

But she is scarcely idle. Even if she will be hospitalized after surgery, she typically is not admitted until the morning of surgery. Before that, she undergoes any necessary tests and physical examinations as an outpatient, and may have a hospital preadmission interview to sign paperwork and give insurance information.

Her gynecologist or surgeon tells her what she has to do to prepare for surgery. She may have to shower with a special bacteria-killing soap, take laxatives or enemas, or follow a certain diet. Unless she is having just a local (skin-numbing) anesthetic, she may not eat or drink anything after midnight. It is especially important that her stomach be empty if she will be put to sleep with a general anesthetic; otherwise, the stomach contents could back up when she is unconscious, causing her serious lung problems.

On the morning of surgery, she goes to the presurgery area and is prepared for the operation. She signs the consent form for surgery if she has not done so already, and talks to the doctor or specially-trained nurse who gives the anesthetic. She may also receive a sedative medicine to relax her.

At some point, an IV (intravenous) line may be started. This tube, usually inserted into a vein in a hand or arm, makes it possible to administer fluids, medications, and blood, if necessary, and to give the short-acting drug which induces, or begins, general anesthesia.

In the operating room the woman is scrubbed and draped so that only the surgical area shows. This preparation helps protect the surgical area from contamination, as do the masks, gowns, and head coverings all the surgical personnel wear.

If the woman is scheduled for a "regional" anesthetic which numbs the lower region of the body, she receives directions to curl up on the operating table. The anesthesia is begun through a narrow catheter (tube) carefully inserted through the previously numbed skin over the backbone into the space around the spinal nerves. When this takes effect, she will no longer be able to move or feel the area below the block. This cannot be done for breast surgery because a regional anesthetic to paralyze that area would affect the lungs and heart also. She may be given sedative medication through her IV so that she dozes through the procedure or cannot remember it afterward.

Before a general anesthetic is started, the woman may have lots of small things placed on her, such as electrode patches to monitor her heart and a sensor placed around her finger to check if she is getting enough oxygen. If she is not asleep already from the sedative, the doctor or nurse giving anesthesia will tell her when the quick-acting general anesthetic is injected into her IV. Within a few seconds, she will be soundly, dreamlessly asleep. It may be hours before she wakes up, but it will seem like a second.

The IV anesthetic lasts only a short time, however. For a surgery lasting longer than a few minutes, a large tube is inserted through her mouth and down her throat after she is asleep. Through this, she receives a mixture of anesthetic gases and oxygen to keep her deeply unconscious but breathing well. The tube will be removed by the time she wakes up.

During the operation, the surgeon/gynecologist may use scalpels and scissors, an electrocautery wand to burn off areas, or a laser beam. Even with a laser, the doctor still has to cut through the skin first.

After the operation, the woman is transferred to the post-anesthesia recovery room where she wakes up gradually after a general anesthetic or regains feeling and movement below the waist after regional anesthetic. If she is scheduled to stay in the hospital, she is wheeled on a gurney to her hospital room where the nurses will help her transfer into bed. If she goes home, she should receive *written* discharge instructions about medications, activities, precautions, and follow-up care.

RECOVERING FROM SURGERY

Depending on the anesthetic and sedatives she received and on how her body reacts to them, a woman may be instantly alert or remember almost nothing for the first day or so. But, sooner or later, she will notice tubes, bandages, and sensations.

Tubes

She may feel temporarily that she has tubes dangling every-where. She may still have her IV for fluids, antibiotics, and possibly pain medicine. If she does not need continuous IVs, the nurse detaches the IV bag and tubing and caps the end of the catheter near where it is inserted in the skin. The tubing is hooked up again only when necessary, (for instance, for an antibiotic medicine that needs to be given every few hours). The rest of the time, the woman is free of the IV bag and tubing. This is called a "heparin lock"; something has to be injected into the catheter after each use so that blood does not clot and close it off, and that something is often a tiny dose of an anticlotting medicine called heparin.

For a few days, tubes of some sort may drain extra blood or tissue fluid from the surgical area so it does not build up, cause discomfort, and strain the incision. A tube may provide a simple pathway only or it may be connected to wall suction or a portable suction device. These devices are typically plastic containers (lemon-sized bulbs, flat cylinders) which can be opened, emptied, and then compressed with the hands; as they gradually decompress, they create gentle suction. A dangling drain can be attached to the woman's gown with tape or a safety pin. If the woman leaves the hospital with the drain(s) still in place, a nurse teaches her the very easy care needed. The doctor will pull out the drain when it no longer removes much fluid. This is a peculiar sensation, rather like having a long worm removed from under the skin. It helps to take a deep breath first and then slowly exhale while the drain is being pulled. The tiny incision where the drain was inserted closes immediately.

After major surgery for a gynecologic cancer, a woman can expect a Foley catheter, a tube inserted through the urethra (opening to the bladder) to drain urine. A small inflated balloon keeps the Foley in the bladder; when it is time to remove the catheter the balloon is deflated and the catheter slips out. The Foley is connected to a portable drainage bag. This means the woman does not have to contend with bedpans for a few days, because the urine drains out continuously. Some women complain of mild irritation from the catheter and may take a little while to relearn how to urinate normally after it is removed.

Sometimes, after abdominal surgery, the woman may have a narrow tube in her nose. This NG (nasogastric, meaning nose to stomach) tube may be attached to a suction source to remove gas and stomach juices until the digestive tract—pulled and pummeled by surgery—begins functioning again. Even without an NG, the woman may have to wait a few days before beginning liquids and then moving on to solid food.

Anesthesia barely fazes some women, but leaves others feeling nauseated, sleepy, and "not quite all there" for a day or more. The woman can request medicine for nausea.

Bandages and scars

The doctor ordinarily closes the surgical incision and either covers it with a bulky bandage at first or leaves the special tape strips (steri-strips) or stitches open to the air. The steri-strips fall off by themselves in about two weeks, and the doctor removes any stitches of the kind that are not absorbed by the body. Sometimes staples are used instead of stitches. These are removed with a staple remover about a week after surgery. Only rarely, the incision is left open to heal from the inside out and then the doctor orders irrigations or special dressings.

Doctor and nurses will inspect the skin around the incision site to be sure that it is clean, with natural skin color except for initial bruising, and without pus drainage. They look for signs of infection and also for any large collection of tissue fluid or blood which may need to be drained. The woman should continue to check the area after she goes home and seek immediate medical help if anything looks or feels significantly different.

No matter how gorgeous an incision looks to the surgeon, it usually looks a lot less beautiful to its owner. In fact, the swelling will go down, the bruising disappear, and the scar fade. However, scars heal differently for every woman. Most of them get "uglier" with the normal healing process before they begin fading. Some scars eventually become almost invisible, while others—no matter how careful the doctor may have been—build up thick "keloid" tissue. Many women feel that rubbing vitamin E oil along the incision reduces the scar.

Surgery and pain

Studies indicate that nearly half of all people who get routine pain therapy after surgery still have moderate to severe pain. *Routine pain therapy does not stop pain!* Most people expect to have pain after surgery, but studies have shown that pain can actually slow down the healing process and be a cause of postoperative problems. There are new methods and medications that can control postoperative pain.

For example, the doctor may order a **PCA** (patient-controlled analgesia) pump, which delivers IV pain medication directly into the vein when the woman presses a button. Following the doctor's orders, the nurse pre-programs the pump to deliver a small continuous stream of medication and/or give a set dose at certain intervals (1 mg of morphine no more often than every 15 minutes, for instance). The woman does not have to wait for the nurse, and often uses less medicine because she can always "stay ahead of the pain."

The pain medicine given in the first days after surgery may be a narcotic or a powerful non-narcotic. Common routes for pain medicines are: into the vein with an IV, under the skin or into the muscle with a shot, through a tiny tube into the space around the spine (an epidural), or by mouth. Using narcotics for a few days after surgery does not turn a woman into a drug addict. They do make some women feel woozy, however, and they slow down the intestinal tract, so constipation is possible.

Nondrug treatments include massage, hot and cold packs, electrical nerve stimulation (TENS), relaxation, music or other distractions, and imagery.

Adequate pain control not only keeps the woman comfortable, but helps her do what she needs to do to recover from surgery. It makes no sense for her to "tough it out" and refuse pain medicine—and then develop a blood clot or pneumonia because it hurts her too much to walk around, deep-breathe, and cough.

RECOVERY "DO-IT-YOURSELF"

There is a lot of "do-it-yourself" in recovering from surgery. General anesthesia insults the lungs and temporarily paralyzes the little hairs that line them and sweep out any impurities. In addition, when the woman lies down on her back, the lungs have to expand against gravity. All this puts the lungs at risk for developing little collapsed areas, so that they do not exchange oxygen and other gases—or cool the body—as effectively as they should. Any collapsed areas (atelectasis) can become a haven for lurking bacteria.

To prevent serious lung problems, the woman should breathe very deeply several times an hour while she is awake. If she is breathing correctly, filling her lungs to their depths, her diaphragm and abdomen will move out as she inhales and in when she exhales. She can check this movement by placing her hands flat on the abdomen, resting the thumbs on the bottom ribs on each side.

To help her breathe more effectively, a woman may be given a plastic gadget called an incentive spirometer. She inhales through a tube (rather like sucking on a large straw) and this makes balls or some other device rise in a chamber so that she can gauge how deeply she is breathing. Seeing the concrete evidence of improvement inspires her to throw in an extra practice now and then—the "incentive" part.

Effective coughing moves any "junk" out of the lungs or at least keeps it from settling in and causing trouble. Holding a pillow or the hands firmly over the incision splints the area and makes it much more comfortable to cough. A woman can often trigger a cough by taking three slow deep breaths in through the mouth and then holding the last breath.

Our bodies are built to move. They work much better when they do and get into trouble when they do not. At first, when the woman is still confined to bed, she can turn from side to side and exercise her legs and arms, moving them in small circles or contracting and relaxing them. This helps keep her blood moving so it does not pool and form a clot.

As soon as possible, however, she should get out of bed and begin walking—a few steps at first and then more. It gets easier quickly. Walking

— helps expand the lungs

— brings blood to the surgical site and begins gently stretching the tissues for prompt healing and greater comfort

— keeps the blood from forming clots

— helps get the digestive tract moving again (and is the best remedy around for the gas "cramps" that can make a person utterly miserable a few days after abdominal surgery)

— protects the skin from bedsores

— feels good

Once a woman is on her feet, it is not too difficult to walk; getting out of or into bed is the challenge. After enough surgeries to qualify me for "frequent-user upgrades," I know the secrets: it is *much* easier if one takes a deep breath beforehand and then moves while breathing out; this automatically relaxes the muscles so they do not tighten up and complain. The other technique is to move in one piece as much as possible. To help herself do this, the woman plans beforehand what she is going to do, and then uses her arms, the bed control, and the nurse as needed. A wheelchair, if one is available, makes a handy companion the first times out: it provides a broad base to lean on and a seat if she gets tired. An IV pole works well if it moves smoothly and does not tip easily.

RADIATION

Radiation therapy devices control the immense energy provided by atoms in transition and focus it to destroy local nests of cancer cells. Radiation can be used to treat a primary tumor or an area where a tumor was removed but which may still contain some stray cancer cells, such as the breast after a lumpectomy. It can also work well on a small metastasis made up of cells known to be sensitive to radiation, such as a bone "met".

The radiation can come from a machine outside the body, as in **external radiation therapy**, or it can be delivered from an **internal radiation** source placed inside the body.

What is radiation, anyway, and how does it work?

Every atom tries to be electrically stable with the positive electrical charges at the core of the atom exactly balancing and holding in place the electrons, the negative charges orbiting outside the core. If there are too many negative charges to hold onto, these extra electrons (ions) rush away from the atom in a stream or ray of energy. This can happen because certain atoms are naturally unstable: certain kinds (isotopes) of the elements uranium or cobalt, for example, are always in transition (radioactive) because their electrical charges are unbalanced. Or an ordinarily stable atom can purposely be made unstable in a specially designed machine.

If radiation rays reach the body, they collide with and disrupt the DNA in the body's cells and change the electrical balance in the molecules of the cells or the cell environment. The cells can die or they can mutate; if they mutate but are still able to divide, they can pass along this mutation to daughter cells. If many cells get moderately damaged, the uncontrolled ionizing radiation can itself cause cancer (as occurred years after the atom bomb was dropped on Hiroshima).

In contrast, radiation therapy targets small local clusters of cancer cells for total destruction: the cancer cells either die immediately or are so damaged they can no longer divide. The rest of the body, which could not survive even a moderate dose of radiation given to the whole body, tolerates a very large dose given to a small area quite well. Radiation oncologists, however, still have to work to protect the normal cells of the body.

However radiation is delivered, there is some natural protection for the body in the fact that the cell's DNA is most exposed when the cell is dividing, so that the fast-dividing cancer cells are the most vulnerable. Thus, while a lethal dose of rays will kill some normal cells in its path because they happen to be dividing, it will kill many, many more cancer cells.

External radiation

External radiation machines either use a naturally-occurring radioactive material (often a cobalt isotope) or, increasingly, make a stable isotope radioactive. In the machine, the electrons streaming from their source accelerate as they pass across some kind of high-energy field. The high-speed electrons then strike a positively-charged target, which breaks them up into even smaller "pieces" and focuses them in one direction: the radiation beam.

Depending on how fast they are going, these packets of electrical energy can be made up of "pure energy," like X-rays and gamma rays, or larger "particles" of energy, like electron, alpha, and beta rays.

LOCAL TREATMENTS FOR CANCER ❖ 95

The "pure energy" X-rays and gamma rays can penetrate to the deeper tissues before releasing their payload of energy. Unable to penetrate so deeply, the lower-voltage "particle" rays work at skin level or just below. Most of the machines used now have an extremely high-energy field and produce either X-rays or gamma rays. However, the linear accelerator, a machine used frequently, can also be set with a lower energy field, producing an electron beam, if that is needed.

The radiation therapist selects the rays that work at the depth of the tumor. The beam is aimed to hit the cancer area while avoiding any vital organs near it. For instance, radiating a breast straight on could cause significant damage to the nearby lungs and heart, so the radiation is aimed at the breast "tangentially," from different angles. (Much of radiation oncology is physics—or maybe billiards!)

The total amount of radiation to be given is divided over daily doses, so that the normal cells which are in the way, and cannot escape entirely (like the skin), have a chance to recover somewhat between doses. The amount of radiation is expressed in interchangeable units called **rads** or **centigrays** (cGy). A woman might be scheduled to get a total of 4,500 rads, divided into doses of 150 rads every weekday for six weeks.

Still another strategy is to protect nearby areas with shields that block the radiation. These may be ready-made or may be custom-fit for the woman, and are put in place every day before the treatment.

Healthy tissue resists radiation much better than weakened tissue does. Thus, the radiation therapy (RT) staff will encourage the woman to maintain very good nutrition. It is also important that she stay at a stable weight during therapy so that the treatment field does not change. She is also asked to keep the skin in the path of the radiation beam clean, gently dried, and lubricated with a product the RT department recommends.

Before external radiation starts, the woman meets with the radiation oncologist at the hospital to learn about the therapy and undergo a full physical examination. She may undergo imaging tests, such as CT or MRI, so that the radiation oncologist has all the necessary information about the tumor and the exact location of her vital organs before setting up the treatment field.

The radiation oncologist then may work with a radiation physicist and/or dosimetrist to discuss the most effective and safest angles and doses for the radiation beam. Together, they work out a radiation "prescription" for the woman.

The woman then comes to the hospital for **simulation**, a dry run of the treatment. No actual radiation is delivered during simulation, but the unfamiliar and often exceedingly "high-tech" machines can be unnerving. Simulation can be a lengthy process, as the radiation oncologist and technologists mark the skin to show the proposed field, assess angles, decide on and maybe construct shields, take regular X-rays to see if they've got it right, and so on.

Because it is crucial that the radiation machines treat exactly the same area each day, the technologists will mark the skin with either marking pens or tattoos to show the radiation field. The woman is told not to wash off any felt-tip pen markings, but they may need to be touched up frequently. They tend to sweat off or rub off on clothes (so clothes that need to be dry-cleaned should be avoided) and they also make some women feel uncomfortably like a marked beef at the butcher shop.

If tattooing is used, tiny purplish dots of dye are injected under the skin; it feels like pinpricks. Only a few tattoos are needed to mark the boundaries of the radiation field, but they are permanent, so that a doctor can always tell where radiation has been given. There are strict limits to how much radiation can be given safely to one area.

Either the same day as the simulation or soon thereafter, the woman has her first actual treatment. This involves a few minutes of setting up, in which the technologist helps her get into exactly the right position, with foam pads placed under her head and knees, perhaps, and skin bared in the treatment field. Any shields are positioned.

The technologist then goes to a computer console in another room, but can still see the woman through a window. Alone in the room, the woman lies still but can breathe normally for the minute or two the radiation is actually given.

There is no pain or other physical sensation, although some women claim they feel warm, or cool where the radiation goes, which makes it easy for them to visualize the rays demolishing the cancer cells.

After the complete dose is given the technologist returns and readjusts the woman and the machine if radiation is being given from more than one angle. *The woman is not radioactive in any way at any time when she is undergoing radiation from an external machine.*

And that is all there is to the treatment, which may be repeated every day: usually some waiting, then a few minutes for set-up, and a couple of minutes of radiation. The radiation oncologist will see the woman about once a week, and may order periodic blood tests or imaging studies to keep track of her progress.

What are the common side effects? Severe (but temporary) fatigue is common—and surprising to many women. This occurs not only because the body has to work to repair the cellular damage from radiation, but also because of the wearying daily trips to and from the hospital. It is more severe if the woman is not eating well. Fatigue usually begins a few weeks after treatment begins.

Temporary skin damage, like a sunburn, is common in the treatment field. This begins a few weeks after treatment starts: radiation attacks the fast-dividing living cells beneath the surface skin layer of dead cells, and it takes a few weeks for the affected cells to reach the surface.

The deeper-penetrating X-rays and gamma rays go through the skin without releasing much of their energy there, so skin damage is usually fairly mild; the shallower beta or electron rays cause more skin damage. The "sunburn" turns to tan and ordinarily fades within several weeks, although some people experience a permanent change in pigmentation. If damage is greater, the skin may become "weepy." Because weepy skin can be an entry way for germs and infection, radiation may be postponed for a few days or other treatment prescribed. Fair, sensitive skin is no more likely than other skin to be damaged. After radiation, the skin and the underlying tissues often feel thicker and firmer.

Each radiation therapy department has its own list of acceptable skin products. Some unacceptable products might contain aluminum or another substance that might deflect radiation, for instance, or intensify it.

Other possible side effects from external radiation depend on the area being treated, such as nausea or diarrhea if any of the intestinal tract is in the field of radiation. Specific side effects are discussed in the chapters on the individual cancers.

Internal radiation

The other way to receive radiation treatment is from a radioactive source that is placed inside the body and continues to emit energy for a specified time. Each source is a radioactive isotope, which continues to decay—lose electrons and emit radiation at a certain known rate—until the oversupply of electrons is gone.

Occasionally, a radioactive isotope is injected into a woman's blood vessel, and travels through her body while it continues to decay. These rays have not been accelerated and energized in a machine so they cannot go very far or escape through the skin. The woman can come and go as she wishes, and the radioactivity poses no risk to anyone else.

When a sealed source of radiation is placed in the body, the treatment is called **brachytherapy.** The treatment plan for a gynecologic cancer might include inserting an empty applicator into a body cavity (such as the uterus) while the woman is in the operating room. Later, in the hospital room, the container is "afterloaded" with a sealed source of radioactive material, brought to the room in a lead-lined box and inserted with special tongs.

The filled applicator is left in place, emitting its rays, for a certain number of days and then is removed. Because the body cavity is not closed completely on all sides, it is an inadequate barrier for the rays. Thus the woman is considered radioactive during the whole time the loaded applicator is in place. That means she remains in her hospital room with a "Danger: Radioactive" sign on the door, so that no one else is exposed unnecessarily. Visitors and health professionals follow very strict guidelines about how close they can be to her, and for how long, and they may use lead screens to shield themselves. Her body wastes are monitored for radioactive material and the nurses use special techniques to dispose of them.

Some of the same precautions apply when tiny radioactive seeds are afterloaded into minute tubes threaded through the skin and directly into the tumor area. The seeds and tubes are removed in 36 hours or so. As soon as any radioactive source is removed, the woman is no longer radioactive.

Typically, the woman hospitalized for brachytherapy feels very bored, quite isolated, emotionally strange (an "untouchable") and, depending on the applicator, somewhat physically uncomfortable. She may be on strict bedrest, if there is any chance that the applicator could be dislodged with movement.

Occasionally, radioactive seeds are injected directly into the tumor and allowed to decay naturally without ever being removed. Her radiation oncologist will tell the woman the precautions to use to protect other people.

However a woman receives radiation treatment, she will have many questions for her healthcare professionals. Like every other woman undergoing local therapies for cancer, she has the right to answers—in words she understands.

Kerry McGinn

Chapter 8

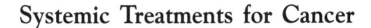

Systemic Treatments for Cancer

Unlike the local therapies for cancer, the systemic therapies —chemotherapy, hormonal therapy, and biological therapy— work throughout the whole body system, moving through the blood stream and beyond to sniff out and destroy cancer cell "strays." They work on local tumors too, but usually not as effectively as the local treatments.

CHEMOTHERAPY

" . . . *And so, of course, you'll need chemotherapy.*"

I don't cry easily but, as my surgeon said that to me over the phone, the tears started streaming down my face. I was scared because I had to acknowledge that there might be cancer cells loose in my body—and I was almost equally terrified by the whole prospect of "chemo."

That night I wrote the first poem I had written in years. Chemo became, for me, a "sky-wrenching" downpour that would flush any cancer cells out of my body. The last part of the poem went like this:

> *Umbrellas are not much use in a storm like this.*
> *It will be a long wet trudge home*
> *Until I'm dry again.*

"Long trudge" says it fairly well for me. I won't pretend I loved chemotherapy, but I tolerated a few months of treatment to get "home" again to my goal of long-term good health. For me, in fact, chemo was not as bad as the horror stories and my imagination had painted it.

Chemotherapy is a different experience for every woman. How she responds to chemo depends not only on the regimen itself—there are all kinds and combinations of drugs and ways of receiving them—but also on how the woman's body and mind respond. While chemo hits some women really hard, and many feel flu-ish part of the time, plenty of others breeze through it with a little tiredness and an occasional nap.

In the last few years many chemo "courses" have become shorter. Effective new medications, products, and techniques help relieve side effects. All of this makes the process easier. As scary as it is to wait for that first chemo dose, it makes sense to adopt a "wait-and-see" approach.

Why use chemotherapy?

Cancer chemotherapy is the use of drugs to kill cancer cells throughout the body. The doctor may recommend it:

- ◆ If it is *known* that cancer cells have spread from the organ where they started. In case of known distant metastasis, chemotherapy can relieve current symptoms or prevent/postpone future ones.

- ◆ If it is *reasonably suspected* that cancer cells might have strayed. **Adjuvant**, or assisting, **chemotherapy** means therapy given in addition to surgery and/or radiation to kill any microscopic metastases that *might* be lingering in the body after all the known cancer has been removed.

- ◆ To decrease the size of a solid tumor so that it can be treated with a local therapy, or as control or palliation if local treatment is not possible.

Obviously, if there is no detectable disease to start with, as with adjuvant chemotherapy, doctors cannot see immediate results from chemotherapy. In general, however, doctors hope for **complete remission**, where no more disease can be detected in the body, whether for a brief time or for long enough to be considered a cure. There can be **partial remission** in which the detectable disease (such as the size of the tumor) decreases by at least 50%. Even **stabilization** of a cancer at a level where it is not causing major symptoms can significantly improve the quality of a woman's life.

How chemotherapy works

Because cancer cells divide more often than most normal cells do, they are more vulnerable to drugs that interrupt the cell cycle.

The side effects of the drugs occur because the other body cells, especially those that normally divide often, are not immune. However, healthy normal cells bounce back much better than dysfunctional cancer cells do. The science (and art) of giving chemotherapy lies in killing as many cancer cells as possible without permanently damaging too many healthy ones.

There are four classifications of chemo drugs, called the four "A's," and each one works differently. **Antimetabolites** attack as the cell is dividing, and starve it by giving it a fake nutrient. **Alkylating agents** bind with the cell's DNA during any phase of the cell cycle to prevent the cell from dividing. **Antitumor antibiotics** (not to be confused with the kind of antibiotics used for infections) infiltrate the DNA itself so that the cell cannot grow. **Vinca alkaloids** interfere with the formation of the chromosomal "spindles" necessary for cell division.

Almost all chemotherapy regimens combine two or more drugs on a certain schedule to maximize the effectiveness of each agent. This fighting on all fronts combines noncycle-specific drugs, which attack at any time during the cycle, with cycle-specific agents. This combination approach can also "confuse" the cancer cells so that they do not develop a resistance to the individual drugs.

A course of chemotherapy usually consists of the same cycle of drugs repeated two or more times. The course may last from two to twelve months, depending on the type of cancer and the treatment protocol. Typically, each cycle lasts a few weeks and includes time for giving the drugs, waiting for them to work, and then allowing the body to recover and rest somewhat before the next cycle starts.

The oncologist planning the cycle considers the strengths and weaknesses of each drug to decide what to give when. For instance, if drug A, given on day one of the cycle, is known to take eight days to "set up" the cancer cells so that they are at their most vulnerable to drug B—drug B would then be given on day eight.

Each chemotherapy cycle is expected to kill a percentage of cancer cells everywhere in the body. Between cycles, the cancer cells that are not killed continue to divide, but before they recover too many of their numbers, the next cycle attacks. Thus, if one cycle kills 75 out of every 100 cancer cells, 25 will still be left. The remaining cells may rebuild to 27 before the next cycle of chemo destroys 75% of the remainder, leaving 7 cells to face the next onslaught. The idea is to get the cancer cells down to a number the body's own defenses can handle.

Chemotherapy drugs are strong medicine, and there is a fairly narrow line between the amount that kills cancer cells and the amount that can kill the person. However, doctors need to give doses that are strong enough to be effective. This means that any chemotherapy must be prescribed and administered by someone—usually a medical oncologist—who knows the drugs, their toxicities, and their side effects thoroughly.

Receiving chemotherapy

The first appointment includes a history, a physical, and plenty of discussion—but usually no chemotherapy. The oncologist talks about the goal of therapy, the potential benefits, the course and cycle being recommended, the drugs and what they do, the risks and side effects. The course advised depends on the results of the history and physical, the records from pathology and any surgery or radiation therapy, laboratory and imaging tests, and the statistical chances that chemotherapy can make the specific situation better. Then the woman goes home to think about it.

If she chooses to go ahead with chemo and will be receiving treatment in the doctor's office, it makes sense for her to bring someone with her the first time to see how she reacts to the medicines—and just to hold her hand. Ordinarily, however, even if she does experience side effects, they will not appear until several hours later.

What might a sample chemo appointment be like? The woman has a "complete blood count" drawn, either beforehand or in the doctor's office. She may take a prescription antinausea pill and may see the oncologist for a brief physical exam and to talk about how treatment is going, often once per cycle.

The oncologist or oncology nurse inserts an IV catheter into a hand or arm vein and either "pushes" (injects with a syringe) or drips one or more chemo agents from an IV bag. When this is finished, the IV catheter is removed, the woman sits in the office for a few minutes to be sure she does not develop a reaction to the drugs, and then goes home.

A sample cycle for one common regimen for breast cancer has her receiving two drugs injected through a vein, a process that takes a few minutes, on the first and eighth day of her 28-day chemotherapy cycle. She also takes a specified number of chemotherapy pills at home every day from the first through the 14th day, then spends the last two weeks of the cycle recovering.

Another woman, who has ovarian cancer, also has a 28-day chemotherapy cycle, but she spends the first four days of each cycle in the hospital receiving continuous IV chemotherapy, and then goes home to recover for the next 24 days until the next cycle starts.

Still another woman, with metastatic cancer, may get a continuous tiny infusion of one chemotherapy drug dispensed by a small pump she carries around all the time, and which she brings into the oncologist's office to be refilled. The idea behind this technique, used most often with metastatic cancer when other therapies have not worked, is to use small, constant "zaps" without giving the cancer cells time to recover.

Chemotherapy "routes"

Chemotherapy drugs can be swallowed as pills or another oral form, injected under the skin or into the muscle, given directly into a vein or artery, or infused into a body cavity. Depending on the most effective route for each drug—how it needs to be given to work best and most predictably—it can be given in the hospital or the doctor's office, or can be taken by the woman at home.

A common route is through the vein. This gives the drug immediate access to the circulatory system where cancer cells can hide, and the drugs can go anywhere in the body that the circulatory system reaches. Also, some chemotherapy drugs are deactivated if they are taken by mouth and have to go through the digestive tract, or it is uncertain how well and quickly they will be absorbed.

Some women have large veins in their arms, and have no problems receiving drugs intravenously. Other women may have veins that make it difficult to start and keep IV access. Or the woman may be receiving a chemotherapy agent that is especially rough on the veins, or can cause major local damage if it reaches the tissues surrounding the vein. Even a woman with "good" veins may be at risk when receiving the most damaging of these, the vesicants.

The woman who either has poor arm veins or is scheduled to receive a vesicant or similar drug may need longer-lasting access to a large central vein in the chest. There are all sorts of access devices that can last for several weeks, months, or even years. They can be used to give IV medications and to draw blood for blood tests (see chart on page 106).

Occasionally, the oncologist wants the chemotherapy to target an organ that is connected to a large artery. For a liver metastasis, for instance, chemo might be infused into an artery and go directly to the liver. This kind of **intra-arterial chemotherapy** is given with a special pump to overcome the blood pressure in the artery. In this case, chemotherapy is being used more as a local treatment than a systemic one.

Intraperitoneal chemotherapy, which is sometimes used in ovarian cancer, infuses the chemo into the abdominal cavity

Access to a Central Vein

Peripherally-inserted central catheter (PICC): long catheter inserted into arm vein, threaded up through arm to central vein.

Advantages: easy insertion by specially-trained nurse; requires no surgery to insert or remove. Easy to access: remove cap and begin therapy.

Disadvantages: not appropriate for long-term therapy (over 6 weeks or so); catheter must be flushed every few days, and site dressing changed; catheter visible on arm.

Most useful: if woman's arm veins "give out" near end of chemo.

Non-tunneled central catheter: catheter inserted directly into central vein near collarbone.

Advantages: no surgery to insert. Can have two or three separate "lumens" (channels) if needed. Easy to access.

Disadvantages: not appropriate for long-term therapy (more than a month); catheter must be flushed and site dressing changed; catheter visible on upper chest.

Most useful: if woman's arm veins "give out" near end of therapy and she needs multiple IV access.

Tunneled central catheter (Hickman, Groshong, etc.): catheter inserted in skin and then tunneled through tissue for several inches before it enters central vein.

Advantages: can be used indefinitely. Can have several lumens. Easy to access.

Disadvantages: minor surgical procedure to insert. Catheter must be flushed regularly and site care given. Catheter visible on chest.

Most useful: long-term use for woman who needs frequent IV access for therapy and for blood tests.

Implanted port (PortaCath, LifePort, PASport etc.): small metal or plastic port, stitched in place under skin, connected to catheter. Some ports rest under the chest or abdominal skin with the catheter inserted directly in a central vein. Others are implanted in the upper arm with catheter threaded through arm vein to a central vein.

(continued)

(Continued)

Advantages: can be used indefinitely. Port is under skin so that, except when port is being used, no catheter shows above the skin and no skin care is necessary. A few larger ports have more than one lumen.

Disadvantages: minor surgical procedures when port is implanted and removed. More difficult access: needle stick, using special technique and supplies, necessary to access port through the skin; must be done each time the port is used and to flush port once a month or so when it isn't being used. (The port can remain accessed for about a week at a time.) Small scars from insertion, removal. Port can show as round bump under skin.

Most useful: woman undergoing long-term therapy who needs IV access only once or twice a month. There are also several small ambulatory ("carry around") or implanted pumps to deliver continuous small doses of chemo.

Possible complications with any central line include infection, vein irritation, and blood clot.

through a special access chamber on the abdomen or chest. Since the chemo stays in one place, bathing the organs in the abdomen, the side effects are confined to that area and the drug can be given in very high doses.

Side effects of chemotherapy

Almost everyone who undergoes chemotherapy suffers some degree of fatigue. The fatigue tends to follow the chemo cycle and gets better during the recovery phase, but it also tends to get somewhat worse with later cycles. Because many people feel "wiped out" for at least a day after IV chemo, it makes sense for a woman to schedule treatment so that she can have a couple of days of "down time" afterwards (Friday afternoons, for instance, so that she can rest over the weekend before going to work Monday).

No one is absolutely sure why there is fatigue. It could be because the whole body is working overtime to dispose of dead cancer cells and rebuild healthy cells. Also, the whole psyche is struggling to cope with the changes cancer is making—more hard work. The woman is often not eating well and may not be getting much exercise. During the later cycles, she may be somewhat anemic, if chemotherapy affects her red blood cells. All of these factors combine to cause fatigue.

My favorite general recommendations for the woman beginning a course of chemo are

1. Be very kind to yourself and listen to your body (take a nap, do not drag yourself to an event)

2. Get some kind of exercise as often as possible

3. Schedule a treat for yourself during the recovery period in each cycle to serve as your carrot on a stick (a simple overnight trip, perhaps)

Many women find that fighting fatigue is counterproductive, and that it works better to relax more (some use relaxation training), ignore anything that does not absolutely have to be done, and pace their activities.

Besides general fatigue, the woman may develop more specific side effects because those cells in the body that normally "turn over" often become targets for chemotherapy. Each drug has its own pattern of which kinds of fast-dividing normal cells it attacks, but the cells most often affected are those in the bone marrow which make blood cells for the body; in the hair follicles; along the digestive tract; and in the ovaries.

There is *no* correlation between the number and severity of side effects a woman experiences and how well the chemo is working. Therapy can be completely effective for the woman who sails through treatment.

Bone marrow side effects

How chemotherapy affects the marrow in the large bones of the body is the side effect that worries doctors most. The bone marrow produces the white blood cells that protect the body, the platelets that help blood to clot, and the red blood cells that deliver oxygen everywhere in the body. The white blood cells and platelets turn over very quickly in the body, lasting only a few days, and thus are especially vulnerable to chemotherapy. The red cells, on the other hand, divide every several months—so that their numbers usually dip significantly only after several months of chemotherapy.

Each chemotherapy drug has a known **nadir**, the number of days after it is administered before the white blood count and the platelets reach their lowest point and start rebounding. Different drugs and dosages affect the bone marrow differently, and that is one of the factors oncologists balance when they are combining chemo drugs.

The oncologist usually orders a complete blood count at the beginning of each cycle and sometimes at the nadir to see what is happening. The woman will probably be told to report quickly any signs of infection or bleeding, especially at nadir. Other than that, she ordinarily will not need to pay much attention to what is occurring in her bone marrow, because there is normally a wide safety margin in the number of white blood cells and platelets in the body.

However, if she has an extreme drop in neutrophils, a specific kind of white blood cell that protects the body against infection, she is considered **neutropenic.** This means that she is at definite risk of infection. Some doctors will prescribe "just in case" antibiotics until her white blood count climbs to a safer level; at the first sign of any infection, she may be hospitalized for IV antibiotics. (Unfortunately, there are no safe white blood cell transfusions.)

A new strategy with some chemo regimens known to affect the bone marrow seriously is to give injections of **colony stimulating factor** (G-CSF, usually). This biological agent stimulates the bone marrow to produce more white cells faster so that there is a lesser and shorter dip.

An extreme drop in platelets (**thrombocytopenia**) puts a woman at risk for bleeding—anything from nose bleeds to bleeding gums to unexplained bruises under the skin. It is often treated with platelet transfusions until her own platelets bounce back.

Since the whole red blood cell life cycle is rather leisurely, it takes the red cells longer to dip, but also longer to recover on their own. If severe anemia occurs because of decreased red cells, usually after a few months, the woman may feel extremely tired or short of breath. Severe anemia is treated with blood transfusions; the doctor may prescribe iron pills or other medication for a lesser problem.

Hair loss

While doctors worry about the effects of chemotherapy on bone marrow, most women are more concerned about the possibility of losing their hair. Not every chemo drug targets the fast-dividing hair cells, but plenty of them cause some women to lose some hair, and a few cause almost everyone to lose all or most of her hair. Her oncologist should inform the woman about how the specific drugs she will receive are likely to affect her hair.

This temporary **alopecia** (hair loss) may affect not only the scalp, but also the eyebrows and eyelashes, pubic, and underarm hair. The hair may start regrowing near the end of chemo or soon afterward and the silver lining to this cloud is that even normally straight, limp hair often regrows thick, lustrous, and curly. This lasts for about two years, and then reverts to its former texture. Many a woman, asked about her gorgeous hair several months after chemo ends, has had to give primary credit to her oncologist!

With the drugs that cause major alopecia, the scalp tends to become tingly and "strange-feeling" two to three weeks after the drug is given. The hair begins falling out a little at first and then in large clumps. Almost no woman is really prepared for the loss.

If a woman knows she is going to receive one of these drugs, it is smart to get her hair cut as short as possible first; that way the handfuls of hair on her pillow or in the shower are smaller and a little less devastating. Some women put a strip of tape across a strip of hair before it is cut, and then tape or sew across the strip to make bangs to wear under a scarf or turban.

Washing her hair very gently, combing it without pulling it, avoiding harsh hair products, and using a satin pillowcase to avoid friction on the scalp may postpone hair loss. If the hair starts falling out, many women wear a cotton scarf or turban in bed to collect the hair, and may consider shaving the scalp.

It is easier for the woman who plans to wear a wig to begin shopping for one while the salesperson can see her natural hair color and style. Some shops specialize in hairpieces for people undergoing chemotherapy; addresses should be available through the Yellow Pages or from the oncologist, local American Cancer Society unit, or support group. Other women prefer scarves (cotton are usually most comfortable and stay on best), turbans, hats—or going proudly bald.

Some chemo drugs are unpredictable. Cyclophosphamide (Cytoxan), for instance, causes a few women to lose all their hair, a larger group to experience considerable thinning, and barely affects another fairly large group.

If there is almost no chance of the cancer spreading to the scalp, the oncologist may allow the woman to wear a "cold cap" over her scalp for a few minutes before the drug is given, and for about 45 minutes afterwards. The theory is that the cap, which cools the scalp dramatically (this feels decidedly strange), discourages the chemotherapy drug from settling there. However, this only works with the borderline hair loss chemo agents, and may not work even then.

One way of improvising a cold cap is to sew a double circle of cloth into a "mobcap," with a drawstring and an opening into which the woman can put several small refreezable icepacks.

Many women who do not lose their hair still favor a short haircut to disguise hair thinning, and they treat their hair very gently. Others find they can cover patchy hair loss well with a longer hair style.

Along with hair loss and changes in hair texture, some women experience temporary complexion changes. For women undergoing cancer treatment who have beauty questions, the American Cancer Society, together with the Cosmetic, Toiletry, and Fragrance Association Foundation and the National Cosmetology Association, has set up a nationwide program called *Look Good, Feel Better.* Every participant receives free a large packet of skin care and makeup products. Then, depending on the local program, she may get an individual makeover (including wig styling, if appropriate) or a group session. Information is available from the local ACS chapter.

The digestive tract

The cells lining the digestive tract from mouth to anus turn over about once a week—which makes them prime targets for several chemotherapy agents. Women undergoing chemo may have no problem at all or may experience anything from occasional mild queasiness to nonstop vomiting, often beginning several hours after receiving IV chemo. It is fairly common, too, for women to complain of a funny taste in the mouth, loss of appetite, food aversions (just the thought of a particular food turns the stomach), or mouth sores. Either diarrhea or constipation is also possible.

In 1991, a new drug called **ondansetron** (Zofran) revolutionized the treatment of severe nausea and vomiting from chemotherapy. This drug, given intravenously a few minutes before the chemo agent and then every several hours afterwards, has tamed some of the most notorious chemotherapy drugs for many women. Even one dose given in the doctor's office may be enough to make nausea no problem, and a new pill form has just arrived on the market. However, the drug remains very expensive.

Currently it is easier to prevent severe nausea than the mild queasiness that affects some women taking chemo pills for two weeks out of every four. There are antinausea medicines women can take as pills, suppositories, or even injections, and many oncologists at least mention marijuana as a possible treatment. In addition, different women swear by different personal remedies, such as herbal teas, acupuncture, seasickness wrist bands, self-hypnosis, relaxation or visualization, or simply keeping something—carrot stick, ginger snap, cracker—in the stomach all the time.

Women sometimes find it helpful to suck on a hard candy to mask the "taste" of intravenous chemo. Since it is crucial to stay as well-nourished as possible during chemo so that the body can do its share of the work, women may have to use considerable ingenuity to stay on a balanced diet. Blender drinks were my ace in the hole, but I wish that the book *Nutrition for the Chemotherapy Patient* with its tempting recipes had been available then (see Resources). A pamphlet, *Eating Hints: Recipes and Hints for Better Nutrition During Cancer Treatment*, can be ordered free from the Cancer Information Service.

Even if she does not experience nausea or vomiting, many a woman develops a real aversion to any food she eats the evening of a chemo day. It makes sense for her to avoid eating her favorite foods then, at least until she finds out whether this is a pattern for her. Something light, like broth and crackers, often works best.

Stomatitis can be a very serious side effect of chemo and women taking chemo agents known for causing inflammation and sores in the mouth may be able to prevent problems by rinsing their mouths frequently with warm water containing salt and baking soda. There are also special mouthwashes to numb and heal the mouth if it becomes inflamed. One nursing research study suggests holding ice chips in the mouth while getting an IV chemo "push," on the same principle as the cold cap for the scalp.

It is an excellent idea to see a dentist for tooth cleaning and repair *before* starting chemo, and to practice careful dental hygiene during the course. Any other dental care during chemo should be coordinated with the oncologist. Dental problems can increase bad tastes in the mouth and the risk of stomatitis; they can also be the source of serious infection when the white blood count is low. (My dentist recommended that I rinse with Listerine twice a day. Thank you, no! As I discovered quickly, alcohol-based mouthwashes are excruciatingly painful on a mouth that is even slightly raw and they just dry it out more.)

The woman may develop changes in bowel habits from the chemotherapy drugs, other medications she is taking, and/or changes in her activity and diet. For constipation, she can increase fluid intake, dietary fiber, and activity. All medication for either constipation or diarrhea needs to be approved by the oncologist first.

The reproductive tract

A few chemotherapy drugs commonly used in treating women's cancers attack the fast-dividing cells in the ovaries of premenopausal women. This is a side effect but, in the case of the cancers influenced by female hormones, it may be medically desirable too.

That is no reason for the woman to be thrilled, however. It is common for her to stop menstruating a few months after treatment begins, and to experience menopausal symptoms such as hot flashes, night sweats, and vaginal dryness. Women not too far past menopause may experience some of these symptoms too.

Sometimes the woman begins menstruating again after treatment ends—often with a very irregular pattern at first—but the closer she is to the normal age of menopause, the more likely it is that the changes are permanent. She is usually discouraged from taking hormone replacement therapy, for fear of nourishing any stray cancer cells (see Chapter 13).

Other side effects

Every chemotherapy drug has its individual fingerprint of known side effects. One drug zeros in on the heart, while another may cause tingling in the feet. Some of these only occur at a dosage—either one-time or cumulative—that is too high for the woman's body and is considered toxic; others can happen with any dosage. Some toxicities can be prevented if the woman follows directions exactly (like drinking lots of fluids to protect the bladder with the drug Cytoxan). Many side effects —but not all—go away after chemo finishes, or even between doses.

The woman needs to find out from her oncologist the most common and serious side effects of any chemotherapy drug she is taking and if there is anything she can do to minimize them. For more information about getting through chemo, she may want to read Nancy Bruning's book, *Coping with Chemotherapy* or NCI's *Chemotherapy and You* (see Resources).

HORMONAL THERAPY

Some women's cancers depend on a supply of female hormones in the right balance so that they can grow and thrive. The idea behind hormone therapy is to change the hormonal environment of cancer cells anywhere in the body so that they starve.

Doctors are trying strategies—sometimes with considerable success—which include manipulations with female hormones, weakened female hormones that fool the cancer cells, "antihormones" that block female hormones, and male hormones. Because breast cancer is the only women's cancer in which hormonal therapy is used with any frequency, this treatment is discussed more thoroughly in Part Two in the chapters on breast cancer.

Of course, these hormone manipulations can and do cause symptoms. Women who are premenopausal or recently postmenopausal appear to be more susceptible because their own hormones are more active. Different hormone medications can cause PMS-like symptoms, menopausal changes, or masculinizing changes such as a deeper voice, acne, and facial hair.

BIOLOGICAL THERAPY

Biological therapy (biologic response modifiers) is a relative newcomer in cancer treatment. It is not new at all in the treatment of diseases, however, since every vaccination against measles or polio follows one basic biological therapy strategy: teaching the body's own immune system to attack something that should not be there.

Biological therapy can use highly purified proteins to wake up the body's defenses or make them work together better. Other biological therapies try to increase the numbers of defender cells, make the individual cells more effective, or mark the cancer cells more clearly as targets. **Interferon** and **Interleukin,** for instance, are two examples of proteins that occur naturally in the body and can be grown in large quantities in the laboratory. They are being investigated in clinical trials against some forms of cancer, but have not shown much promise yet in women's cancers.

The colony stimulating factors (CSF), sometimes used to push the white blood cells to recover faster after chemotherapy, are one example of a biological response modifier. Researchers are currently experimenting with **monoclonal antibodies,** laboratory copies of the normal antibodies that attack specific kinds of cancer cells. They hope that eventually these antibodies can be harnessed to carry chemotherapy or radioactive compounds directly to the target cells: "smart bombs" on the cellular level. But there are problems. Monoclonal antibodies may attack the wrong cells, for instance, or the body may start seeing the biological therapy proteins as foreign and attack them. As with chemotherapy, side effects can make the patient miserable, or even be life-threatening.

At the moment, biological therapy is more promise than delivery in the women's cancers. Many oncologists and cancer researchers are convinced, however, that this is where tomorrow's cancer victories will come from.

CLINICAL TRIALS

A clinical trial is a study done under stringent conditions to evaluate a new therapy. The new treatment is tried because there is reasonable hope that it will be more effective than current therapy. Clinical trials, done after extensive animal studies, can be the source of treatment breakthroughs—or may show that this therapy is a blind end.

Clinical trials usually randomly assign patients to either a group receiving the experimental treatment or to a second "control" (comparison) group receiving the standard treatment or a placebo. Until the study is over, patients do not know who received what. If there is no standard therapy available for a particular condition, the treatment group is compared with people who receive no treatment.

Cancer clinical trials are carried out in three phases. A Phase I trial tests the experimental treatment in a few patients to find out how to give the therapy most effectively, how much can be given safely, and whether there are side effects that have not shown up in animal studies. Since less is known about the treatment at this early stage, a Phase I trial is the riskiest. The only patients allowed in this phase are those with metastatic cancer who do not have other treatment options.

Phase II studies build on the Phase I information to look at how the proposed therapy works in different kinds of cancer. Finally, Phase III studies use patients in all stages of cancer to compare the experimental treatment with standard therapy to see which is more effective, and to try variations in dosage and timing. All treatment in a clinical trial is provided free.

Phase I trials are ordinarily carried out at major cancer centers with hospitalized patients. By the time the treatment reaches Phase III trials, however, the researchers know a great deal more about the treatment. Thus, Phase III trials may be carried out at a cancer center or out in the community through the Community Clinical Oncology Program (CCOP) of the National Cancer Institute. CCOP, with clinical trials in many states, gives researchers a much larger pool of potential partici-pants. In addition, it allows many more cancer patients to be part of a study if they so wish, and it moves research findings more quickly and smoothly into standard practice.

Historically, most cancer patients have not participated in clinical trials. For many women, however, this can be a way to help not only themselves but generations of women to come. Every successful anticancer agent we have now came out of clinical trials, and finding out that something *does not* work is equally important information.

PAYING FOR IT

Cancer treatment is expensive. In addition, many a working woman has to take time off work for surgery or other therapy and may lose salary. How does she cope?

For the woman in a hospital, the social worker, discharge planner, or financial counselor can provide information about financial aid available and help her make her way through the insurance thicket. In the doctor's office, one of the office staff should have basic information. Health insurance, Medicare or Medicaid/Medi-Cal usually pays many or all of the medical bills, but the woman needs to read and ask questions about her particular policy.

If available, sick leave benefits from work or disability insurance (private or state) can help with living expenses. U.S. Federal Government disability payments come through the Social Security Administration for those who are totally disabled or expect to be totally disabled for at least one year; many women with cancer will be back at work long before then.

It is vitally important to get any insurance paperwork filled in and filed as promptly as possible. The woman who either does not find out what she needs to do, or—in the midst of everything else going on after a cancer diagnosis—forgets to do it, may miss out on coverage she could have received.

A free pamphlet, *Cancer Treatments Your Insurance Should Cover*, is available from the Association of Community Cancer Centers (see Resources). The American Cancer Society may also have information about financial resources for cancer treatment. Clinical trials that pay the cost of all treatment, often including transportation, may also be an option.

Many people in the U.S. are unhappy with the current state of health insurance, and changes could happen at any time. In the meantime, one of the best sources of information about insurance for the woman with cancer is the National Coalition for Cancer Survivorship, 1010 Wayne Avenue 5th Floor, Silver Spring MD 20910; 301-585-2616.

Kerry McGinn

Chapter 9

❖

Complementary and Unorthodox Therapies for Cancer

Neither physical recovery nor life extension is the test of the value of spiritual approaches to cancer. The test is the effect they have on the living experience of the person involved.

—Michael Lerner

Unproven or unorthodox cancer therapy is controversial—to say the least. To some, mostly those with cancer, unproven treatments offer hope for a better and perhaps longer life. To critics, unproven treatments are often a cruel hoax, and an expensive one to boot. The major idea that I hope this admittedly brief chapter will provide is this: not one of the therapies described here—or that is reported in any other lay or professional literature—has been scientifically proven to cure cancer. But for many people, some of these forms of therapy could be incredibly helpful as complements to conventional cancer therapy. People need to choose judiciously from among the unorthodox therapies.

Unorthodox treatment methods are not for every person who has cancer—or at least, not every form of therapy is "right" for every person with cancer. For example, I cannot imagine my father using imagery or relaxation techniques even though he suffered with pain, nausea, and vomiting during his battle with lung cancer. I wish he could have found relief through some of these techniques, but for him "that stuff was just too far out."

I have been privileged to be with many people who have cancer and have seen some pretty unbelievable things first-hand. I have watched men and women survive against all odds—or at least survive long enough to achieve some hoped-for goal. For some, the quality of their survival was most important. My own father survived much longer than the statistics gave him, and he didn't do anything special like imagery or nutritional therapy. He always said he was "too stubborn to just give up and die." And he had things he wanted to get finished before he died.

Lorraine was faced with a cancer of unknown origin that was fairly widespread even when it was diagnosed. I gave her the Simontons' book *Getting Well Again,* and she found a group that helped her develop skills in guided imagery. She lived for five years, at least four and a half years longer than the statistics gave her—much of the time without symptoms or problems from her cancer. During that time, she worked as a docent at the local art museum, was involved in several charity organizations, and helped found a cancer support group in my hospital.

Jane had late-stage ovarian cancer at diagnosis. She was a young, ambitious, determined woman. Despite the prediction that she had less than six months, she lived more than three years, married, and helped other women deal with the side effects of chemotherapy. A young man with lymphoma had a tough time coping with the side effects of radiation and chemotherapy. He had every chance for cure, but the treatment bordered on more than he could—or wanted to—handle. He joined Lorraine's group, discovered artistic talent he did not know he had, and has since married and hosted several one-man shows of his art.

Ascella had metastatic breast cancer but she wanted to see her daughter graduate from high school. She went through heavy-duty chemotherapy but also went to a health spa in Lourdes. She did see her daughter graduate and she enjoyed her life. My college roommate and friend, Cindy, had a very vicious form of skin cancer (melanoma) and her prognosis was dismal even when she was first diagnosed. But Cindy was a fighter. She found a clinical trial program that gave her extra months, during which she got to spend valuable time with her teenage daughter, resolve some issues in her marriage and, probably most important for her, find a dream job that gave her the chance to prove herself and be fulfilled in her art.

With all this evidence, I cannot deny the impact of the interaction between the mind and the body on the body's ability to heal itself and fight disease.

There is a whole host of terms that get used interchangeably when speaking of treatments. For the sake of consistency, the terms and definitions used here reflect those agreed to for the U.S. Congressional Report, *Unconventional Cancer Treatments* (1990). Generally, the terms used reflect the degree of acceptability that a particular form of therapy has within the medical establishment. "Mainstream" and "conventional" treatments refer to those that are widely used in major American cancer centers. These treatments include surgery, radiation therapy, chemotherapy, hormonal therapy, and biologic therapy. The "unconventional" approaches are those that fall outside of mainstream cancer care. "Complementary" therapies complement or add to the use of conventional approaches. Sometimes the complementary therapies are also called "unorthodox" or "unconventional," though the term "unconventional" is probably the more neutral. "Alternative" refers to treatments that are further outside the mainstream. "Adjunctive" therapy is closer to mainstream, and includes psychosocial approaches like support groups, psychotherapy, imagery, and hypnosis.

There are at least a hundred known unconventional treatments, and infinite variations within each major category. Unconventional treatments can be simple or complex and range from slight modifications to drastic changes in the patient's lifestyle.

The best unconventional treatments are those that improve quality of life, promote general health, and engage the "patient" in the treatment in helpful ways. The worst exist for the financial gain of the practitioner. A lot of unconventional treatment plans have both good and bad elements—which makes for a good deal of confusion on the part of the patient and health-care professionals alike.

Therapies can be "open" or "closed." Open therapies are those in which the nature of the treatment—how it works, its theory, and so on—are openly revealed. In closed treatments, some major part of the therapy plan is not available for scrutiny. Closed therapies increase suspicion about the practitioner's motives.

Practitioners of unconventional treatments vary in their competency and the care that is taken during the treatment. The specific treatment can be open and ethical, but the practitioner may be unqualified to provide care. Americans spend an estimated $10 billion each year on unproven cancer therapy. Typically, treatments last just over a year. Some cost as much as $20,000 annually, but most cost far less. Insurance will cover some forms of unconventional therapy (in part or fully); costs are more likely to be reimbursed if the treatment involves drugs.

Over 50% of all people with cancer try some type of unproven therapy during the course of their cancer. Most do not tell their doctor they are using an unproven treatment—a secret that can be dangerous if the treatment has side effects. And alarmingly, 17% of people in one study who had used unproven cancer treatment selected that treatment *before* getting conventional cancer therapy. For these people, a delay in conventional therapy could have decreased the chance of successful treatment.

WHO USES THESE FORMS OF TREATMENT?

Contrary to popular belief, it is *not* the uneducated, poor person who gets duped into trying unconventional cancer treatment. Generally, people who use unconventional therapy are among the more educated, informed, and affluent healthcare consumers.

People don't need to go to Mexico or the Bahamas to get unconventional treatment either. Medical establishments in

Europe, Japan, and China are more open to unconventional therapies, so they are easier to find in those countries. In America there is also some backlash against the slow-moving FDA drug approval processes—evidenced most recently in demonstrations by AIDS activists urging a speed-up of approval for new AIDS drugs. However, only about 2% of all Americans who use unconventional therapy went outside of the United States to find it.

Another factor is that cancer is treated much more aggressively in America than in European and Asian countries. This is particularly important for women. In France, for example, more emphasis is placed on preservation of sexual organs. As a result, French doctors recommended lumpectomies and partial mastectomies much earlier than these surgeries were advocated in the United States. Many Latin doctors share the same concerns. An American woman is two to three times more likely to have a hysterectomy than a woman with the same diagnosis in England, France, or Germany. This preference for gentler cancer therapies leads the French to greater acceptance of therapies like homeopathy.

Homeopathy treats diseases with very dilute doses of substances that would produce symptoms like the disease in a healthy person; in the U.S., homeopathy is sometimes used as a more general term that includes the use of "natural remedies." There are signs that use of homeopathy is increasing in the United States: the American market for homeopathic drugs is about $100 million each year. Certainly, medicines with no side effects are attractive to anyone facing illness, especially if that illness is cancer.

In Germany, people with cancer have more choices of therapies than in any other modern country. Popular choices there include naturopathic, herbal, homeopathic, spiritual, and conventional cancer treatments.

In Great Britain, choices are influenced by the British healthcare system and ease of access to unconventional therapies. When conventional therapy is used, it is likely to be much less aggressive than would be recommended in the United States.

Why do so many people opt to use unproven methods of cancer treatment? Maybe one of the most important reasons is that they offer an alternative to what some people characterize as the "slashing, burning, and poisoning" methods of conventional treatment. Most unproven cancer therapies promote the use of nontoxic and/or natural substances or healing methods. Supporters of these methods claim success based on anecdotes of cure or control—stories about the cure of a few people. This lack of evidence from clinical trials methods is probably the major objection the scientific community has to unproven therapies.

American medicine is rarely "user-friendly." Many people really want to be actively involved in getting well, and in the U.S. at least, patients are all too often the last to be consulted about treatment plans. An office visit with a doctor here, even when the doctor is seeing a woman with a new cancer, lasts an average of 16 minutes. Doctors spend, on an average, from one to three minutes giving information (though most doctors believe they spend seven times that long). The "patient" spends about eight seconds asking questions. This is in great contrast with the generous amounts of personal attention given by practitioners of unconventional therapies.

WHAT IS UNCONVENTIONAL CANCER THERAPY?

There are some currently accepted treatment modalities that were once considered quackery, and there is every chance that some "alternative" forms of cancer treatment will some day be accepted therapy—or at least be accepted as complements to traditional cancer treatment. Over the years, NCI has tested many unconventional agents including laetrile, vitamin C and hydrazine sulphate.

The U.S. House of Representatives asked the Office of Technology Assessment (OTA) to develop a clinical trial to study the effect and safety of Immuno-Augmentation Therapy (IAT). This resulted in the creation of a panel—and funding of $2 million—to develop criteria to assess unconventional cancer treatments. NCI is prepared to help unconventional practitioners document the effectiveness of their therapies. An amendment to the National Institutes of Health budget gives its director the authority to permit research on unconventional therapies by licensed doctors.

Most unconventional cancer therapies fall into these categories:

♦ metabolic and dietary

♦ herbal

♦ megavitamin

♦ psychological/psychosocial

♦ physical

♦ traditional or folk medicine

♦ spiritual healing

♦ pharmacological (using drugs or special preparations)

Different practitioners advocate variations and sometimes combinations from these categories, which are discussed in more detail below.

METABOLIC AND DIETARY THERAPY

Cancer treatment is generally much more effective if the person is well-nourished, so diet is tremendously important during cancer treatment and recovery. There are many claims for different nutritional therapies but since most doctors and nurses are not experts in nutrition they may not be able to adequately explain the pros and cons of dietary therapies. While scientific evidence is still incomplete, healthcare professionals generally recommend a balanced diet, often with multivitamin supplements—which include vitamins C, E, and A, and some minerals like zinc, to enhance cell renewal and healing.

The majority of people with cancer use some form of metabolic or dietary therapy—with or without conventional cancer treatment. The theory behind metabolic therapy is the belief that body toxins and wastes interfere with healing, and therapy focuses on removing toxins from the body. Practitioners believe cancer results from degeneration of the liver and pancreas, as well as the immune system in general. The interaction of the lungs and blood vessels—the body functions that provide oxygen to all body cells—is also disrupted. By clearing the system of the toxic end-products of chemicals we ingest and avoiding ingesting new ones the cells receive the nutrients needed for health.

Dietary therapies focus on the nutrients a person takes into her body. Most dietary cancer therapies are vegetarian. Treatments usually require that the patient's diet include specific foods. Some of the more common diets promote grapes, raw foods, and wheatgrass extract. Some dietary regimens include detoxification. Mainstream medicine does not recognize detoxification at all, but it is a vital component of many unconventional programs.

Actual regimens vary from one practitioner to another, but typical metabolic therapy plans include special diets, detoxification by colonic cleansing (enemas or high colonics), and regular doses of vitamins, minerals, and enzymes. Coffee enemas and high colonic irrigations using wheatgrass or other substances are used to "detoxify" the liver. Though most clinics offering metabolic therapy are in Mexico, there are a few in the United States, Europe, and Canada. In 1991, Michael Landon used metabolic and nutritional therapy as a primary treatment for cancer of the pancreas and described his treatment, including coffee enemas and carrot juice supplements, in detail on *The Tonight Show* a few weeks before he died.

Metabolic therapy was first advocated by Max Gerson in Germany in the 1920s and his diet was the best known nutritional therapy until the introduction of macrobiotics. It is derived from a combination of Gerson's research and European folk medicine. The **Gerson diet** begins with a raw, vegetarian diet, modified with some cooked foods, and still later with animal products. The patient drinks vegetable and fruit juices every hour, has several types of enemas, and drinks several glasses of fresh calf's liver juice or carrot juice daily. Gerson brought his treatment to the United States and continued using it until his death in 1959. A modified version is promoted by his daughter at the Gerson Institute in Bonita, California and the Gerson Clinic in Tijuana, Mexico.

In 1980, American actor Steve McQueen drew media attention when he opted to go to the Kelley Clinic at Plaza Santa Maria (south of Tijuana) for treatment. The Kelley theory is that cancer is caused by a pancreatic enzyme deficiency. Dr. Kelley, a dentist, developed the Kelley Enzyme Test and the Kelley Index of Malignancy—questionnaires used to analyze tumors and prognosis. The Kelley regimen is a nutritional program based on vitamin and enzyme supplements and computerized metabolic typing. Kelley no longer practices, but his plan is still used in several forms by his followers.

Macrobiotics is probably the most widely used nutritional approach to cancer in the United States. Its proponents offer both preventive and curative claims. Macrobiotic therapy is based on the traditional Eastern concepts of balance and harmony—the balance of opposite and complementary energies, *yin* and *yang*, which in healing strategies extend to body functions. According to specific macrobiotic theory, there is a "mother red blood cell" in the intestine from which all body cells and organs derive. Intake of foods balanced in yin and yang qualities promotes health and counteracts disease. Deeper aspects of the yin-yang balance also bring in the spiritual aspect of life. Macrobiotic diets, derived from a traditional Japanese diet, are largely low-fat, complex carbohydrate, vegetarian diets —including only whole grains, some specially cooked vegetables, and miso, a soybean product believed to prevent cancer development. The major hazard of macrobiotic therapy is, strangely enough, malnutrition.

The program advocated by Dr. Virginia Livingston and used at the **Livingston-Wheeler Medical Clinic** in San Diego integrates diet, nutritional supplements, and immunotherapy. Treatment includes immune-enhancing vaccines (Bacille Calmette-Guerin), a vegetarian diet, and coffee enemas. Dr. Livingston claimed to have discovered a microbe that causes cancer and a vaccine to counteract it. The Livingston diet evolved from the Gerson diet, and can include megavitamin therapy. However, the Livingston-Wheeler therapy is totally dismissed by mainstream practitioners. A recent study found that survival rates did not differ between people going through the Livingston-Wheeler program and people receiving conventional cancer therapy in a university cancer center. Actually, people getting conventional therapy had *better* quality of life throughout the study period. More Livingston-Wheeler patients had negative side effects like decreased appetite, pain, and breathing problems.

The major problem faced by people who follow metabolic regimens is related to colonic cleansing. The colon (bowel) can be damaged or punctured by the enema tube during the procedure, resulting in irritation and/or infection. The bowel tissue can be overloaded with fluid, cutting off blood flow to these tissues. Enemas can pull important electrolytes (potassium, for example) out of the body. The resulting deficit of electrolytes can cause heart irregularities and death.

Keith Block, M.D., of the University of Illinois School of Medicine advocates a middle ground approach of combining unconventional and conventional cancer treatments. While his specialty is internal medicine, he has done advanced research into the nutritional and behavioral aspects of cancer and has developed an approach to cancer care and treatment based on a philosophy of compassionate caring for others. Dr. Block was a member of NCI's Unconventional Cancer Treatments Advisory Panel and his work is widely followed—though not necessarily promoted—in the mainstream medical community.

Dr. Block's model of care has six basic elements: biomedical, biopsychosocial, biochemical, biomechanical, medical gradualism, and the use of diagnostic and therapeutic tools that are minimally invasive. He uses the most effective and least invasive procedures first. More aggressive tools are introduced later, if and when they become necessary. He uses laboratory evaluations to show the activity and aggressiveness of cancers; antagonists, which combat the side effects from conventional therapy; and agonists, treatments or specially developed drugs that increase the effects of conventional cancer treatments. Block claims to design treatment plans that use conventional and unconventional therapies specific for each patient. He promotes self-care to the extent that an individual is capable, urging patients to consider what they need, how they respond to challenges, what they experience as stress, and how they learn. These elements of each person's psyche are considered in the entire treatment plan.

Other important parts of Block's regimen are physical conditioning and diet. The nutritional component of the Block program has evolved from macrobiotics. The dietary recommendations are similar to the low-fat preventive diets endorsed by the American Heart Association, the American Cancer Society, and the National Cancer Institute. The major difference is that this "preventive" diet is continued after the diagnosis of cancer. In the diet, 50–60% of nutrients are drawn from complex carbohydrates. Fat intake, mostly from vegetable sources, ranges from 12–25%, and the rest of the daily caloric intake comes from protein sources. The diet uses exchange lists, similar to diabetic exchange lists, based on whole cereal grains, fruits, nuts and seeds, vegetables, legumes, and limited amounts of certain fish and poultry. Megavitamin supplements are not emphasized, though vitamin supplements, where there is evidence that they are helpful, are encouraged. Specific nutrients like vitamins A and E and trace minerals are used to bolster immune functions impaired by malnutrition, the effects of conventional treatment, or the cancer itself. Block also uses some natural supplements like echinacea and garlic to boost immune function and counter the side effects of treatment.

HERBAL THERAPY

There are over 3,000 different plants that have been used worldwide throughout history in the treatment of diseases, including cancer. Traditional herbal practices use a whole plant or crude extracts of the plant. Traditional Chinese healing practices combining herbs with acupuncture and other techniques are used by people in the United States for pain management, to control side effects, and to improve the quality of life. Chemicals from some fungi—especially edible and inedible mushrooms—are known to affect tumor growth and stimulate immune activity. The shiitake mushroom in particular has been intensely studied.

Chaparral tea has been used as a folk remedy for leukemia and cancers of the kidney, liver, lung, and stomach. Native Americans in the southwestern United States use chaparral for many illnesses including cancer. Tea is made from tiny leaves and twigs on the bark of the creosote bush that is found in the southwestern desert. Chemicals derived from the creosote bush have been found to have some antioxidant properties, which may promote healing. A study of chaparral tea was completed in 1970 at the University of Utah. In a few patients it seemed to produce a slight antitumor response, but the methods used in study were not described well and its results have not been duplicated in other studies.

Essiac is an herbal preparation developed in Canada based on a Native American folk recipe. Rene Caisse, a nurse, was the sole proprietor of Essiac from 1920 to 1970. The story goes that she got the recipe from an Native American woman and began to use it on a family member who had cancer. She found it to be effective and began to make it available to others, calling it "essiac" which is her name spelled backwards. Before she died in 1978 she gave the formula and marketing rights to the Resperin Corporation of Ontario. Resperin provides Essiac to people with cancer through a special agreement with the Canadian Federal Health Offices.

Essiac supposedly contains four ingredients: Indian rhubarb, Sheepshead sorrel, Slippery elm, and Burdock root. The proportions are not known. NCI's Natural Products Branch reports that breakdown products from each ingredient are known to show some antitumor activity. The mixture, as supplied by Resperin, was tested in two trials at the Memorial Sloan Kettering Cancer Center in New York and found to have no effect on tumors *and* to be toxic in high doses. The Canadian health system reviewed the results of Essiac treatment on 86 patients.

Only one of the 86 felt better after Essiac therapy, and four had an objective, measurable response. Four were stable, and the rest had no benefit, could not be evaluated, or had died.

Currently, Essiac is not approved for marketing in Canada, but it is available to certain patients in certain conditions—primarily when no other treatment is available. Practitioners using Essiac discourage use of conventional therapy (radiation, chemotherapy) with the preparation.

The **Hoxsey therapy** was developed when Harry Hoxsey's grandfather noticed that his horse's tumor disappeared after the horse had grazed in a field filled with herbal wildflowers. Grandfather Hoxsey used a preparation made from the wildflowers on a family member who had a tumor and believed that the tumor vanished. The original recipe was passed to Harry Hoxsey from his father, and the first clinic was opened in Dallas in the 1920s. By 1950, the Hoxsey clinic was one of the largest private cancer centers in the world and had branches in 17 states. After multiple clashes with the FDA, the Dallas clinic closed in the late 1950s. A Tijuana clinic, under the direction of Hoxsey's nurse, has continued to use variations of the Hoxsey remedy since 1963.

According to Harry Hoxsey, chemical imbalances cause mutations that eventually result in a "vicariously competent cell" that is cancer. Normalization of body fluids creates an unfavorable environment for these cells and they eventually die. His remedy corrects the abnormal blood chemistry and normalizes cell metabolism. Hoxsey's regimen can be used internally (taken as a pill or liquid tonic) or topically (applied to the skin.) Nutritional supplements and dietary restrictions are also part of the overall treatment plan.

The mixture has not been tested for antitumor activity; though a few of its ingredients show minimal antitumor effects, most ingredients had no antitumor effects at all. Hoxsey's nurse claims an 80% cure rate, and the 20% who fail, she says, do so because they have a "bad attitude." No clinical trials have been done, though a review of medical records has been published. This review showed that of 71 patients, more than half had died, and in 25% of these patients, there was no proof that they ever had cancer. One in ten had been given conventional treatment (chemotherapy, surgery, and/or radiation) before going to the clinic.

Mistletoe preparations are available in several forms. They have been mainly used in Switzerland, Germany and other European countries, and less commonly in the United States. Trade names include **Plenosol** and **Iscador:** both are fermented extracts combined with metals like silver, copper, and mercury. In the early 1980s, forty thousand people were using Iscador, and it is currently available in Switzerland, Germany, the Netherlands, the United Kingdom, Austria, and Sweden. It is not approved for sale in the United States, but American doctors can order it from European manufacturers. The Lukas Klinik in Switzerland uses Iscador with conventional therapy, homeopathic preparations, a vegetarian diet, artistic activities, light exercise, baths, oils, and massage.

Crude mistletoe extracts and Iscador have been studied with mixed results. Some antitumor effects have been noted in some animal studies. There seems to be some increase in immune functions related to Iscador, but that could be caused by normal reactions to bacteria and other ingredients in the preparation. Proponents claim that Iscador increases both the length of survival and the quality of life, that it stabilizes disease, causes tumor regression, and improves a patient's general condition.

A nurse tells me that she has been following a woman for several months who gets chemotherapy and also uses a ground mistletoe preparation. The woman's blood counts are more stable that would normally be expected and she does not have problems with nausea and vomiting. As an experiment, the nurses in the clinic asked this woman to stay off mistletoe for just one cycle of chemotherapy. Sure enough, her white blood cell count dropped much more than usual and she had more nausea and vomiting than she had experienced when she was on the mistletoe. Needless to say, the woman continues to use her extract!

Pau d'Arco is an herb that is available in healthfood stores. American companies market this herb in capsule, tea, and loose powder forms. Pau d'Arco is also called taheebo, lapacho, ipes, ipe roxo, and trumpet bush. It is grown in South America and is a popular folk remedy for various forms of cancer and other diseases, including malaria. It is reported to be a "strengthening and cleansing agent." Research studies have focused on one of the chemicals derived from it: lapachol. Proponents cite an unpublished study as evidence of its antitumor effect and its ability to enhance the immune system. Its major danger is its ability to cause blood clotting at doses given in cancer treatment.

MEGAVITAMIN THERAPY

Megavitamin therapy is one of the more common forms of alternative cancer treatment. Dr. Livingston promoted megavitamins as a way to make up for unknown, but harmful vitamin deficiencies. Practitioners of megavitamin therapy believe extra large doses of vitamins increase the body's ability to destroy cancer cells. But megavitamin therapy most likely does not offer much. The human body seems to "know" what vitamins it needs, and the rest are removed from the body, mostly in urine. Some people say that Americans, because of their extraordinary overuse of vitamins, have the most expensive urine in the world! In some cases overuse of vitamins can be harmful. Some vitamins interfere with the action of conventional chemotherapy. For this reason, it is important for the doctor to know about a person's use of vitamin therapy.

PSYCHOLOGICAL APPROACHES

Mental imagery, or **visualization,** is useful in the management of cancer. During "gentle imagery" a woman focuses on imagining peaceful, pleasant scenes. Gentle imagery is often used with relaxation, meditation, and hypnosis. In "guided imagery" a woman visualizes the symbolic destruction of cancer cells. Imagery can be used to reduce pain and stress, and maybe even to change the course of disease. It is a major component of the total program described by the Simontons' in *Getting Well Again*.

Imagery in healing can be traced to ancient cultures. Historical records from Babylonia, Assyria, and Greece document the use of imagery to chase disease from sick people. Imagery is also a part of Freudian psychoanalysis, and some kinds of imagery are used in biofeedback, Gestalt, and desensitization therapies. Imagery is useful in changing bodily processes, emotional status, self-image, physical performance, and behavior.

Imagery is a mental picture of a reality or a fantasy. It can include all five senses—sight, touch, hearing, smell, and taste. In guided imagery, a person intentionally creates an image that she chooses, and through this image, communicates with her body processes. Some sort of relaxation exercise is usually the first part of guided imagery, followed by action imagery and end-result imagery—imagining what the desired end result will be.

Guided imagery used by a woman with cancer might go like this: the woman uses a simple relaxation exercise, such as silently repeating the word "relax," to let go of muscle tension. When she is relaxed, she pictures her cancer in any way it appears to her and then images her form of treatment. For example, chemotherapy might be seen spreading itself through her blood and being picked up by the cancer cells. (My friend Lorraine imaged the chemotherapy as piranhas eating up the cancer cells.) The woman then images her cancer shrinking or being destroyed, and her white blood cells removing dead cancer cells from her body. Lastly, she sees herself healthy and her body free of disease.

Meditation is any activity that keeps attention pleasantly focused in the present moment, clearing the mind of daily events and problems. Its purpose is to raise self-awareness, a first step in regaining control of the mind. This self-awareness and mental control are important tools in self-healing. There are different approaches to meditation; most attempt to achieve a state of absence or suspension of logical thought and emotional process. People who advocate meditation believe it recharges the immune system and helps it to function more effectively.

Hypnosis, another form of tapping into mental processes, is becoming more accepted as a complement to conventional therapy for relaxation and pain control.

The study of **psychoneuroimmunology (PNI)** by the medical establishment has given legitimacy to these complementary therapies. But it was quite a different story in 1978 when the Simontons were ridiculed for their belief in imagery techniques. This is a perfect example of turnaround in conventional wisdom regarding unconventional cancer therapies. Evidence that mental imagery works is only recently becoming accepted. Growing scientific exploration in psychoneuroimmunology examines the connection between the mind and the body—particularly the effects of mental processes on hormone production and on the nervous and immune systems.

Many people with cancer find that mental training including visualization and relaxation helps them cope with the side effects of cancer and cancer treatment. Nurses often teach and use relaxation, imagery, and music therapy to help people decrease the nausea and vomiting caused by some chemotherapy drugs. Even when these techniques cannot increase the quantity of life, they contribute to the quality of life.

Diversional activities might be considered a sort of cousin to imagery and relaxation therapies. Humor therapy, leisure activities, recreational therapy, and music and art therapies are all used in various settings to help people cope with cancer and its treatment. Cancer treatment can cause long hospital stays and social isolation. As the woman is physically and emotionally separated from friends and family, she may have decreased physical and emotional motivation to take part in leisure pastimes. All of these things take their toll.

Music has been used for teaching, celebration, and self-expression. It has also been used to summon and encourage soldiers in battle. During World War II, music was used to calm shell-shocked soldiers (some women with cancer feel shell-shocked too!) Since that time, the use of music as a therapy has steadily grown.

Ever since the invention of the phonograph in the 1800s, music has been used in hospitals to induce sleep. There is a relationship between the tempo of music and responses of the human nervous system; relaxing music with a repeating rhythm reduces anxiety. Music has a positive effect on the sensory and emotional reaction to cancer pain—possibly because it stimulates the release of endorphins, the body's natural painkillers. It can reduce anxiety during medical procedures. As a universal form of communication it bridges age, culture, language, and education. Some women enjoy playing musical instruments, which can be a satisfying way to fill time or a wonderful gift to share with others. For information about music therapy, contact the National Association for Music Therapy, 8455 Colesville Road, Suite 930, Silver Spring, MD 20910.

Laughter and humor have only recently been recognized as important parts of the coping and healing processes. There is a relationship between humor and increased immune system activity that seems to help prevent infections. Norman Cousins described his use of humor to relieve pain and other distressing problems in his book Head First: The Biology of Hope. People who enjoy humor also have better morale and a sense of well-being. Not only does humor help relieve anger, anxiety, and tension, it can actually be of physical benefit! It improves breathing, heart and blood vessel functions, muscle and bone structure and function, hormonal production, and immune function.

Art therapy is being used to help adults and children cope with cancer. It can help women understand themselves better, make changes in their behavior, and express their feelings in a safe, nonthreatening way. Art can provide diversion and relaxation, and support self-esteem.

PHYSICAL APPROACHES

Physical treatments provide an accepted, supportive role in conventional cancer treatment. Exercise and mobility are key components in a holistic cancer care program. Rehabilitation concepts, including physical and occupational health, are at last considered crucial in comprehensive cancer care. Programs like the American Cancer Society's "We Can Weekend" combine physical exertion—hiking, climbing, swimming, canoeing—with group work, peer support, and counseling.

Exercise is important. So often, people with cancer are advised to "take it easy" and "get plenty of rest." Certainly fatigue is a common cause of decreased quality of life for many people living with cancer and cancer treatment. But unnecessary bedrest and prolonged immobility results in a *loss* of energy and function. Our bodies work on a "use it or lose it" principle. Unless muscle groups are stimulated and used, they waste away and the woman gets weaker and weaker.

In several studies, many people started exercising while going through cancer therapy or after therapy. Women using exercise during chemotherapy for breast cancer found an increased sense of control and an increase in their functional abilities. Women who exercise have less tension, anxiety, depression, and fatigue, and actually have increased feelings of well-being. Exercise can also help control the nausea caused by chemotherapy and radiation. My friend with ovarian cancer makes it a point to walk her dogs a couple times each day. The only bad result is that she looks so good and so healthy that her doctors have trouble believing she is in pain. But, she says, without her walks she would have more pain and, most importantly, would lose the companionship she enjoys with her dogs.

Be aware, however, that there can be risks associated with exercise during the stresses caused by cancer and cancer treatment. For this reason, exercise programs should be started only after appropriate screening, a medical check-up and review of the noncancer-related health factors such as heart, blood pressure, and orthopedic problems (knees, ankles, back, etc.). Symptoms that would prohibit a woman from taking on an exercise program—and would warrant further evaluation—include:

- ◆ an irregular or resting pulse of more than 100 beats per minute

- ◆ frequent leg pain or cramps

- ◆ chest pain

- ◆ rapid onset of nausea during exercise

- ◆ dizziness, blurred vision, feeling faint

- ◆ bone, back, or neck pain that is new

- ◆ fever

- ◆ shortness of breath

A walking program is the simplest—and perhaps the best—exercise. Shoes should be designed for walking or jogging with a cushioned mid-sole and skid-proof outer sole. They should lace up and have smooth, soft, areas inside that will not cause blisters or sores. Clothing should be comfortable. In winter, a hat or hood will prevent heat loss. Other expensive equipment is not needed. The pulse rate is the best indicator of the amount of work the body is doing. When walking, count the pulse for six seconds and add a zero to get the beats per minute. To benefit from exercise, the pulse should be increased to the "training range" and kept there for 10–20 minutes.

TRAINING PULSE RANGE

Age in years	Suggested training pulse rate	Pulse, 6 sec.
<20	140–150/minute	14 or 15
20–30	130–140	13 or 14
30–40	120–130	12 or 13
40–50	110–120	11 or 12
50–60	100–110	10 or 11
60+	90–100	9 or 10

(Winningham, 1991)

Touch

Touch is the most sensitive of our five senses. We all have it, and we can all use it to improve the quality of our lives. During illness, touch is sometimes forgotten or neglected. Historically, the fear of contagious diseases prevented people from the benefit of touching another person. We have all seen pictures of the study where sad little monkeys cling to a cloth-wrapped metal substitute in an effort to touch something resembling their own species. Unfortunately, many people with cancer have been denied the physical comfort that can be provided by touch. Today, people with AIDS are very aware of the need for, and frequent lack of, touching another person.

Massage has been described as a therapy for illness since the fifth century B.C. and offers nurturing and relaxation that can be a special complement to other cancer therapies. Massage is the kneading, manipulation, or application of methodical pressure and friction to the body. It has five basic strokes that are used in sequence on the skin, muscles, tendons, and ligaments. These basic strokes are:

1. Effleurage: superficial or deep gliding, long, rhythmic strokes that warm the muscles; the whole hand moves over the body toward the heart.

2. Petrissage: kneading with the fingers and thumb of each hand in C-shaped motions to stimulate the muscle.

3. Friction: circular movements with thumbs, fingers, or heel of the hand to penetrate deeper muscle layers or work around joints.

4. Tapotement: quick, vigorous, rhythmic strokes like tapping, cupping, slapping, or pummeling to stimulate muscles.

5. Vibration: shaking movements with fingers or the hand to stimulate or relax muscles.

Though scientific evidence favoring massage as a complement to cancer therapy is sparse, the effects of one human touching another, with care and concern, offer both the caregiver and the patient a truly meaningful experience. The benefits derived from massage include relaxation, reduced swelling, decreased stress, relief of fatigue, improved sleep, and decreased pain.

Therapeutic touch is a relatively new version of "laying on of hands." Touch healing is described in the New Testament but it has been used by women healers for centuries; some believe its origins rest with survivors of Atlantis. Native Americans use forms of therapeutic touch that amazingly resemble those found in Tibet, South America, and Africa. Today this technique involves a systematic protocol pioneered in America by Dolores Krieger, Professor of Nursing at New York University. Krieger's methods assume that the human being is an open system and that illness represents an imbalance in a person's energy systems. The healer is charged with rebalancing these systems. The three phases in the process include "centering," "assessing," and "rebalancing." During centering, the therapist/healer meditates so that her thoughts are opened to input from her client. Then during the assessment phase she tunes in to imbalances in the energy fields around the client's body. Finally, the energy fields surrounding the body are smoothed out and redirected during rebalancing. The process usually takes no longer than twenty minutes. Therapeutic touch has been effective in relieving postoperative and generalized pain, improving red blood cell levels, and decreasing anxiety, stress, and headaches in many people.

Reiki is a formalized laying on of hands in which "master" status is given to only a few practitioners; it is expensive to achieve. Reiki can be a beautiful addition to healing processes, but it is not an essential skill. It has origins in ancient Tibet, traveled to China and Japan, and was brought to the United States in 1938. Reiki practice uses formal physical positions in a sequence for applying energy over specific energy centers, called *chakras*, of the body. Reiki is learned and mastered through a series of three steps or degrees. The beginning degree opens the woman healer's ability to channel her energy and teaches her the healing positions. The second degree involves learning Reiki as a distance healing process, and the third and final degree allows the healer to be known as a "Reiki Master" and to teach others.

Laying on of hands is a way of applying life-force aura energy to relieve pain, speed healing, regenerate, and calm. It can be useful in helping women cope with the distressing symptoms of cancer and its treatment. It can be done by the woman herself: she does not necessarily have to find a healer, though the human to human bond and sharing process is also a meaningful component of the healing process. The energy transferred by laying on of hands can be totally positive and beneficial, and harms no one. Anyone can do this type of healing to help herself or others.

Laying on of hands and Reiki healing can seem a little spooky. But skilled, intelligent women, many of them nurse colleagues, use and enthusiastically endorse these healing techniques. A group of nurses at the University of Iowa College of Nursing have established a network of nurse healers. Their stories are amazing and wonderful. Patients with illnesses or problems that seemed impossible to control were helped by these healing forces. Pain, nausea, and vomiting problems were allayed by these energy forces, making a big difference in the quality of life. Many practitioners are looking for ways to document the effects of these techniques. Some believe that the energy forces activate parts of the immune system, allowing the body to fight cancer, infection, and other stressors more effectively.

Traditional Eastern Healing

Acupressure, an East Asian healing technique, includes the Japanese form called **shiatsu,** and **reflexology.** Acupressure is a form of massage that uses energy channels called *meridians*, and it can be useful in pain and stress management. Acu-points, or *tsubos*, are thought to be points of decreased electrical resistance that follow the body's energy paths. These paths form the meridian system. Stimulation of the tsubo, the meridian, or a portion of one or more meridians can improve energy flow, in turn affecting organs distant from the area being stimulated; this can have a positive impact on physical health, stress levels, and the emotions.

Shiatsu addresses mind, body, and spirit and like other Asian healing therapies, implies a significant role for psychosomatic components in the development of disease. According to shiatsu theory, no one meridian is affected in isolation. A change in one can cause a number of other changes in the quality of others. Shiatsu can be an effective form of health promotion and disease prevention.

The 5,000 year old science of **acupuncture,** which evolved from acupressure, uses needle insertion to relieve pain and open energy flow. Acupuncture is performed by licensed practitioners, while acupressure can be done by lay persons. Both were derived from the Chinese *Nei Jing,* the oldest written medical text (dated about 300 B.C.) which is now being combined with Western medicine. The basic tenet of Chinese healing is to strengthen the "ki"—the flow of life force—which in turn balances energy flow to create well-being. The meridians described under shiatsu are the channels that carry ki through the body and connect the yin and yang functions. The chakra system in Reiki (and Native American healing) and the meridians used in acupressure, acupuncture, reflexology, and shiatsu are similar in that they are all energy channels.

Research shows that endorphins are produced when acupoints are pressed, warmed, or needled. It is probable that acupressure causes hormonal changes and also stimulates the immune system.

SPIRITUAL APPROACHES

Spirituality and religion are words and ideas that get used interchangeably, but they can be very different things. Not all people who have a sense of spirituality consider themselves to be religious. Spirit and spirituality relate the essence of a person to her world and give meaning to existence. Spirituality and health have been intertwined from early times when priests and shamans were the first healers. Spiritual well-being can be the cornerstone of health, integrating one's inner resources—the physical body, rational mind, emotional psyche, and intuitive spirit. A 1971 White House Conference on Aging defined spirituality as "the human belief system that pertains to humankind's innermost concerns and values, which ultimately affects behavior, relationship to the world, and relationship to God—however the individual defines the order of the universe."

The days and months after a diagnosis of cancer are a time filled with concerns about life and death. People try to find the meaning of their eventual death, the meaning of the cancer experience, and the meaning of the life remaining to them. Very early, people come to realize that facing cancer and cancer treatment is going to be a huge challenge. To meet the challenge and put out the effort needed, it is natural for people to look for meaning in what faces them. In an especially interesting study, six major themes evolved that relate to how a person interprets the meaning of the cancer experience and which activ-ities, life experiences, relationships, values, beliefs, and philosophies people look to for meaning:

- ◆ seeking an understanding of the personal significance of the cancer diagnosis—"Why me?"

- ◆ looking at the outcomes of the cancer diagnosis

- ◆ reviewing of one's life

- ◆ changing one's outlook toward self, life, and others

- ◆ living with cancer

- ◆ rekindling hope

Support during the search for meaning comes most often from personal faith and social support. Social support involves relationships with others that are expressed as care and love. Faith helps people cope through renewal of an inspirational contact with their religion and/or God, or a deeper aspect of themselves. In turn, hope develops as a result of renewed faith. For many, formal religion is not important in this process, but most people say that their idea or feeling about God has always affected their lives. This idea of God represents a person's spirituality, it includes religion but is not limited to religion only.

There are countless spiritual approaches to healing. They generally share a common precept that the healer must gain access to a hidden reality in order to share the power and wisdom of the universe with others in need. For example, a healer in India maintains that she communicates with the universe through a link provided by a Hindu saint. In a tribal culture, a different but similar spiritual link might be made; it could involve a sacred plant, a rock, or quartz crystals. Sometimes, spiritual healing is referred to as shamanism and its practitioners as shamans. In shamanism, conflict, pain, and suffering are part of ordinary reality. The goal of shamanism is to attain an experience of nonordinary reality (shamanic ecstasy)—that is, moving beyond time and becoming one with the universe. The shaman helps people move between ordinary and nonordinary reality, and in doing so, experience deeper harmony within themselves and heal pain.

The practice of **laying on of stones and crystals** is fascinating. Quartz crystal and gemstones are used for healing in Native American culture, South America, Africa, Europe, and Egypt, and India. Legend has it that people on the lost continent of Atlantis used clear quartz crystals as their major source of energy, and healing was powered by crystals and gemstones.

Native American shamans and medicine women in several tribes use crystals and turquoise on various parts of the body to tap into this wisdom. Today, crystal work and laying on of stones are being used to release physical disease and work with the emotional sources of physical illness. Healers work to change the electrical field, or aura, that surrounds the body. This aura is made of eight levels of energy or light and four bodies that surround the body. The etheric double is the first of the four bodies and is closest to physical. Moving outward from the skin, other levels are the emotional body, the mental body, and the spiritual body. Gemstones of different colors are coordinated with the different energy levels. The chakras or energy centers are activated by laying on stones located in the etheric body. Each chakra has unique characteristics and healing uses. Even though individual chakras can be targeted, laying on of stones is most often done to bring the whole woman into balance.

A central part of all spiritual healing processes is helping the woman accept and love herself. Louise Hay believes that illnesses, which she calls dis-eases, are the result of emotional and mental stresses. Cancer, Hay says, is "probably" caused by deep hurt and longstanding resentment, deep secrets or grief that eats away at the self, and carrying hatreds. Hay believes that "dis-ease" can be cured by reversing mental patterns. She describes metaphysical causation, "the power in words and thoughts that create experiences" as crucial in creating and healing dis-ease. The mental work of releasing and forgiving are healing processes. Old thought patterns should be replaced by healing affirmations. For cancer, Hay suggests the affirmation:

> I lovingly forgive and release all of the past. I choose to fill my world with joy. I love and approve of myself.

Some people interpret Hay's message to mean that the person with cancer is to blame for causing the cancer, or, if they do not get well, they are to blame for the failure. The confusion may rest with a lack of universal interpretation or definition of being "well" or being "healthy."

Healers from the ancient shamans and medicine men and women to Dolores Krieger, O. Carl Simonton, and Jeanne Achterberg have a definition of wellness different from the conventional medical one. Wellness and health are not necessarily the same as absence of disease, and getting well does not necessarily mean getting cured of the cancer. On the contrary, healing can mean finding a balance between the physical, emotional, intellectual, and spiritual dimensions of one's condition.

PHARMACOLOGIC AGENTS: DRUGS AND SPECIAL PREPARATIONS

Vitamin C is an example of a drug that is available and used in conventional therapy but is also used in an unconventional way by some practitioners. Nobel Prize winner Linus Pauling advocated vitamin C for the treatment and palliation of cancer. He advocates the use of vitamin C as a complement to conventional therapy to support the patient's natural defenses. While the recommended daily allowance (RDA) for vitamin C is 45 mg (0.045 gram) per day, Dr. Pauling and others recommend doses up to 10 gms/day oral or intravenous in the treatment of cancer. The oral dose starts at 1–2 gms/day and gradually increases to at least 10 gms. Proponents of this approach admit they do not know the best dose. Researchers are looking at the role of vitamin C in preventing cancer and preventing its spread once it has developed.

Antineoplastons are being developed and promoted by Stanislaw Burzynski, M.D., at the Burzynski Research Institute in Stafford, Texas. At least ten types of antineoplastons, available only at Burzynski's Houston clinic, are given orally or intravenously, mostly orally. The clinic charges from $135–685 for a day's therapy, in addition to room, board, diagnostic tests, catheters, and pumps used for IV therapy. An initial deposit of $5,000 is required.

Burzynski says that antineoplastons are a "totally new class of compounds" and describes them as urinary peptides that reprogram cancer cells. The National Cancer Institute will study antineoplastons in clinical trials when a synthetic form is available. Despite funding from NCI from 1974 through July of 1977, no form of antineoplaston has come to the FDA for approval.

Most patients begin with small doses that eventually increase to an optimal level—which is not clearly defined. Some patients also get low-dose chemotherapy with antineoplaston therapy. So far the treatment seems to be nontoxic, but a small percentage of people on antineoplaston therapy have reported some side effects. There are no reports of serious side effects in the literature; however, articles about antineoplaston appear in lay magazines and not scientific, peer-reviewed literature. One magazine article claimed that 46% of the people taking antineoplaston for colon cancer had a total remission. Burzynski says clearly that antineoplastons are not effective for all cancers. Most successes are reported to be in the treatment of cancers involving the bladder, brain, breast, prostate, and bone. They may also be effective for ovarian cancer. Burzynski asserts that most people taking his treatment have a positive response. On the other hand, two NCI trials completed in 1983 and 1985 showed no increase in survival rates and no apparent effect on tumors associated with two antineoplastons.

Hydrazine sulfate was popularized as an antitumor drug in the 1970s. A few studies demonstrated some tumor response, and patients reported they felt better. The major effect seemed to be improved nutritional status. It has since been proposed as a treatment to prevent the weight loss and muscle wasting that occur with may forms of cancer. In the early studies, hydrazine sulfate was also associated with an increase in survival time. Based on these studies, it is being tested for its effects on nutritional status and the effects of nutritional status on the progress of various forms of cancer.

Dimethyl sulfoxide (DMSO), a chemical solvent, is sometimes combined with other agents—particularly vitamin C and laetrile—to treat cancer. DMSO is not believed to be able to kill cancer cells. Its promoters claim that it dissolves the protein shell around cancer cells and thereby restores the abnormal cell to normal. Healthfood store literature promotes DMSO in the management of symptoms of tuberculosis, herpes, and arthritis. One form of DMSO has been approved by the FDA for the treatment of bladder inflammation (cystitis).

Cellular treatments, also called "live cell therapy," "cellular therapy," "cellular suspensions," "glandular therapy," and "fresh cell therapy," involve injecting or swallowing processed tissue from animal fetuses (usually sheep, cow, or shark). The type of cells given correspond to the organ or tissue that is affected by the cancer. Its users claim that the injected cells travel to similar organs and stimulate that organ's function. The known side effects and dangers result from allergic reactions and infection. Cellular therapy is not widely practiced in the United States. It was developed and popularized in Switzerland in the 1930s and moved to Tijuana in the late 1970s. It is now available in perhaps five clinics.

Laetrile has become the best known unconventional cancer treatment development over the last twenty years. By the mid-1970s at least 70,000 people were using it for cancer prevention, cancer treatment, and pain control. By 1977, its use was legalized in 22 states. It has lost some appeal since studies at the Mayo Clinic seemed to disprove any positive effect, but it is still available at cancer clinics in Mexico.

Amygdalin, laetrile, Laetrile (brand name), sarcarcinase, nitriloside, and vitamin B-17 are all chemically similar substances used for laetrile treatment. The active ingredient is found in the pits of apricots and other fruits and its use is based on two theories about the cause of cancer. According to one theory, cancer is caused by "trophoblastic" cells—cells that are normally present during pregnancy to protect the fertilized egg from being rejected by the mother's body, which for some reason are present in the body of the person with cancer. The second half of the theory is that cancer is a disease caused by a vitamin deficiency—a lack of the vitamin laetrile. Proponents of laetrile believe that it kills cells selectively, affecting only cancer cells and leaving normal cells alone. Claims made in the 1970s reported that laetrile had antitumor effects. Now most practitioners use laetrile as a part of a regimen that may include other agents like DMSO, vitamins, minerals, amino acids, enzymes, oxygen, and cellular therapy.

Laetrile naturally contains of at least 6% cyanide and is toxic in large doses. Combining it with some other foods actually causes the release of more cyanide. There are also wide variations found in the potency of sampled laetrile containers, and some bottles have been found to be contaminated by bacteria and viruses.

Immuno-Augmentative Therapy (IAT) is not a widely known form of unconventional therapy. It was developed in the 1970s by biologist Lawrence Burton, who practiced out of a clinic in New York State. In 1977 he founded the Immunology Researching Centre, Inc. in the Bahamas. In 1987, a clinic opened in West Germany and another in Mexico in 1989.

IAT is based on the theory that restoring optimal immune function allows the immune system to find and destroy cancer cells. These immune functions then serve as a natural weapon to control carcinogenesis. Advocates of IAT claim that it can control or stabilize most cancers and cause others to regress.

Treatment consists of daily self-injections of processed blood products, to be administered for the rest of the person's life. The complete regimen can include other drugs, especially steroids. Practitioners suggest that large tumors be removed surgically before the start of IAT, but they discourage chemotherapy and radiation therapy.

In conflicting reports of the same study one group of researchers determined that the study was evidence for the efficacy of IAT, while a second group analyzing the same data decided that no valid deductions could be made from it about the effect of IAT. This is typical of the differences between mainstream and unconventional practitioners. Negotiations to arrange a clinical trial for IAT have fallen through several times, and to date no clinical trial is planned.

Oxymedicine uses hydrogen peroxide and ozone to destroy tumors. These oxygen treatments are not widespread in the United States but there are clinics in Mexico and Germany. Oxygen treatments are usually used to complement other therapies. For example, the Gerson clinic in Tijuana added ozone enemas to its regimen. Oxymedicine is based on the idea that a buildup of manmade toxins from foods, food additives, and environmental pollution is the major cause of degenerative diseases, including cancer. Therefore, the appropriate treatment is to detoxify the body and reverse the disease with dietary changes. A second premise is that tumors thrive *without* oxygen and are killed by substances that increase oxygen to the tumor site.

Ozone, a gas, is administered by direct infusion into the rectum or muscle—often in an infusion of blood. In most regimens a pint of blood is removed from the patient, treated with oxygen, and then returned to the patient. Hydrogen peroxide in dilute forms is given by mouth, through the rectum or vagina, into the veins, or added to baths. Advocates believe that the peroxide oxidizes toxins, kills bacteria and viruses, and stimulates immunity.

Shark Cartilage is the basis of a relatively recent development in cancer treatment. On a recent trip to my hometown in Iowa I visited a friend's mother who has been dealing with ovarian cancer for several years. Even though she lives in a small town and does not travel much, she had found *The Newsletter of Advanced Natural Therapies and Alternatives*. She asked my opinion of what is currently in vogue in natural therapies—shark cartilage pills.

The rationale for shark cartilage, according to an article in *Alternatives*, is that "sharks rarely develop cancer, either in clear open waters or in water highly polluted with carcinogenic chemicals. The key to their resistance seems to lie in their boneless skeleton."

It turns out that the fact that sharks do not actually seem to get cancer has been of interest to researchers at the National Cancer Institute for several years. A 1983 study showed that shark cartilage contains a substance that interferes with the development of blood vessels that feed tumors, which in turn limits tumor growth. Other studies support at least some further investigation of the mechanisms that prevent sharks from developing cancer. Even without definitive study, many people promote the use of shark cartilage in humans as a means to prevent the development of cancer or slow its progress after it has developed.

Shark cartilage is available in healthfood stores and from mail-order outlets as pills or capsules. While it is supposed to be non-toxic, the woman who first told me about its use had to stop using it. She said the pills made her "sick to her stomach" with cramps, nausea, and vomiting. As soon as she stopped taking the pills, the symptoms stopped. *Sharks Don't Get Cancer* by Lane and Comac (Avery 1992) offers a review of events and research that seek to demonstrate the effectiveness of shark cartilage in the treatment of cancer and other chronic diseases.

PROGRAMS USING UNCONVENTIONAL THERAPIES

Many complementary therapy programs use combinations of different therapies. A common goal of multifaceted programs is to help individuals with cancer learn how to form a partnership with the healthcare team. For example, dietary changes, massage and therapeutic touch, and guided imagery are key components of several formalized cancer support programs. **The Wellness Community**—started in Santa Monica, California, in 1982 and promoted by Gilda Radner—now has centers in many cities across the United States. It offers mutual aid groups that focus on positive emotions and mental activities, and self-help skills that increase the possibilities of recovery. Some programs offer one-to-one sessions with a psychotherapist and other varied group activities. Services are free and programs are supported through community and corporate donations.

Dr. Bernie Siegel, author of *Love, Medicine and Miracles*, founded a program called **Exceptional Cancer Patients (ECaP)** in New Haven, Connecticut in 1978. The program includes individual and group support, and uses dreams, drawings, and images to increase awareness of each person's healing potential. Psychotherapy is available as are books, and video and audio recordings. There is only one center, but training sessions have allowed at least 160 people to develop ECaP-like groups in other locations. Patients are charged for all sessions.

Commonweal was established in 1976 by Michael Lerner, Ph.D. It is located on 60 acres of the Pacific coast near Bolinas, California, north of San Francisco. It is a nonprofit corporation supported by foundations and public agencies as well as individuals. Commonweal offers ten programs, including family consulting services, a children's training institute, projects in Patient-Centered Medicine, and the Commonweal Cancer Project. The Commonweal Cancer Help Program helps people seek "physical, emotional, and spiritual healing in the face of cancer." Commonweal offers intense, week-long sessions for groups of up to eight participants. These sessions are geared to help participants cope with stress, resolve fears and decrease anxieties, and improve their quality of life. The program includes informational, spiritual, and lifestyle components. Small group work, massage, yoga, training in relaxation, meditation, imagery, dream and journal work, and nature walks are important parts of the program. The staff are respected members of various health and healing disciplines, including a cook who is a "master of vegetarian cooking" and nutrition educator. The basic fee for the workshop is over $1,000 per person, and financial help is "available on a limited basis for those for whom the fee is a barrier to participation."

The **Cancer Support and Education Center** in Menlo Park, California (formerly the Creighton Health Institute), offers several services designed to assist physical and spiritual healing, improve the quality of life, and help others fight for life. The center offers seminars consisting of group work, individual, couple, and family counseling, nutritional consultation, and massage. The basic program is a two-week program for a person with cancer and a spouse or friend for a fee of about $1,500 (as of 1992).

❖　❖　❖

Most women want help finding legitimate, acceptable ways to improve their health, however each individual defines it. But the fear generated by a cancer diagnosis and feelings of helplessness can make a woman easy prey for anyone promising a cure. How can a woman, faced with so many decisions, find and integrate the best unconventional therapies with her conventional cancer care? How can a woman find rational, responsible complements to her treatment plan?

Conventional therapies go through heavy scrutiny in order to pass two major tests: 1) have they been proven safe when provided by a competent practitioner? and 2) have they proven effective? Women trying to separate facts from fantasy in cancer therapies need a healthy dose of skepticism. Keep in mind that

— No single test done once can definitively diagnose cancer.

— There is no agency that approves or verifies claims in advertisements before they are printed. Authorities can take action only after an advertisement has appeared.

Beware of testimonials that sound too good to be true, because they probably are. Common characteristics of quack advertisements are claims of

♦ a quick and painless cure

♦ a "special," "secret," "ancient," or "foreign" formula, available only through mail and/or one supplier

♦ testimonials or case histories from satisfied users as the only proof that the product works

♦ a scientific "breakthrough" or "miracle cure" that has been held back or overlooked by the conventional medical community

Before buying or signing up for a product or program, check it out with

- ◆ your doctor, pharmacist, nurse, or another healthcare professional
- ◆ the Better Business Bureau
- ◆ the local consumer office
- ◆ the state's Attorney General
- ◆ the Federal Trade Commission
- ◆ the Food and Drug Administration
- ◆ the Postmaster or the Postal Inspection Service

(HHS Publication No. 85-4200)

Pamela Haylock

Chapter 10

Feelings

When they hear the words "You have cancer," some women begin to cry—and do not stop for days.

I could not cry at first. I wanted to, and this big lump of unshed tears in my throat and chest was nearly choking me. Even watching sad movies and peeling onions (I tried both) would not start the tears flowing. I had to make the immediate decisions before I could relax into tears.

That was simply my individual emotional timetable. It is common for the woman diagnosed with cancer to experience fear, sadness, anger, perhaps guilt. She may agonize over who she is, how she looks, what is going to happen to her. But she will do it on her own timetable.

This is partly because she is who she is, with a background and set of circumstances that are hers alone. But it is also because the timetables for cancer therapies are so different. One woman may finish diagnosis and treatment within a week, and another may still be undergoing therapy months or even years later.

Thus, one woman may feel an emotion much earlier or later than another woman—and both of them are quite normal. That is why this chapter and Chapter 21, Feelings After Treatment Ends work together. What is not in one chapter is discussed in the other.

NUMBNESS AND DENIAL

The doctor says, "You have cancer." The woman may hear the first few words and then little else. This normal protective mechanism saves the woman from the full initial shock of what is happening. She talks, and moves, and drives home—and may even say "Oh, I'm just fine, thank you"—but inside she is numb. None of it feels *real*.

Sometimes, that cushioning sense of unreality persists during treatment: "This is not happening," "This is happening, but it won't make any real difference in my life."

Some women continue in this state for years, and never confront the cancer. In fact, if the treatment is minimal and the prognosis excellent, the cancer may never have to make any real difference in their lives. But some women may be truly expert deniers who never notice the elephant in the living room, or may be totally distracted by other events happening in their lives.

Others may bargain unconsciously during therapy: "I'm doing what I'm supposed to do, as hard as it is. Such good behavior means that I deserve not to have this in my life anymore." Then, when treatment is over, these women reward themselves by putting cancer out of their minds forever.

Indeed, it is possible for a woman to choose to live as if the cancer makes no real difference in her life (although she may be ambushed by painful feelings years later). On the other hand, this means she loses the opportunity for it to make a real difference in her life. She misses the cloud—but also the silver lining.

The silver lining is that cancer is a chance to change and grow. "Business as usual" so often does not work after a cancer diagnosis that many a woman has to try business as *unusual*. Cancer has a way of shaking up the status quo.

A woman may discover that she likes the new ways better. She may have ignored her own needs for years as she cared for others, but now she must listen to herself more. She may discover, as many women do, that in daring to face the possibility of her own death, she learns to spread her wings. She can see what is important, set new priorities, have more fun, and be less afraid of what other people think. I love the sweatshirt that proclaims on the front, "Rule #1: Don't sweat the small stuff" and on the back, "Rule #2: It's *all* small stuff."

At the same time, life has a sweeter edge. Many a woman experiences a "honeymoon" with life: never has she felt so in love with the world around her. Holding on to this fresh delight is one of the challenges of long-term cancer survivorship.

Of course, there may be easier ways to learn these lessons!

REGAINING CONTROL

When the numbness wears off, the woman may feel more helpless than she ever has in her life. Everything is spinning out of control; her once somewhat-predictable life is orderly no more. What goals? What personal calendar? What sense of independence and autonomy? She may feel utterly dependent on people she did not meet until last week who now say she must do such and such if she wants to save her life.

This is the perfect time to remember the famous Serenity Prayer:

> God grant me the serenity
> to accept the things I cannot change,
> the courage to change the things I can,
> and the wisdom to know the difference.

Indeed, there are some factors about a woman's experience with cancer that are out of anybody's hands. All she can do is accept that and not waste her energy fighting what cannot be changed. Just doing something—anything—does not help, because her feeling of control is soon revealed as an illusion.

There are sensible steps a woman can take to establish some real control. She can get information from her doctors, books, and other sources. She can assemble a cancer care team she trusts and think of herself as a contributing team member rather than a universal victim. She can gather as much support from family, friends, and others as she needs. She can stay as healthy as possible, eat well, and get some exercise, so that she feels stronger, more able to do what she must do. She may choose to research and use complementary therapies to help make herself feel better.

And she can start looking at herself as a cancer survivor or a cancer victor—or even a cancer "thriver." The National Coalition for Cancer Survivorship contends that survivorship has several "seasons," but that being a cancer survivor begins at the moment of diagnosis. So, right from the beginning, the woman can start saying, as cancer survivor Melinda Sheinkopf does in *Coping* magazine (Summer 1992), "Listen, Cancer, maybe it is your job to take years from my life. I really don't know. But I know it's my job to see you don't take life from my years."

EXPERIENCING FEELINGS

Some people believe that to be cancer survivors, they must think positive all the time and squelch any negative thoughts. Not true. Susan Diamond, L.C.S.W., a social worker/psychotherapist who leads a support group for women with breast cancer, hates that "positive attitude bullshit. It makes women think they can't admit to their very scariest feelings, even to themselves. Then, if they harbor fears, concerns, and anxieties —and have no way to put them out on the table and deal with them—the women become immobilized and wonder why."

Feelings are energy, power. But if we repress painful, difficult feelings, eventually we spend our lives guarding an emotional volcano, terrified lest it erupt and overwhelm us and everyone around us. But released and expressed, in a safe manner, those same emotions become energy for us to use.

How do we let emotions free in a safe manner? Acknowledging and naming feelings, at least to ourselves, is the first step, though often not an easy one. Trying to sort out strong emotions may be quite new for us. Susan Diamond advises: "Make the unspoken spoken. This has the effect of making it smaller and more manageable."

There are many ways to do this, and not all of them require talking (or even words). We can consciously think about what is happening and what we are feeling: "What's going on here? This feels like the way I felt when . . . . "

Our unconscious minds will do much of the work for us if we let them. Thus, some women meditate regularly, begin a journal of their experience, write poetry about it, or examine their dreams—and wind up exclaiming, "Where in the world did *that* come from?" Others use their hands or bodies creatively to show their feelings and begin finding a place for them: drawing perhaps, or sculpting, or dancing.

For many of us, making the unspoken spoken means talking about it. Some find it helpful to compare notes with other women in the same situation: a mentor or a support group. Discovering that other women have similar strong emotions helps validate and legitimize our own feelings. This doesn't mean that everyone has identical emotions, of course. Our feelings are our own, but it is reassuring for a woman to know that she is not crazy, that there is a very broad range of normal emotions. Such a group is a safe place for learning new ways to make our feelings work for us.

Many women seek counseling or psychotherapy. If emotional distress is disabling, especially if extreme anxiety or deep depression lasts more than two weeks, it is urgent that a woman see a therapist. The chief signs of depression are continuous empty, very sad feelings (sometimes with suicidal ideas) combined with major changes in eating or sleeping habits. Depression may show itself in severe restlessness or agitation.

Some women sensibly choose psychotherapy or counseling because their distress makes them miserable. Others want to gain something positive from their experience with cancer and want support and guidance. A competent, caring therapist or counselor (preferably one familiar with cancer patients) can help a woman sort through painful feelings safely, begin integrating her cancer experience into her life, and perhaps make her life more satisfying than it ever was before. Seeking counseling in no way means a woman is crazy or weak; rather, it means she has the sense to make use of available help.

At some point in their cancer journey, many women draw on spiritual resources to cope with painful feelings. Whether it is against the background of a lifetime of organized religion, or a new search for meaning in this crisis, women often find comfort and hope in personal prayer, talk with clergy, spiritual reading and/or membership in a church. Feeling the presence of a Higher Power makes them feel less alone and vulnerable.

On the other hand, some women lose faith after the cancer diagnosis, questioning or blaming God. Harold S. Kushner's book, *When Bad Things Happen to Good People* is a thoughtful guide for a woman asking spiritual questions.

Brisk physical exercise and/or deep relaxation are both strategies for coping with distressing emotions. Reading about feelings may help, as can talking them over with a partner, friends, or family.

And, since most women do not want (or need) to spend every minute dwelling on feelings, distractions of any kind can be a godsend. Hobbies, a movie, a trashy novel, a visit with a friend in which cancer is never mentioned—all these keep a woman aware that life exists apart from cancer. I found that spending a few hours a week working intensely on "cancer stuff" in my support group freed me to focus on everything else most of the rest of the time.

The woman with a sense of humor will find it comes to her rescue now. Laughter cheers her, broadens her perspective, makes her more attractive to be with, and may actually stimulate her body's defenses. Cancer is serious, but her experience with it does not have to be perpetually grim.

DEALING WITH FEAR

It is fairly common for a woman to feel an intense blast of fear soon after diagnosis. She may also find her fear lessens while she undergoes treatment: she is "doing something," and has a sense of greater control with a weapon in hand. Thus it is typical for fear to become more severe again as the woman finishes treatment and no longer feels "protected."

What do we fear? Death, of course. Indeed, some people with cancer will eventually die of the disease. What is absolutely certain is that every person with cancer will eventually die of *something*, someday—as will every person who never gets cancer. Death is a fact of life.

Given the choice, however, most of us try not to think about dying. We cram our feelings about death into an emotional closet deep within. A cancer diagnosis wrenches open that closet door. We can try to ignore feelings and fears that tumble out, or try to cram them back into the closet, but avoiding something so obvious takes a huge emotional toll.

It is far easier to look at death, to put a name and shape to it; it is the nameless things that go bump in the night that terrify us the most. Becoming more familiar with what happens when we die lets us put death in its proper place. So, we can talk about death, read about it, consider it at our own pace, and express our feelings about it. This is not morbid and does not make us die any sooner.

However we come by it, that fundamental awareness of death gives a context to our life. Cancer lets us look at death squarely while we still have time to change the way we live, to make our lives what we want them to be.

Most of us fear protracted, painful dying. Most patients and even many health professionals do not realize that cancer-related pain can be treated effectively now for almost everyone —if health professionals use all the information and techniques available to them. Every day, as an oncology nurse, I see advances in treating pain and, especially, erosion of the belief that cancer must mean pain. As a nurse I cheer; as a cancer patient I am comforted.

Many of us fear treatment: either what we are going through now or our ability to muster the will and energy to go through it again if necessary. We may have such specific fears as "What will become of my young children if cancer comes back?" All of these fears are real, normal, and legitimate.

Taking back control over them involves acknowledging that they exist, shedding some tears, talking about them, and taking action when appropriate: drafting a will, or making a backup plan for the care of any young children. It seems to be human nature to postpone this kind of practical "housekeeping," perhaps because of unspoken fears that if we plan for trouble, trouble will come. In fact, however, having our affairs in order allows us to relax and get on with life.

DEALING WITH ANGER

Many women have been brought up afraid to feel intense anger. Our feelings are supposed to be positive, moderate, gentle—in a word, "ladylike." It is okay for us to be peeved, but God forbid that we connect with any deep rage within. Our culture and political systems, too, tend to gloss over female anger. As a result, many women spend their lives performing emotional contortions to "prove" that black is really white.

We may be so accustomed to doing this that we cannot tell what we are feeling anymore. We cannot separate anger from sadness, for instance. Sometimes, when we cannot tolerate one emotion in ourselves, we substitute another less painful one. "Will I die?" might become "I can't *believe* that the doctor didn't call back." Or if we cannot face anger at someone perceived as powerful in our lives (would the doctor stop caring for me? Would the person I love stop loving me?), we may turn our anger on those perceived as less powerful—such as ourselves—and feel sad or guilty.

Anger is one of the most energetic emotions: it screams for action. Once a woman knows what she is dealing with, she needs to find something to do with this force, other than turning it against herself in the form of depression. Even if she cannot resolve the situation, she may be able to channel the energy elsewhere—through physical exercise or joining a cancer political action group, for example.

DEALING WITH GRIEF

Only a leaden lump could go through a cancer diagnosis without feeling deep sadness. Our normal response to any loss is to grieve for it, and cancer brings about inevitable losses—physical losses, of course, and perhaps financial losses. We lose the way things were, and our "innocence" of disease and our own mortality. Often we must change our dreams to fit a new reality.

We cannot sweep our losses under the bed and ignore them, or they will turn into monsters, lying in wait to bite us. So the woman before a mastectomy, for instance, needs to look at her breast and cherish it fully, appreciating what she is losing; afterward, she can mourn what is gone. Even years later she may feel an occasional pang of sorrow, and this does not mean she appreciates any less the fact that she is alive and healthy.

But the good thing about the changes of cancer is that while we lose, we also gain. Good things begin happening to crowd out the sorrow. Time—and seeking out the good things—are the best cures for the grief of cancer.

FEELING RESPONSIBLE FOR CANCER

Human nature wants a universe that makes sense. We feel safer if life is ordered in a way we can control, so that we can avoid things that cause problems. That means we want a cause for every effect, including cancer. When the effect is cancer and when no obvious cause is known (like smoking for lung cancer), we keep looking anyway.

Lacking a clear villain outside, many people become convinced that cancer comes from within us, that we are responsible for it. (As the old Woody Allen line puts it, "I don't get angry, I grow tumors instead.") A common perception is that only "nice" people—"nice" because they have repressed strong feelings—get cancer, despite the fact that most nice people do not get cancer, and plenty of decidedly un-nice people do. The New Age extension of this thinking is that if we get cancer it is because we somehow *need* it—that cancer fills some kind of emptiness within.

This kind of thinking may comfort the onlookers and help them deal with their own terror of developing cancer. They may believe that if they deal with stress better or express their emotions more effectively, they have "cancer-proofed" themselves.

But this all backfires if we get cancer. We may feel blamed and shamed and responsible for the disease. What did we do *wrong*? How did we fail? The woman with a cancer diagnosis may not only berate herself for emotional "failings," but may also have to cope with "friends" who try to get her to see the error of her psychological ways.

Cancer patient Treya Killam Weber did the same kind of smug theorizing when her mother was diagnosed with cancer. After her own diagnosis, she acknowledged in a speech entitled "What Kind of Help Really Helps": "When my mother was sick, I was motivated by fear and a desire for self-protection. When I got cancer myself, my theorizing was initially fueled by the 'you create your own reality' philosophy, which generated guilt about my past and a feeling that others must think I had failed in some way by getting cancer. This philosophy also bred the magical hope that if I could find 'the cause,' I could correct it, root out the mistake, cleanse my past, change my future and, hopefully, thus cure myself. This philosophy also implied that the only proof of success at creating my own reality would be if I got well physically."

This touches on the negative side of the theories about feisty "exceptional patients" in such popular books as Bernie Siegel's *Love, Medicine and Miracles*. These books offer hope because they say that patients who fight the disease psychologically can get well despite enormous odds. But the other side of this viewpoint is that a patient can feel undeserved guilt if the cancer gets worse. ("I just didn't try hard enough, wasn't exceptional enough.")

What will people looking back from the 25th century think about some of our current psychological theories about cancer? Will they consider them pioneering work, or laugh at them as we do now at earlier "sensible" theories that a child's blindness was caused by the sins of the parents, epilepsy by demonic possession, TB by an "artistic temperament"?

We do not know what causes many cancers or makes some people live and others die after developing them. Our emotional states and coping styles may indeed influence our immune system response somewhat, but there seems to be much more involved in a normal cell turning cancerous and growing into a tumor than a person's mental attitude.

When it comes to cancer, I see "responsibility" as the "ability to *respond* as best I can." But I also believe that there is much about cancer that we do not know and much that is totally beyond human control.

If a woman finds it personally helpful to consider that her cancer arose from her own inner need or was a lesson she needed to learn, that is fine—for her. And it is always helpful, of course, to care for our emotional health. We can use a cancer diagnosis to see where we can make good changes. But it makes no sense at all to blame ourselves.

FEELING GUILTY

Many a woman strives to get an "A" in the "cancer experience" —whatever that means to her. She sets up expectations for herself which may or may not be realistic and helpful, and then feels guilty if she fails to "perform." If she expects to work throughout treatment, for instance, she may blame herself if she has to take time off. Ironically, if she feels fine during chemotherapy and continues working, she may feel guilty because she is not being "kind enough" to herself!

Why do we torture ourselves like this?

Are we the products of our upbringing as females? Is this a Judeo-Christian religious legacy? Do we feel that if we don't suffer enough—and guilt can be very effective suffering—and pay our "suffering dues," we will not get well?

It helps to step back and look at what is happening—and then to laugh gently at ourselves for getting caught up in such tangles. We are doing the very best we can under very trying circumstances. We deserve to *appreciate* and *love* and *cherish* ourselves.

HOW WE SEE OURSELVES

How we think of ourselves is our self-image or self-concept. It is our sense of who we are. We continuously (but usually unconsciously) monitor how well our behavior, feelings and appearance match this internal picture. Our self-image includes, but is not limited to, our body image: how we "see" our physical selves. For better or worse, cancer almost always changes this image.

In our society, few women have learned to love and value themselves simply because they are what they are. Most of us attach conditions to our sense of self-worth, many of them holdovers from our growing up ("Oh, I just love you because you're such a giving person . . . " or "Can't you do anything right?" or "A truly feminine woman always . . . "). We internalize these messages—some of them useful, others quite harmful—from our families and friends, religion, culture, and the media, and they become our self-image.

Given the choice, many of us prefer not to examine this image of ourselves too closely. To do so is scary and unsettling. Although the image may not "fit" perfectly and although it may pinch or even hobble us, we hold on to it.

When cancer comes along, suddenly we may see ourselves as *un*healthy, not in control, *un*feminine, *a*sexual. A woman who viewed and valued herself because she was a hard-working, productive, and efficient attorney, now can barely move from the couch. Or she may have seen herself as sweet, loving, and giving, and now is so filled with anger that she could explode.

While we may never have fit our old self-image, now the mismatch is so obvious that it is impossible to ignore. Although some of the changes are temporary and treatment-related, others are permanent. Being so at odds with that old familiar self makes us feel uncertain and lost.

Some women cling desperately to the old image. No matter how exhausted, a woman may drag herself to work every day during treatment to prove to everyone else—but mostly to herself—that she is perfectly healthy and in control, and that nothing has changed. To her, preserving a sense of normalcy is worth any price. (Unfortunately, many women have no choice but to work throughout treatment.)

Other women, instead of changing themselves to fit the precancer self-image, prefer to put their emotional energies into crafting a self-image that fits them better. Many cancer survivors echo Chris' sentiment: "I wish to God there were an easier way, but it took cancer shaking me by the scruff of the neck to get me to look at myself. I was trying to live up to something that wasn't me at all. I realized that my self-image was just going to have to learn to live with me, rather than the other way around."

The idea is to save what is "us," broaden and enrich our definitions of what is acceptable and lovable, and discard the constricting limits of the old image. Like a truly comfortable walking shoe, an authentic self-image does not bind or distort—it allows us to move forward without pain.

We don't have to start from scratch and we can take all the time we want. In fact, we may discover the pleasures of an evolving self-image, one that grows with us. Some aspects of the old self-image do not need to change at all. If I have always viewed and valued myself as a fine seamstress, for example, cancer does not alter that at all.

A woman may preserve certain parts of her image but express them differently. Perhaps she continues to feel that having a sense of control is healthy for her and necessary to her vision of herself. Instead of managing a tight time schedule, however, she maintains that sense of control during treatment by obtaining information, participating as a decision-making member of her healthcare team, and persisting in a healing package of therapies for herself. After treatment, she may choose an entirely new way of expressing this part of herself.

On the other hand, after a cancer diagnosis she may recognize that, for her, the need to be in control goes far beyond being a healthy, normal coping technique. As she learns to acknowledge the "uncontrolled" parts of herself, a woman may replace some of that need for control with more self-acceptance and spontaneity.

Our concepts of what a "real woman" is need to be expanded and deepened. Culturally, women tend to see themselves as caretakers and to define their self-worth in terms of what they do for other people. Nurse-psychotherapist Diane W. Scott, Ph.D., who specializes in therapy for women with cancer, claims that men with cancer tend to relax and let the women in their lives cosset them, make them special foods, and make the process easier for them. Women with cancer, on the other hand, keep "protecting" others: keeping painful news from them, continuing "business as usual" (career, being a wife and/or mother, or whatever), making it as easy as possible for everyone else, despite the cost to themselves. Even if women allow themselves to let down a little during treatment, they may expect themselves to be up and doing the moment treatment ends.

But, somewhere along the way, a woman may begin to question this picture. At some point, out of necessity, she puts her needs first and discovers that the world does not fall apart. Perhaps she becomes aware of some simmering resentment in herself. She talks with other women with cancer and finds a broader definition of acceptable "womanly" behavior.

How assertive can a "feminine" woman be? During cancer treatment women often discover that they must make their needs known, directly and forcefully. Their very lives depend on it, and there is neither time nor energy to shilly-shally. Support groups often model techniques for clear communication with doctors (and others) and offer opportunities for women to rehearse these approaches in a safe environment. When they sees how effective this kind of communication is, some women will not settle for less after cancer treatment ends.

The way society tells it, a woman with a "women's" cancer is less a woman. She has scars or missing organs and no longer fits the narrow definition of "femininity." But many women with cancer know differently—and they come to realize that it is society's definition that is lacking.

Womanliness is a concept that should include rather than exclude. To fill its own needs, society has given women a limited picture of what "real" women "should" be. Cancer offers us the opportunity to experience some energizing anger, and then come up with a better definition.

COPING WITH BODY CHANGES

All the philosophizing aside, how does a woman cope with losing a breast, her hair, and svelte figure all within a few months? Some losses may be temporary, but that is small comfort to the woman with handfuls of hair on the floor of the shower.

First, she can acknowledge the loss. Even if she is an ardent feminist, and convinced intellectually that what our bodies look like has nothing to do with our inner value, it is normal and human to mourn the changes.

It is very hard not to feel alone when we look different. This does not bother some women at all, but others feel much happier if they can either disguise the differences or join other women in the same situation.

To disguise the difference—and even make it a plus—a woman who has lost her hair might use bright scarves, experiment with a frivolous wig, or attend a "Look Good, Feel Better" session. She may feel less invested in appearance as usual, and this can translate to a sense of freedom and daring in her fashion statements. Some women develop a whole new "look" for themselves after a cancer diagnosis. Or, a woman may just relax with other "baldies" in a support group, take courage from their shared strength, and learn from their experiences.

Kerry McGinn

Part Two

Breast Cancer

Breasts.

Two mounds, mostly fat and glandular tissue, that perch on the large chest muscle. They can nourish babies, bring pleasure to a woman and her lover, fill out clothes—and cause many a woman endless worry.

When a healthy woman is asked what disease she fears most, chances are she will answer, "Breast cancer." It is not the deadliest cancer women get (lung cancer is) and it is not the most common life-threatening illness (heart disease is), but breast cancer has a hold on women's fears that no other disease can match.

However, most women *never* develop breast cancer. Even with family histories of cancer and several personal risk factors, most women do not get the disease.

On the other hand, most of the women who *do* develop breast cancer do not have any particular known risk factors beyond the fact that they are women growing older. The woman who says, "No one in my family has breast cancer, so I don't need to worry," is fooling herself. There is no cause for women to panic about breast cancer—but there is ample reason for every woman to take care of herself.

When it comes to their breasts, many women feel panicky, helpless, hopeless. Every time there is another scary newspaper story about breast cancer statistics, they *know* they will get breast cancer; it is simply a matter of when. They feel so much at the mercy of forces beyond their control that they cannot begin to take action—even if they had some idea what to do.

Some of this sense of vulnerability may have little to do with medical facts. Physically, the breasts are soft, yielding, exposed and "out there" on the chest—but it may be that the greater vulnerability has cultural roots.

Traditionally a young girl grows up defining much of her self-image/body image in terms of external cues rather than from the inside out. Do her breasts look like the breasts in vogue during her adolescence? How do other people (family, friends, lovers) react to her breasts? And these external cues keep shifting. Depending on what year it is, the woman's breasts should be bigger or smaller, pointier or higher or droopier. Is this the year of Twiggy or Dolly Parton?

The breast has several functions—and there is plenty of misinformation available about each of them, which means more possibilities for a woman to question her self-worth. Did she stop breast feeding because she "didn't have enough milk"? Does she fail to reach orgasm from breast stimulation? Do her blouses bunch over her breasts?

Add the breast cancer statistics to the equation, and it is small wonder that many a woman with perfectly healthy breasts feels off balance. It doesn't help that some doctors insist that only the things doctors can do, like professional breast exams and mammography, make a real difference in breast health, and that the woman should just "trust the doctor" to take care of her.

But there is plenty we can do. Whether or not there is a breast cancer diagnosis, it is possible to reclaim our own breasts, establish our own standards of what they should be, learn to live comfortably with one or no breasts, and make a genuine difference in protecting our own breast health.

First, we ask who is telling us about how our breasts should look and function, and by what right? Often there is a profit motive, as with fashion changes. Sometimes there is a social agenda. For instance, society may extol bigger—and supposedly more "feminine"—breasts when economic factors push women to stay home and nurture a family. And, were it not for society's confusion about women, would the same slang word—"boob"—mean both breast and . . . dunce?

Once we recognize what is happening, we may feel an energizing anger, or may laugh at ourselves for listening to such silly messages. We are so much more than a pair of mammary glands.

Caring for our breasts means getting accurate information. What is going on in there? What can we do to protect ourselves? What can we safely ignore? And, when do we need to take prompt action? A doctor, nurse practitioner, breast health center personnel, or other health professional can teach a woman how to examine her breasts effectively. Books, pamphlets, magazine articles, or videotapes can give her general information.

Finally, we can gather the best possible breast health team. The team includes the woman herself, knowledgeable about what she can do to protect herself. It includes the doctor or nurse who examines the woman's breasts thoroughly and regularly. After the woman reaches 40 or so, the team adds routine mammography to the program.

Most breast changes are not cancer. But because breast cancer is by far the most common women's cancer and because breast health issues cover so much territory, they have received one section in this book. The following four chapters run the gamut: from what is inside the normal breast to the different kinds of breast cancer, from how a woman can examine her breasts effectively to what it feels like to undergo—and complete—breast cancer therapy.

Kerry McGinn

Chapter 11

Questions About Breasts

Why should a woman learn about her breasts? If she knows something about how they are constructed and how they function, she can understand better what goes wrong with them—and how much goes right. She can examine her breasts more effectively if she knows what she is feeling. Also, a working knowledge of breast terms gives her a language to share with health professionals.

The breasts include more than what fits into a bra. Breast tissue extends from the collarbone to the "bra line," from the breast bone to the middle of the armpit (axilla), and from the skin to the chest muscle. Breasts contain no muscle of their own. They vary in shape, size, coloring and skin texture from woman to woman, and in the same woman at different times in her life.

In the middle of each breast is a nipple—which may protrude a little or a lot, be flat against the skin, or even be inverted ("tucked in") and still be functional and normal, as long as that is the way it has always been. Nipples contain spongy tissue that fills with blood and becomes taut in response to touch, cold, a baby's suckling, or even a baby's cry. The pigmented area around the base of the nipple is called the areola, which means "ring of color." Montgomery's tubercles are the visible pores or tiny lumps on the areola which are openings for the oil glands that lubricate the nipple and areola during breastfeeding.

Each breast is divided into 15–20 sections, rather like the sections of a halved grapefruit, called lobes. Cooper's ligaments are bands of strong, flexible, fibrous tissue that separate the

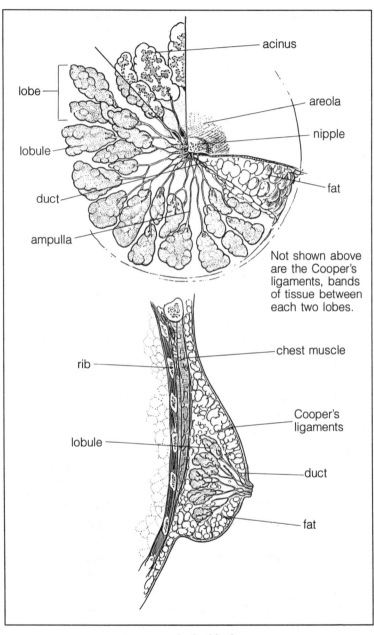

Not shown above are the Cooper's ligaments, bands of tissue between each two lobes.

Anatomy of a healthy breast
(*courtesy of* Breast Cancer Digest, *National Cancer Institute*)

sections, passing from the chest muscles, between the lobes, to the skin. They give the breast its support; as they stretch with age, the breast droops. A lacy filigree of tiny fibers forms a network throughout each breast. Doctors interpreting mammograms look for any place this architecture of fibers has been disturbed.

Fat cells, found between and around the lobes, cushion and shape the breast. The fat cells, fibrous tissue, and other parts of the breast that are not involved in producing, transporting, and storing milk are called the stroma. The working part of the breast is called the breast parenchyma, which is where most serious breast problems occur.

How does the breast work? Within each lobe are lobules (little lobes) that look rather like tiny bunches of grapes. When a mother breastfeeds her baby, the tiny gland cells lining the acinus (sac) at the end of each "grape" follow the body's recipe to extract from nearby blood vessels the ingredients they need to make milk. For a few days after birth, the gland cells extract the right amounts of water, sugar, fat, protein, and salts to make colostrum, the best fluid for a newborn baby. As the baby grows a little older and needs a different kind of nutrition, the body's hormones instruct the gland cells to use different proportions of the same materials.

After the gland cells extract and combine the right ingredients, the milk is squeezed into the acinus and from there into a small duct, or passageway. Small ducts join to become larger ducts, transporting the milk to an ampulla (reservoir) under the areola where it stays until it is time for the baby to nurse.

The breasts are supplied with many blood vessels that bring the ingredients for milk, hormonal messages from the rest of the body (brain and ovaries especially), and the chemical energy for the breast to do its work. The lymph system, the body's second circulatory system, removes wastes from the breast, recycling when possible; thus fluids and tissues that can be reused by the body are swept into the lymph system and eventually back into the blood supply. Lymph vessels connect the two breasts and also drain each breast by way of channels through the axilla, along the breastbone, and up past the collarbone. Along the lymph channels are lymph nodes, filter stations that trap cells that cannot pass through; an occasional one is a cancer cell.

The nerves in the breast, concentrated around the nipple, send only one-way messages—that the breast is being touched, perhaps—to the brain. Any reply from the brain comes as a hormone message through the bloodstream. If a baby starts suckling, for instance, the breast nerves send a message to the brain, which then releases a hormone through the blood stream to "let down" the milk.

Each month, from adolescence to menopause, a woman's breasts prepare for a possible pregnancy. Throughout the menstrual cycle the hormone **estrogen** flows to the breasts from the ovaries and the adrenal glands, but it reaches its peak during the middle two weeks of the cycle, counting from the first day of the menstrual period. Estrogen, the "buildup" hormone, pushes the breast cells to prepare for possible milk production and transport.

When the ovary releases its ripe egg at midcycle, it begins releasing the "secretory" hormone **progesterone** as well. The breast cells begin rehearsing their functions of secreting (producing) and transporting milk. The blood supply increases to the breast to meet the additional needs of the working breast and some extra fluid—basically blood minus the blood cells—seeps from the tiny blood vessels into the breast tissue. A woman may feel this extra fluid as a sense of fullness, tenderness, and sometimes discomfort.

If no pregnancy occurs, the breasts begin their monthly cleanup after the menstrual period. The extra fluid returns into the body's general circulation via the lymph system. The body reabsorbs unused extra cells and secretions so the whole process can start over again. This relatively quiet period after the period is the best time to examine the breasts.

If pregnancy does occur, preparations for producing milk accelerate. The gland cells multiply, lobules enlarge, ducts lengthen, and blood and lymph vessels become larger. By the end of pregnancy, under the influence of the hormones, the glandular tissue in the breast has crowded out almost all the fat tissue.

After pregnancy (and lactation if the woman breastfeeds), a massive cleanup begins as the cells and structures revert to their prepregnancy state. The lymph system recycles what can be recycled and gets rid of any debris.

A woman's breasts change throughout life. The basic structures are present from before birth, but need the hormonal stimulation of adolescence to begin growing and developing. With pregnancy and/or lactation, the working tissue crowds out the stroma. After pregnancy and lactation, however, the parenchyma decreases dramatically. The woman may feel as if she has no breasts until the stroma builds up again.

As a woman grows older and especially after menopause, the proportions of parenchyma and stroma inside the breasts keep changing until there is almost no working tissue left. Since fatty tissue shows up clearly on mammograms and working, glandular tissue often does not, mammograms tend to become easier to read as women grow older.

WHO GETS CANCER OF THE BREAST?

Like every cancer, breast cancer develops from a series of mutations in the body genes, particularly those that control how often the cell divides. Many breast cancer researchers now point a finger at a specific growth-promoting gene, called the **HER-2/neu oncogene,** located on chromosome 17 in cell DNA.

About 30% of women with breast cancer have been born with or have acquired abnormal quantities of this gene, which can promote runaway cell division. Many women with too much HER-2/neu never undergo the additional mutations necessary for cancer, but they remain more at risk than the average woman. If breast cancer develops, it is likely to be quite aggressive. But 70% of women with breast cancer still have normal amounts of HER-2/neu oncogene. Researchers are looking for further clues in other genes, such as p53 (see Chapter 2).

What causes genes to mutate so that a woman develops breast cancer? We do not yet have a clear villain (such as tobacco smoke for lung cancer). We do know that being a woman and growing older are the two major risk factors. Although men occasionally develop breast cancer, as do women under 25, it is very rare.

FAMILY AND PERSONAL CANCER HISTORY

Many women worry about breast cancer because they have a relative with the disease. In fact, women are often at much less risk because of family history than they think. The questions to ask are these: How close is the relationship—sister, mother, aunt, or grandmother? (The relationship need not be through the mother's side to increase risk.) How old was the relative when breast cancer was diagnosed—before or after menopause? Did cancer develop in one breast or both? What type of breast cancer was it? How many relatives and/or generations? Have people in the family developed colon or ovarian cancers? They are two kinds of cancers that tend to cluster with breast cancer in family patterns.

The woman whose only cancer history is a grandmother who developed breast cancer at age 75 may be at minimally increased risk for cancer. This tends to be the garden-variety type of cancer to which all women become vulnerable as they grow older.

However, the woman whose mother and two sisters all developed aggressive cancer in both breasts before menopause may face a very high risk of developing the disease herself. Researchers believe that, in some "breast cancer families," abnormal amounts of HER-2/neu and/or other genetic flaws may be transmitted from generation to generation. What this does is to move the timing of a first genetic mutation forward many years; the cancer may never develop, but the woman is born with a headstart she wishes she did not have.

Not every female in the family inherits this legacy, since we have two parents and receive genetic information from both. Researchers are working now on diagnostic tools accurate enough to tell from noncancerous breast tissue who is at risk. Meanwhile, women with a substantial family breast cancer history can obtain information from a medical geneticist or other cancer risk counselor; these professionals are often associated with a medical school or large hospital. Some women in this situation seek prophylactic mastectomies, preventive removal of the breasts during early adulthood to avoid breast cancer.

If she has a personal history of breast cancer, a woman faces a higher than average risk of developing a second, unrelated breast cancer—although the great majority of women never do. Women with cancers of the ovary also run an increased risk of breast cancer.

Women treated for breast carcinoma in situ who keep their breasts have a risk of about 1% a year of developing invasive breast cancer. If a woman is diagnosed with a benign breast condition in which the individual cells are atypical but not abnormal enough to be cancer, her risk of later cancer significantly increases.

DIET, FEMALE HORMONES, AND OTHER FACTORS

Many researchers are convinced that diet is a major factor in causing the genetic mutations necessary for breast cancer, and believe that low fiber and high fat—any kind of fat, animal or plant—may be the culprits. Worldwide, the higher the average amount of fat in the diet, the higher the breast cancer rate. The theory behind the fiber connection is that fiber from fruits, vegetables, and grains helps move food waste products, including some suspected of causing cancerous changes, quickly and easily through the digestive tract before they have a chance to cause problems. Obesity is also related statistically to breast cancer: the more fat a woman carries, the more she is at risk. Adequate amounts of such nutrients as selenium and beta carotene seem to protect a woman somewhat.

Early findings from an ongoing Harvard study of almost 90,000 nurses appeared to question the connection between a high-fat diet and breast cancer. However, the women in the study with the lowest fat intake still consumed about 32% of their calories in fat. Later results (1992) from the study found no apparent change in the risk between women who took 25% of their calories as fat and those with a much higher fat diet. But while 32% and 25% are well below the average 42% fat intake in the U.S., they are still higher than the 10–20% fat intake of societies with very low breast cancer rates. Many researchers contend that, rather than a gradual decrease in risk as the amount of dietary fat goes down, there is an abrupt cut-off at about 20% fat intake: fat intake has to be 20% or so, they say, to make a real difference. High-fat diets and obesity both tend to increase the amounts of the female hormone estrogen in the body, and this may be a crucial factor in any diet-cancer link.

For years, researchers have backed away from doing large, long-term studies of a diet with very low fat intake, citing difficulties in getting sizable groups of women to participate. However, a 20% fat diet study is now on the drawing board, partly because women have become more militant and committed to finding out whether dietary fat really does make a difference.

Whether or not hormone medications, ordinarily taken either as birth control pills or after menopause, play a role is not known. Women who have been treated for breast cancer are usually not given female hormones because, in theory, these might nourish any stray cancer cells that are already there and are responsive to hormones. (This makes sense, but researchers lack evidence about whether or not this actually happens.) However, this does not mean hormone medications *cause* breast cancer.

How long and how consistently a woman experiences ovarian hormonal cycles seems to correlate with her risk. The woman who began menstruating young, goes through menopause late, and has never been pregnant faces a relatively high risk of the disease. Women who have had both ovaries removed in young adulthood appear to be at lower risk.

Childbearing patterns may be a factor. Having a first baby before age 20 seems to offer significant protection from breast cancer. Women who do not have children at all are at a higher-than-average risk; women who have a first child after age 35 are at still greater risk. One reason for this may be that with normal body wear and tear, abnormal cells become more common as a woman grows older; the hormonal "storm" of pregnancy could nourish these cells so that they outgrow the body's defenses. However, the overwhelming majority of women who get pregnant after 35 never develop breast cancer. Breastfeeding and/or number of children do not appear to make a statistical difference.

We just do not have good, solid information yet about hormonal factors and breast cancer. Whether the questions are about hormone pills, pregnancy hormones, increased hormone levels because of a high-fat diet or obesity—or even the safety of meat from animals fed large amounts of hormones—the research is just not yet available.

PREVENTING BREAST CANCER

What does this all mean for the individual woman? She cannot change her family history and she probably will not change her childbearing plans. She *can* change her diet so that she gets lower fat and higher fiber, and she can keep her weight reasonable through both diet and exercise. She can seek current information before taking hormone medications. She can stay as healthy and happy as possible—it may help and certainly cannot hurt.

A controversial large-scale research study, started in 1992, looks at the possibility of preventing or postponing breast cancer by using the drug **tamoxifen citrate** (Nolvadex) on healthy women. Tamoxifen (not to be confused with taxol, the investigational chemotherapy drug from yew trees) acts as a weakened estrogen and is used as "antihormone" therapy by many women who have breast cancer. No one is quite sure how it works, but one theory is that it binds to the hormone receptor sites on many breast cancer cells so that the cells cannot get the "real" hormones they need. It is a bit like setting out swarms of sterile insects to mate unsuccessfully and thus reduce their pest population. At the same time, tamoxifen seems to act like a mild estrogen in the rest of the body, which means that it may protect the bones and heart somewhat.

Sixteen thousand women—with no history of breast cancer but at considerable risk for the disease because they are either over 60 or have other major risk factors—are divided randomly into a treatment group and a control group. Women in one group will take two tamoxifen tablets a day for five years; the control group will take two placebo tablets. Until the study is over, neither doctors nor women will know who took what. If the tamoxifen group develops significantly fewer breast cancers over the five years and afterward, and does not have major side effects from the drug, doctors will have a prevention strategy to offer women at high risk.

Tamoxifen does cause hot flashes and other menopausal symptoms in premenopausal women and carries medical risks of its own. Probably only those young women at very high risk for breast cancer would want to consider this option.

Opponents of the study are concerned about side effects of a powerful drug being used in a healthy population. Too, they worry that this is a "just do something—anything" approach to breast cancer. But many women are eager to participate in a study that may help them personally and should answer some of the scientific questions about tamoxifen.

Information about the tamoxifen clinical trial is available from NCI's Cancer Information Service (see Resources).

MAKING SENSE OF RISK STATISTICS

Currently, the American Cancer Society estimates that one in nine women in the United States will develop breast cancer during her lifetime, up from one in 15 not many years ago. About 180,000 women were expected to be diagnosed with the disease in 1992; about 46,000 will die of it. Breast cancer is diagnosed in about 2% of all women under 50 and becomes considerably more common after that age.

The 11% (one in nine) risk figure says that, under present conditions of risk, a white baby girl born today has an 11% chance of being diagnosed with breast cancer at some time up to age 85. Women with African or Asian roots are at less risk, but this statistical advantage wanes the more generations the family has been in the U.S. and the more acculturated it has become. The situation appears to be similar for Hispanic women, but statistics are lacking. This risk percentage is a "cumulative" figure obtained by adding a woman's risk of developing breast cancer from age 20 to 30, plus that from 30 to 40, and so on.

At no one time does the average woman face an 11% risk of developing breast cancer. She faces a small risk during each segment of time. If she does not develop breast cancer during that segment of time, that portion of risk is behind her forever. It does not get added on to future segments. During the next segment of time, she faces another small risk. Because breast cancer is often related to body wear and tear, however, each segment is a little riskier than the one before.

The 11% figure is outrageous and scarcely reassuring, but is not quite as scary as it sounds. These figures reflect partly the rapid increase in longevity for women, who can now expect to live into their 80s and beyond, into the decades at very high risk for breast cancer. Ironically, if large numbers of women died young—in childbirth, for instance—the breast cancer statistics would look brighter.

The rising rate also reflects an increase in detecting breast cancer earlier. However, many people believe that the increasing rate of breast cancer does indicate that there is more going on. They question whether something in the environment, dietary patterns, or changes in childbearing patterns—or something else entirely—may be making women more vulnerable.

Statisticians warn against a "The sky is falling, the sky is falling!" approach, either for groups of women or for the individual. Statistics often go up for a few years and then decrease just as unpredictably. Too, since a cancer large enough to diagnose has been growing for many years, and since the genetic mutations may have begun decades before, statisticians and epidemiologists try to keep a long-term perspective.

For the woman with a family history of breast cancer or another factor that increases her risk significantly, it is especially valuable to think of breast cancer risk as a series of time segments, each with its small portion of risk. For instance, a condition that "triples" a woman's risk means that, in a decade where she would normally face a 1% risk, she might now face a 3% chance of developing the disease. When she finishes that decade without the disease, that portion of risk is behind her forever. Also, if the risk condition is discovered when she is 45 (for example if a family member develops breast cancer or the woman is diagnosed with a benign condition that increases her risk) she already has several decades of risk behind her. A medical geneticist can use statistical life tables to be much more precise than "triples" or "significantly increases." It also makes sense to remember that statistics tell about groups of women, but say nothing about what will happen to the individual.

BREAST CHANGES THAT ARE NOT CANCER

At least half of all women at some time in their lives experience something about a breast that worries them: discomfort, a lump, or some other change. Probably almost all of these women wonder whether this change could be cancer.

In fact, most of these changes are not cancer, and do not in any way increase a woman's risk of cancer.

Many doctors call any noncancerous breast change by the same generic label: fibrocystic breast disease. But "breast" is about the only accurate part of the term, since many of the changes have nothing to do with either fibrous or cystic tissue and most of them are not a disease at all. "Benign breast changes" is a better term, along with the name of the actual condition, if possible.

Lumping the lumps together is the problem. Dr. Susan Love, breast surgeon and author of *Dr. Susan Love's Breast Book*, divides benign breast conditions into six categories:

1. Normal physiological changes, like minor tenderness, swelling, and lumpiness

2. Mastalgia, or severe breast pain

3. Infections and inflammations

4. Discharge and other nipple problems

5. Lumpiness or nodularity beyond what most women have

6. "Dominant" benign lumps, ones that "stick out" from the normal lumpiness

Once a woman finds out that her breast condition is not cancer, she still wants to know if it could increase her chances of developing cancer later. Prodded by the American Cancer Society's National Task Force on Breast Cancer Control, the College of American Pathologists held a consensus conference in 1985 entitled, "Is 'Fibrocystic' Disease of the Breast Precancerous?" The Board of Governors of the College of American Pathologists later adopted the conclusions as policy.

The pathologists divided the common benign breast changes into three categories, depending on whether they might possibly increase a woman's risk of developing breast cancer later:

1. Nonproliferative changes

2. Proliferative changes without atypical cells

3. Proliferative changes with atypical cells

Nonproliferative breast changes are the most common kinds of changes and they do not in any way add to a woman's risk. Except when the breast is developing during adolescence and during pregnancy and lactation, normal breast cells divide at set times to replace old cells and maintain the breast status quo. In nonproliferative changes, the breast cells stick to their normal schedule of division but the total number of cells may pile up somewhat, perhaps because the old cells are not being disposed of quickly enough.

The glandular tissue of the breast *normally* feels lumpy as it does its work; the breast normally gathers in extra fluid every month, which may stretch nerve fibers and send discomfort messages to the brain. These are not considered breast changes at all.

But what happens to many women over the years is that

the cell cleanup does not keep up with the cell buildup. The breasts may receive a faulty hormonal message, or overreact to a normal message and overprepare. Or the lymph system and other cleanup agencies may fall down on the job a bit. Instead of being efficiently recycled, the extra fluid and secretions may gather into a **cyst**, large or small, which may pop and drain or may persist from month to month. Cysts are the most common kind of breast lump in women before menopause. Some women are prone to form large numbers of them. A cyst can also press on nerve fibers and cause considerable discomfort.

At other times, breast debris builds up in a benign solid lump called a **fibroadenoma**. This is usually rather round, moves easily in the breast, and may feel rubbery. This may need to be removed in a biopsy and examined under a microscope because that is the only way to be absolutely sure of what the lump is. There are several other kinds of nonproliferative breast changes but as long as they fall into this category they do not increase a woman's risk of cancer.

Proliferative changes without atypical cells occur when, for some reason, the cells divide more often than they should but the individual cells themselves appear quite normal. Duct hyperplasia, for instance, means that the walls of the breast ducts and lobules, ordinarily lined with a layer two cells deep, have become thicker. The layer can overgrow slightly, up to four cells in depth, and not affect a woman's risk for developing breast cancer later. If the layer grows to more than four cells deep, however, the hyperplasia is considered to increase a woman's risk slightly, about $1\frac{1}{2}$–2 times the average. Hyperplasia often reverses itself.

In another common benign condition called **sclerosing adenosis**, tiny chunks of benign breast debris can take up calcium salts from the body and "calcify." While these are too small to be felt with the fingers as a lump, they can show up on mammograms as microcalcifications; if these look a certain way and appear in clusters they need to be evaluated, since cancer sometimes shows itself the same way.

Proliferative changes with atypical cells happen when the cells divide more often than they should *and* the individual cells appear abnormal. Possibly the quality control slips when the breast works overtime to make too many cells. These atypical cells can disappear, stay where they are without causing any trouble, or once in a while lead to the ultimate atypical cells: cancer. The more atypical a cell is, the more vulnerable it is to further mutations.

Proliferative changes with atypical cells do increase a woman's risk of cancer moderately, 2–5 times the average, depending on how atypical the individual cells are and how many of them there are.

How are benign breast changes treated? General lumpiness is considered normal and requires no treatment. If a diagnostic procedure is necessary—for a persistent solid lump, some kinds of nipple drainage, or certain changes on a mammogram—and benign changes are found, the doctor needs to describe to the woman what those changes are, especially whether there are any proliferative changes with atypia. With nonproliferative changes, she does not need to do anything except continue a routine breast care program of monthly breast self-exam, regular professional breast exam, and mammography. If there are proliferative changes, particularly with atypia, she can discuss with her doctor whether more frequent professional exams and/or mammograms are advisable.

Insurance companies have been known to deny a woman coverage for any future breast problem because of a benign breast change that is not a disease and in no way increases her risk of cancer. This is not right or reasonable, but it is legal and it happens. While she has to answer direct questions honestly, and her doctor must too, there is no reason to volunteer anything or to mention a nonproliferative nondisease.

What about breast pain? If it continues month after month and causes distress, there is usually a therapy or combination of therapies used for relief: mild analgesic pills, heat or cold, gentle massage or specific lymph drainage massage, a firm bra, dietary changes, distraction, and so on. Two books that contain more information are *The Informed Woman's Guide to Breast Health* and *Dr. Susan Love's Breast Book* (see Resources).

Kerry McGinn

Chapter 12

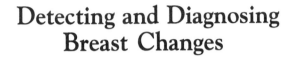

Detecting and Diagnosing
Breast Changes

Until medical science learns how to prevent breast cancer, the best strategy is to find it early. Early detection means that women live longer and may be able to save their breasts as well.

Early detection means being alert to changes in how a breast looks, feels, or functions. Most of these changes are not cancer, but they need to be evaluated.

A breast lump is the most common change, felt with the fingers and/or seen on a mammogram. The cancerous breast lump is ordinarily hard ("rock-like") but it can be as minimal as a soft thickening. Besides a lump, there are other possible signs:

- changes in how the breast appears, such as swelling, dimpling, number of visible blood vessels, skin redness or enlarged pores, nipple alterations

- nipple discharges

- microcalcifications or other findings on mammograms

What needs to be evaluated by a health professional? Any breast change that lasts over a month in a premenopausal woman. In the postmenopausal woman, who is at more risk for breast cancer and no longer experiences the monthly breast changes that come with the ebb and flow of hormones, *any* breast change needs to be checked as soon as possible.

Pain, especially pain that comes and goes with the men-

strual cycle, is usually not the earliest symptom of a breast cancer, but persistent pain definitely needs to be checked.

DETECTING BREAST CHANGES

The "big three" in detecting breast changes, benign or cancerous, are **mammography, monthly breast self-examination
(BSE),** and **regular examinations by a health professional.** No
one method of detection is perfect, but the three work together
as a team. Each method has advantages and weaknesses. Each
finds certain breast changes that the others can miss. The woman who uses all three methods gives herself the best obtainable
breast health care.

Mammography remains the workhorse of breast imaging
techniques, both for screening the woman who does not have
any breast symptoms and for giving information when she does.
It saves many lives by finding very early cancers even before
there is a lump to feel (See Chapter 3).

In specific cases, doctors may order another technique.
Ultrasound, for example, is commonly used if the woman with
a breast lump that can be felt is under 35, or is pregnant or
nursing. It can also help when the breasts show up poorly on
mammograms, or the doctor suspects that a lump is a cyst. Less
often, doctors turn to computerized tomography, magnetic
resonance imaging, diaphanography and/or thermography.

Women—not doctors or mammograms—still find over
80% of the breast lumps that can be felt. Unfortunately, too
often these lumps are found by chance when they are relatively
large. A common scenario has the woman soaping her breasts
in the shower and suddenly feeling this . . . thing.

The idea behind regular breast self-examination is that
after a woman learns what to look and feel for, she becomes so
well-acquainted with her own breasts that she can spot very
early changes. BSE is not an anxious monthly cancer search.
Instead, it means "checking for normal."

What advantages does BSE offer? It involves the person
most concerned with her own breasts and most motivated to

take care of them. It offers continuing surveillance. If the doctor examines the breasts annually in September and a cancerous lump becomes big enough to feel in October, the woman has lost eleven crucial months before the cancer is detected by her doctor the following September.

When a woman examines her own breasts, her fingers feel from "the outside in." But at the same time, her chest wall and other internal structures feel from "the inside out" against her fingers. This gives her an extra sense of her own breasts that no health professional can share.

BSE also does not cost anything and a woman does not have to leave home for it. It is absolutely safe and does not cause discomfort. Plus, many women like the fact that this is a real contribution they can make to their own health.

BSE is available to every woman who has eyes and fingers. That includes women who cannot get routine mammography because they are pregnant, nursing a baby, or too young for mammograms. The American Cancer Society recommends that women begin practicing BSE at age 20; routine mammography is not usually considered necessary until age 40, with one baseline set of films taken sometime after age 35.

For the woman with "dense" glandular breasts that do not show up well on mammograms, BSE may be her best chance of finding an early cancer. And while the woman with lumpy, difficult-to-examine breasts may find it hard to learn BSE initially, it still may be easier for her to detect changes if she examines her breasts every month than it is for the doctor who checks them once a year.

Some doctors minimize the importance of BSE, usually because they think of it as occasional, halfhearted poking and prodding by a woman who does not know what she is doing. But self-examination, used consistently and effectively by women who are well-trained and motivated, is something else entirely. Doctors and women who put all their trust in mammography may miss many breast cancers completely, especially in premenopausal women.

Obviously, I'm a believer. When I found a tiny breast lump with BSE, it did not show up on mammography. My careful and competent surgeon could not even feel it. I finally convinced the doctor to aspirate a few cells through a needle and promptly learned the lump was cancer. Of the four doctors I saw during the next few days—two surgeons, one medical oncologist, and one radiation oncologist—*every single one* volunteered that he or she would not have found the lump: "How in the world did you ever find that?"

My experience is not unique. Roughly a third of the women in my breast cancer support group, mostly premenopausal, discovered our own tumors, which did not appear on mammography and which our doctors had difficulty feeling.

Women often avoid BSE because they do not feel competent to perform it. Everything feels lumpy to them and they do not know "what's what." Even with the best of training, no woman is competent at first; it takes months to "learn" the breasts. Early on, every woman wonders if what she is feeling now was there last month or not. But each month brings increasing expertise and confidence, *if* the woman does not get discouraged and give up too soon.

No woman has to interpret or diagnose what she feels. The only conclusion she needs to draw is whether her breasts have changed or not since the previous exam.

Many women do not practice BSE because they are scared of what they will find. It is natural and normal to be scared, but most of the time there will not be any changes, and a woman will feel reassured. If there is a change, it most likely benign. Should there ever be a cancerous change, the scary thing is *not* finding it. With life and breasts at stake, most women discover that learning BSE—taking concrete action to protect their health—soon crowds out fear and brings peace of mind instead.

PERFORMING BSE

BSE takes about fifteen unhurried minutes once a month. If it is less often, it is harder to "remember" the breast; if it is more often, it is too soon to recognize a change. Women who still menstruate should schedule it about a week or so after their period starts, when their breasts are most at rest hormonally. Women past menopause or who are pregnant or lactating can choose any day of the month that they will remember easily. Those who have undergone hysterectomies but still have functioning ovaries have to listen to other bodily cues; they should try to avoid times when symptoms such as bloating or breast tenderness indicate more hormonal activity.

It is very helpful for a woman to have BSE training, especially with a doctor or nurse who will take the time to "map" a woman's breasts for her. A woman's personal doctor or nurse practitioner, a breast health center, American Cancer Society BSE trainers, or a women's health group can teach her what she is feeling and what is normal for her. Many women get a breast model with simulated lumps to use each month to "reeducate" their fingers before feeling their own breasts.

Each month, a woman can jog her memory with the "seven P's" of BSE:

- *positions* to assume while inspecting and palpating (feeling) the breasts

- *perimeter* (boundaries) of breast tissue to be examined

- *palpation* using pads of the fingers

- *pressures* of the fingers

- *pattern* of the search

- *practice* with feedback

- *plan* of action for breast health

What initially seems awkward soon becomes second nature. There is nothing difficult about the BSE eye and hand movements.

Inspecting the breasts

To examine her breasts visually, the woman first stands with her arms relaxed at her sides in front of a large mirror in a good

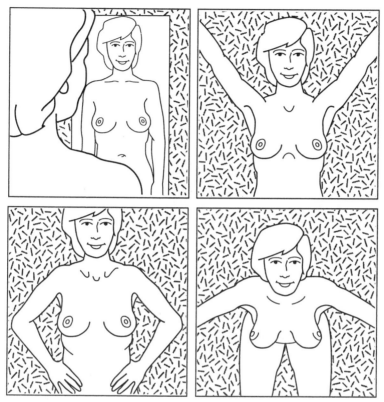

Breast Inspection Process
(this series of illustrations—on pages 193,195, 197, 198, and 199—
courtesy of The Informed Woman's Guide to Breast Health)

light. As she faces the mirror, she looks carefully at her breasts: their symmetry, shape, color, skin texture, pattern of blood vessels, and so on.

Skin over a tumor can appear stretched, shiny, and large-pored; in fact, this condition is called peau d'orange, skin of the orange. A cancer's need for nutrition can lead to increased numbers of blood vessels in the vicinity, and these may show through the skin. Nipples and areolas get special attention: any rashes, discharges, or an "outie" nipple that has become an "innie"?

The woman turns slowly, bringing first one breast forward to examine and then the other so that light and shadow help disclose any changes in breast contour. Then, since other positions do a better job of accentuating any breast swellings or puckerings, the woman raises her arms above her head, with her elbows back, or clasps her hands behind her head. This tightens the chest muscles, elevates the breasts, and stretches the skin. She pivots slowly in this position and then with her hands pressing firmly on her hips. Puckerings, "dimples," and/or changes in the shape or direction of the nipple can result from a tumor pulling on one of the Cooper's ligaments that attach from the chest wall to the skin.

A woman can also bend forward at the hips and check the symmetry of the breasts as they hang down. Most women normally have one breast a little larger than the other, but the two should look relatively similar. Only if the size and symmetry have changed is it significant. The woman with large and/or pendulous breasts can lift each one with the opposite hand so that she can see the underside.

Feeling the breasts

Positions   After she has looked carefully at the breasts, the woman lies down in the best position for palpating her breasts effectively. Many women accidentally discover a breast lump while they are showering—but when a woman is standing up, gravity pulls the breast tissue down so that it bulges at the bases and is difficult to examine. The idea with BSE is to support and spread the breast evenly so that all the tissue can be felt against the firm background of the chest wall.

A small-breasted woman may be able to do this just by lying flat on her back. If breast tissue bulges to the side then, she can place a small pillow behind the shoulder of the breast she plans to examine.

The MammaCare Method, one popular program of BSE training, refines this further. A woman always palpates her breast with the opposite hand. Thus, when it is time to examine the outer half of her right breast, for example, she turns onto her left side, bends her knees, and then lets her right shoulder fall back slightly until the nipple "floats" at the top of

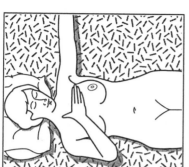 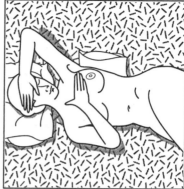

Breast Self-Examination

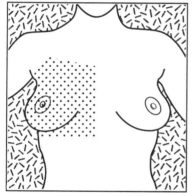

Shaded area is perimeter for BSE

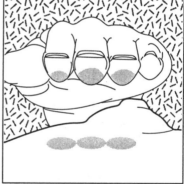

Palpation with pads of fingers

the mound of breast. (A pillow behind her back makes the position comfortable.) She rests the back of her right hand on her forehead.

When she is ready to check the inner half of the breast, from nipple line to breastbone, the woman keeps the examining fingers in place on the breast, so that she does not miss any area, while she pushes the pillow away and rolls onto her back. She holds the other arm out to the side.

Perimeter   The area to check on each breast is bounded by an imaginary line down from the middle of the armpit to the bra line just below the breast, along the bra line to the middle of the breastbone, up the breastbone to the collarbone, along the collarbone, and back to the middle of the armpit. The upper outer *quadrant* (quarter) of the breast is the most common site for breast cancers, but cancer can occur anywhere in the breast area.

Palpation (with pads of the fingers) If a woman applies cornstarch, powder, oil, or lotion to the breast, it is easier for the fingers to glide over the breast and feel any changes. That is why so many women discover lumps when they are soaping their breasts in the shower. If she loses a slippery feel during the examination, she can relubricate the breasts.

After she lies down, the woman places the flat areas of three or four fingers (not the thumb) from the last joint to the end of the finger on the tissue to be examined.

She uses the hand opposite the breast to be examined, and lays the fingers flat and parallel to the chest wall. She moves the pads of her fingers in small, dime-sized circles over all the breast tissue, and does not lift them from the breast between palpations. The pads of the fingers are more sensitive than the fingertips, and using more than two fingers stabilizes the tissue so that a lump cannot skitter away from probing fingers.

Pressures At each spot, the woman makes circles using three different pressures. The light-pressure circle just moves the skin without jostling the breast tissue underneath. The medium-pressure circle presses midway into the tissue, while the deep-pressure circle probes deeply and firmly into the breast, down to the ribs or to the point just short of discomfort. Changes can appear at any depth, and this thoroughness gives a woman the best chance of finding anything that is there.

Pattern of search There are three common patterns of search. Most women find that they become more familiar with their breasts if they use the same pattern each month, but any one of the three, used carefully and consistently, can be effective.

The MammaCare pattern, now recommended by many American Cancer Society BSE trainers, searches the breast in parallel vertical lines. Lying on her side, the woman moves her fingers in their small circles and different pressures along an

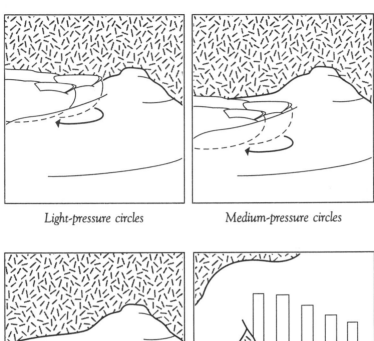

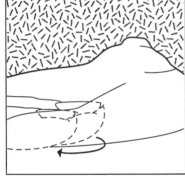

Light-pressure circles

Medium-pressure circles

Deep-pressure circles

Vertical pattern

imaginary line from the middle of the armpit down to the bra line. At the end of that strip, the fingers move inward one finger breadth and start up from the bra line to the collarbone. The fingers repeat vertical strips up and down until the fingers reach the nipple. They are held in place over the nipple as the woman rolls to her back, and then continue their parallel strips until they reach the breastbone.

A second pattern involves examining the breasts along imaginary concentric circles. The fingers begin their journey at the top of the breast, far from the nipple, and then move a

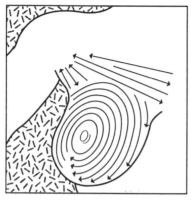

Concentric rings

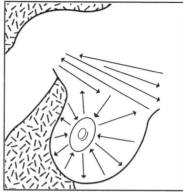

"Clock" pattern

fingerbreadth clockwise or counterclockwise to continue. When that entire circle has been examined, the fingers move inward a fingerbreadth to begin the next, slightly smaller ring, and so on until the nipple is reached. It is very important to feel carefully under the nipple, in the armpit, and along the collarbone for any lumps or changes.

The third pattern divides the breast into twelve sections like a clock, and draws imaginary lines from the nipple to each of the "numerals." The fingers move along each imaginary line making their dime-sized circles: from "12" to the nipple, back from the nipple to "1," over to "2," and down the line to the nipple again. Again, it is crucial to check under the nipple, in the armpit, and along the collarbone.

Whichever pattern she uses, a woman also checks for any nipple discharges. Most doctors are more concerned about spontaneous discharges—the stain on the bra—than with those that are "milked" from the breast, but many recommend that women try to "express" a drop or two of fluid from each breast. Some women normally can, and others cannot.

A good way to do this is to perform BSE small circles around the edge of the areola so that any fluid in the collecting reservoirs is massaged into the nipple area. Then the fingers, positioned on both sides of the nipple, press into the areola and come almost together under the nipple. The fingers are moved around

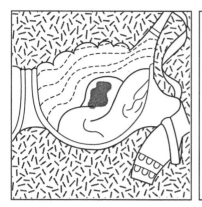

Nipple discharge around bra

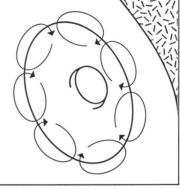

BSE around areola

the nipple a quarter circle and press again from that direction.

Many discharges come from benign hormonal changes. Doctors tend to worry more about cancer when discharges come from only one breast and contain blood (are pink, red, or black). Like any other breast change, any discharge should be investigated.

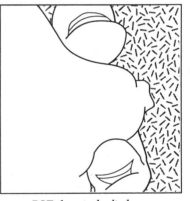

BSE for nipple discharge

Practice with feedback The woman with very easy-to-examine breasts may have her skills checked once by a health professional and then feel quite confident performing BSE. On the other hand, the woman who normally has very lumpy breasts usually finds it takes her much longer to become reasonably familiar with her breasts and comfortable with her skills. Her doctor probably will have similar difficulty: some breasts are just much harder to examine than others.

The good news is that many breasts become much easier to examine after menopause, as the tissue becomes less glandular.

Plan of action BSE is not just an exercise for eyes and fingers, of course. Unless there is also concentrating and questioning going on, it is a waste of time. A woman looks and feels for anything that has changed since last month, and for any obvious differences between right and left sides. She feels for the normal soft fatty tissue, ridgy "corrugated" fibrous tissue, and lumpy normal glandular tissue (rather like partially cooked rice). She checks for any dominant, three-dimensional lump or new thickening and looks for any kind of visible change. Many women normally have a thickened natural "underwire" under both breasts and perhaps some thickening at the upper outer portion of each breast.

What if she finds something? First she checks the same area of the opposite breast to see if there is something similar and presumably normal there. If she discovers something new in one breast, she reports it to a health professional. *Right away*. In most cases, it will be a benign change. In the case of cancer, this prompt action could save her life.

Knowing ahead of time what she will do if she ever discovers a breast change is part of a woman's breast health plan of action. The other part is setting up with her health professional a reasonable schedule for the rest of her breast care. How often she should have mammograms and routine professional breast examinations depends on her age and individual risk factors.

Having a plan gives a woman some sense of control over her breast health. And, this plan of action can truly make a difference.

PROFESSIONAL BREAST EXAMINATION

When it comes to detecting breast changes, a woman contributes her intimate knowledge of her own breasts. What the health professional offers, in contrast, is experience with a wide variety of breasts.

The gynecologist, internist, family doctor, or a nurse practitioner usually carries out the professional exam along with a regular physical. A sensible plan for the woman under 40 with no special risk factors or breast complaints is to have her breasts examined at least every three years, then at least annually after age 40. A breast or general surgeon is an option for the woman with special needs such as frequent benign lumps.

A professional breast examination need not be lengthy, but must contain at least the following elements: a breast history of risk factors and past problems, taken during the first visit; questioning about any current breast concerns; visual inspection under good light, with the woman standing or sitting with arms both down and raised; careful palpation of all the breast tissue, including in the armpits, beneath the nipples, and along the collarbones, while a woman lies down with arms behind her head.

Some health professionals use additional positions or spend time teaching the woman. A few try to extract nipple discharge with a suction device, either to look at or to send to the cytology lab for an experimental "Pap smear"-type analysis.

The examination must be carried out with respect for the woman's dignity and modesty. If the exam does not meet the minimum standards of thoroughness and concern for the patient, the woman needs to speak up and/or change doctors. I had a surgeon once whose idea of an adequate annual breast exam was placing the palms of the hands flat against the breast for ten seconds. I did not agree, told the surgeon so—and took my business elsewhere.

DIAGNOSING BREAST CHANGES

If a breast change is detected, what then?

In the case of a lump that can be palpated but feels as if it could be fluid-filled, a needle can be inserted into the lump and any fluid withdrawn into the syringe—fine needle aspiration. This makes a cyst collapse, and sometimes gets rid of breast pain. A needle biopsy with a wider tru-cut needle may be able to get enough tissue to make a diagnosis (See Chapter 4).

A persistent, dominant lump that can be felt needs to be either removed or followed carefully. This includes the lump that does not collapse after an aspiration and the needle-biopsied lump in which the pathologist cannot find cancer cells. A positive-for-cancer result is considered trustworthy, but with such a small tissue specimen, a negative result needs to be followed up.

For the breast change that can be detected only by mammography, the radiologist and the surgeon can collaborate on a wire localization biopsy or a stereotactic guided needle biopsy.

Nipple discharges can be checked for cancer cells; if they are present or if the doctor is otherwise concerned, an open biopsy can be done of the area under the nipple.

After any diagnostic procedure, the biopsied tissue is sent to the pathologist for examination and diagnosis.

IF BREAST CANCER IS DIAGNOSED

If the pathologist finds very abnormal cells that have not broken through into neighboring tissue—that are confined within a duct, for instance—the diagnosis is carcinoma in situ. But if the highly abnormal cells have invaded neighboring tissue, there is a possibility that they have strayed into the lymph nodes or even beyond.

Thus, with any diagnosis of invasive cancer, both the woman and the tumor go through a thorough workup. For the woman, it is the beginning of the staging process, in which her doctor discovers how extensive the cancer is. To stage the cancer using the TNM information, the doctor needs to know the size of the tumor (T), whether any lymph nodes have cancer in them (N), and whether there is any known metastasis to a distant organ (M) (See Chapter 4, Staging a Cancer).

If the lump has all been removed, the size of the tumor is known. The doctor may be able to feel lymph nodes in the axilla or along the collar bone that are either hard and swollen or "fixed" (attached) to the skin. If not, the lymph node information must wait until the pathologist has some axillary lymph nodes to examine under the microscope.

Occasionally, there is an obvious clue that the cancer has metastasized to one of its common target organs: bones, lungs, liver, or brain. Even if there are no symptoms, like bone pain or shortness of breath, for example, many cancer doctors routinely

Types of Invasive Breast Cancer

Invasive Ductal Carcinoma, NOS: The most common kind of invasive breast cancer (70% of all breast cancer cases). "NOS," or "not otherwise specified," simply means the tumor has no unusual cellular characteristics and does not fall into one of the categories below. Usually appears as hard breast lump.

Medullary Carcinoma: An invasive ductal carcinoma (7% of all breast cancers). It appears to be confined (encapsulated), and often has many small white blood cells. May grow large, but has a better-than-average prognosis.

Comedocarcinoma: An invasive ductal carcinoma (5% of all breast cancers), which fills the ducts with tumor plugs before invading the duct wall. Prognosis is better than average.

Mucinous Carcinoma: An invasive ductal carcinoma (3% of all breast cancers), which contains mucus-producing cells which make the tumor look glistening. Very good prognosis.

Tubular Carcinoma: An invasive ductal carcinoma (2% of all breast cancers), which contains characteristic tubular structures ringed with a single layer of cells. Better than average prognosis.

Invasive Lobular Carcinoma: Arises at the ends of the ducts or in the lobules. Otherwise looks and acts like invasive ductal carcinoma, NOS. Better than average prognosis.

Invasive Paget's Disease: Rare cancer in ducts beneath nipple, originally appears as itching, eczema-like rash around nipple. Prognosis dependent on the individual case.

Inflammatory Carcinoma: Most serious breast cancer (1–4% of all breast cancers) with skin over breast appearing acutely inflamed and swollen because skin lymph vessels are blocked by cancer. Least favorable prognosis.

Prognostic Tests for a Breast Cancer Tumor

Aside from the visual examination of the breast cancer tumor which the pathologist does to see how large the tumor is, what the cells look like, what the blood supply to the tumor is, and so on, the tumor is often subjected to several tests, including:

Estrogen and/or progesterone receptor measurement tells whether and to what degree the cancer cells have "receptors" to the female hormones estrogen and/or progesterone on the outside of the cell. Each hormone "status" is measured as a number, and scores above a certain point are considered "positive." Positive receptor status for one or both hormones correlates with a better prognosis, and a better response to hormonal therapy.

Flow cytometry analyzes the DNA content of the tumor. Tumors which have the normal amount of DNA (diploid) tend to be less aggressive and have a better prognosis than those with abnormal amounts of DNA (aneuploid).

Cell cycle analysis measures the percentage of cancer cells in the "S-phase" of the normal cell cycle, which is when the cell is preparing to divide. The more cells in this phase, the faster the tumor is dividing, so the prognosis is less good.

Abnormal tumor protein analysis looks for tumor proteins, including the enzyme cathepsin-D (low levels associated with better prognosis).

Oncogene levels, growth factors, etc. measure such factors as HER-2/neu oncogene, with high levels of "expression" associated with faster tumor growth and poorer prognosis.

Each day brings word of new prognostic tests to detect and/or measure a factor which could be related to prognosis, so that doctors will know how aggressively to treat an individual woman's breast cancer.

order baseline tests: a chest X-ray to rule out lung metastasis, a bone scan to check the bones, and perhaps a computerized to-mography study of the liver. Many women also undergo base-line blood tests for such tumor markers as CA15-3 or CEA.

Meanwhile, if the whole tumor has been removed, the pathologist classifies the cancer according to what the cells look like, and also examines both individual cells and the whole tumor to get as much information as possible about how the tumor is likely to behave. The tumor may be sent to an outside laboratory for many additional tests (see Table on page 204). All this information from the woman and the tumor is used in making treatment decisions.

CARCINOMA IN SITU: THE IN-BETWEEN DIAGNOSIS

When a pathologist looks at a breast biopsy slide and sees a place where highly abnormal cells have broken through the duct wall, the diagnosis is obvious: invasive cancer. However, if the abnormal cells are still all in one place, confined inside the duct with no evidence of a breakthrough, the pathologist calls it carcinoma in situ (at the site or "in situ"). Other names are noninvasive or noninfiltrating carcinoma or intraductal carcinoma.

"Carcinoma" means cancer, of course, but the condition got its name years ago before pathologists saw it very often. Now some doctors disagree whether this is simply a very early cancer that just has not shown its hand yet or the last stage of benign breast changes. Or, since there is a range in how abnor-mal the carcinoma in situ cells are in different women, could there even be two or more different processes going on?

In any case, by itself, carcinoma in situ does not threaten a woman's life; by definition, it has not left its own neighbor-hood. However, the condition does markedly increase the chances that a woman will later develop either more in situ disease or invasive cancer; statistically, the risk is about 1% per year. The presence of carcinoma in situ says that a significant cell quality control problem exists. As with invasive cancer, how to treat carcinoma in situ is controversial.

Duct carcinoma in situ

With the use of screening mammograms, doctors diagnose duct carcinoma in situ (DCIS) much more often now than they used to. While DCIS may be discovered during a breast biopsy for a lump, frequently the only abnormality is a suspicious cluster of microcalcifications on a mammogram. Like a breast lump, these microcalcifications must be biopsied, and can mean anything from the most benign of changes to invasive breast cancer.

How large the area of DCIS is almost always correlates with how much risk there is of invasive cancer. DCIS typically occurs in only one breast, but it may be multicentric, occurring in more than one area of the breast. If one lesion shows up clearly on mammography, however, the others should also.

Surgeons at one time always treated DCIS with a mastectomy. Now, however, some women with small areas of DCIS who really want to keep the breast may have another option: the area, with a clear margin of normal tissue around it, is removed with a lumpectomy. No lymph nodes are removed, since DCIS, by definition, involves cells that have not left their own neighborhood. The women then undergo close monitoring through BSE, yearly or twice-yearly mammograms, and check-ups every three months or so.

To be eligible for this treatment plan, a woman must have:

♦ an area of DCIS less than 25 millimeters (one inch) in its largest diameter, without any evidence of invasive cancer; pathologists have discovered that areas this small are almost never associated with invasive cancer

♦ an area of DCIS that shows up clearly on mammography; the woman's breasts must be otherwise easy to image on mammography and palpate so that any new problem can be detected promptly

- ◆ no other major risk factors for breast cancer; ordinarily this means no significant family history of the disease

- ◆ full information about the treatment plan and its risks and benefits; she must accept the commitment to long-term follow-up and must be psychologically comfortable with a degree of uncertainty (although at any time she can change her mind and have a mastectomy)

Pathologist Michael Lagios, M.D., of California Pacific Medical Center, San Francisco, helped develop this DCIS treatment protocol several years ago, and has continued working to find any subgroups of patients with DCIS who need more aggressive treatment. He has discovered that when the DCIS cells have a high nuclear grade—are very abnormal, with unusual numbers of chromosomes or other specific changes—they are more likely to recur or to be associated with invasive cancer. Thus, when he finds these changes, he may recommend more aggressive treatment.

A clinical trial is now testing the effectiveness of radiation therapy after a lumpectomy for DCIS. Many doctors, however, do not believe that DCIS cells are as vulnerable to radiation as are the cells of invasive cancer. They also want to keep radiation as an "ace up the sleeve" in case a separate invasive cancer develops later in that breast, since the amount of radiation a woman can receive to an area is limited.

Women who do not meet the criteria for minimal treatment—or who realize that they would constantly feel anxious with it—may be better served with a mastectomy. The woman with a DCIS diagnosis who is interested in breast-conserving therapy can check with a medical center that offers it. Pathology slides and other medical records can be mailed for a second opinion.

Lobular carcinoma in situ

Like DCIS, **lobular carcinoma in situ (LCIS** or **lobular neoplasia)** often occurs at the ends of the breast ducts. While it does not itself invade neighboring tissues or spread beyond the breast, LCIS puts a woman at increased risk for developing invasive breast cancer later on. It is often diagnosed in pre-menopausal women.

There the similarity to DCIS ends. LCIS frequently does *not* show up on mammograms (or as a lump) and is often discovered when the pathologist looks at slides after a breast biopsy for something else. Typically, the condition occurs in both breasts. If it is not in both breasts yet, both breasts are at equal risk for developing new areas of the neoplasia. However, the size and number of areas of LCIS do not appear to affect the woman's prognosis in any way: widespread LCIS in both breasts is no more likely to be associated with invasive cancer than a tiny area.

Traditionally, the treatment for LCIS has been a double mastectomy. The other conventional option has been removal of one breast and a biopsy of the "mirror image" location on the second breast to see if by any chance there was more neoplasia there.

But over thirty years ago, a group of doctors at New York's Columbia University noticed that, of the women who for some reason did not have any breast surgery beyond the biopsy, very few ever developed invasive cancer. Since then, they have been treating LCIS with close follow-up only: professional breast examination every three to four months. The woman performs BSE every month and gets her routine mammograms (LCIS does not show up on mammograms, but a lump or other breast problem could). The invasive lobular carcinomas tend to be relatively slow-growing, and the idea is to find any as early as possible.

Paget's disease of the nipple

This rare condition shows itself with an eczema-like rash around the nipple. Until recently, doctors considered the nipple condition a "beachhead" established by an underlying breast cancer. Now many are coming to view it as another in situ change. While it can be invasive, it often is not; it does significantly increase a woman's chance of developing invasive cancer later, however. Breast-conserving treatment includes removing the nipple and an area under it so that there are clear margins.

Kerry McGinn

Chapter 13

❖

Treating Invasive Breast Cancer

"You have breast cancer. You have three options. You can do nothing—but that is not a good option, or . . . . "

Later, I suggested to my surgeon that a cup of tea might have helped. Or at least a brief pause after the words "breast cancer." But in no way could I quarrel with his immediate emphasis on *options*. The woman diagnosed with breast cancer must choose (and fairly soon) between mastectomy and lumpectomy, with or without radiation. If she opts for mastectomy, she decides whether or not to undergo reconstructive surgery at the same time and, if so, what kind. And that's just for starters.

But "fairly soon" does not mean that the choices have to be made the day or even the week of diagnosis—and they should *not* be made then. Many women, on hearing they have breast cancer, feel an urgent need to take action, to "do something." But this is one time when it is much better to think about it for a few days.

Some women may immediately react with "get rid of it— take off my breast tomorrow." For others, it's "You can do anything else, but you can't take my breast." Whatever that first desperate urge, it makes sense for a woman to resist it, to take the time to find out about all the options, and to think about what each would mean in her life. She may eventually choose to follow her original impulse, but then it will be a real decision with which she can live comfortably and confidently. Waiting two weeks or so after diagnosis before further surgery makes no difference in a woman's prognosis.

Many women rely on their surgeons to offer some guidance, perhaps a strong recommendation one way or the other—and that is as it should be. As oncologic surgeon Peter Richards, M.D., of California Pacific Medical Center in San Francisco, puts it: "I tell a woman about all her options, but if I believe strongly that she should follow one of them, it would be remiss of me not to tell her what I think and why. She's paying for my experience and knowledge. She has to make the final decision, but my recommendations serve as a reference point for her and are part of the data she should have."

However, if both mastectomy and lumpectomy are possible options, it makes sense to also consult a radiation oncologist before making a decision. Surgeons, by their experience and training, may be more likely to recommend mastectomies, radiation oncologists to speak up for lumpectomy with radiation. It is worth hearing what each of them has to say.

LOCAL TREATMENTS: MASTECTOMY OR LUMPECTOMY/RADIATION

As with any cancer, treating invasive breast cancer may involve either or both local treatment (getting rid of any cancer cells in the breast itself), and systemic treatment (destroying any cancer cells that have strayed outside the breast). The local therapies for breast cancer are surgery and radiation. The systemic possibilities are chemotherapy and hormone therapy; biological therapy shows promise but few results as of yet.

During the last several years, doctors have learned that either one of two possible strategies can work equally well to get rid of cancer cells in the breast itself. One strategy involves removing the whole breast (**mastectomy**). The second conserves the breast, cutting out only the obvious area of cancer with a wide margin of clear tissue around it (**lumpectomy**) and then giving several weeks of radiation treatments to the breast to destroy any residual cancer cells.

Mastectomy

Until quite recently, the standard treatment for breast cancer was the **Halsted radical mastectomy**. This surgery, named after the surgeon who developed it in the late nineteenth century, removes the breast itself, the lymph nodes in the armpit, the chest wall muscles, and other lymph nodes. The theory was that breast cancer started in the breast, moved out to all the lymph nodes, and only after conquering the last lymph node did it spread out to the rest of the body. Surgeons followed the dictum, "The more you take, the better off she will be," and tried ever more extensive surgeries. Eventually, even the Halsted radical looked almost conservative. The Halsted procedure left a woman with a long scar down one side of her chest, a "caved-in" appearance, and often lingering disability from the missing muscle.

In time, doctors learned that this kind of mutilating surgery did not make women survive any longer and began pushing for less drastic operations. If there is a mastectomy now for invasive cancer, it is almost always a **modified radical mastectomy**, which removes an island of skin over the breast (including the nipple and areola), all the actual breast tissue, and some or all of the lymph nodes from the axillary area. The chest muscle is left alone. If reconstructive surgery is not done at this time, the area where the breast used to be is flat, but not caved-in; some surgeons leave some extra skin for possible reconstructive surgery later. The scar typically runs horizontally or diagonally from near the breast bone into the armpit.

A prophylactic (preventive) mastectomy or a mastectomy for a small carcinoma in situ removes the same tissues except the lymph nodes and is called a **simple** or a **total mastectomy**. Sometimes, for a prophylactic mastectomy, the surgeon leaves the nipple and areola intact, but cancer can grow there later. Occasionally, if a large invasive cancer has also spread to the chest wall muscle, the surgeon will remove part of that along with the breast and lymph tissue in a **radical mastectomy**.

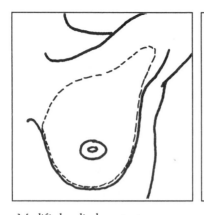

Modified radical mastectomy, area
of breast tissue to be removed

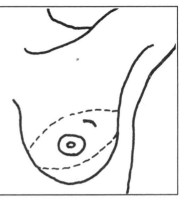

Skin incisions (modified radical)

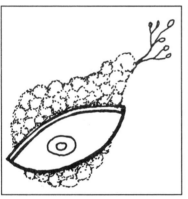

Breast and axillary tissue removed
(modified radical)

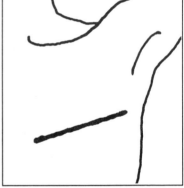

Mastectomy scar (modified radical)
(this series of illustrations—on pages 212
and 213—courtesy of Susan Schoen)

Lumpectomy

A lumpectomy spares most of the breast and cuts out only a
piece of tissue around the cancer. Ordinarily, when a biopsy,
which removes minimal tissue, is followed by a cancer diagnosis, the surgeon wants to cut out a somewhat wider swath of
breast tissue (**wide excision**).

Depending somewhat on how much tissue is removed (but
mostly on the surgeon labeling it), this can also be called a
tylectomy, **segmental resection**, **quandrantectomy**, or **partial**

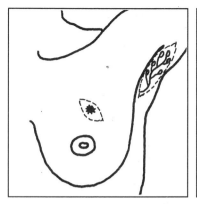

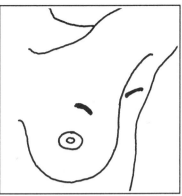

Lumpectomy, breast and lymph node tissue to be removed

Lumpectomy/axillary surgery scars

mastectomy; there are no precise definitions for what's what. Usually the rest of the breast tissue moves over to fill in the empty spot, and the surgery leaves a minimal scar.

Doctors discovered that when they performed a lumpectomy and then simply sent a woman on her way, the cancer recurred in the breast in about 40% of patients, so several weeks of daily breast radiation treatments were added to the regimen. With lumpectomy/radiation, the local recurrence rate is about 10%; with mastectomy, it is about 8%, but the recurrences may be harder to treat.

Many invasive cancers have large areas of duct carcinoma in situ around them. For a time, some surgeons thought they could remove just the cancer itself with a small margin of surrounding tissue and that the radiation would eliminate the rest of the abnormal cells. But cancer showed up again at the same location in over a quarter of these women. The theory is that radiation, which neatly dispatches stray cancer cells and tiny clusters, does not deal adequately with large clumps of abnormal cells. What this means for surgeons is that they must be careful to remove any DCIS around the cancer so that the margins are truly "clean."

If the lumpectomy is performed because of invasive cancer, the surgeon usually also removes some or all of the lymph nodes in the axilla. This involves a separate incision, two to three inches long just below the hollow of the armpit, so that the surgeon has good access to the axilla.

The Axillary Surgery

Most of the immediate discomfort and/or long-term side effects of either a modified radical or a lumpectomy come from this lymph node surgery. The surgeon cannot reach this area without injuring and occasionally severing one or more of the nerves that perceive sensation. Because of the stretching and pulling the surgeon had to do, almost everyone has numbness in the armpit and along the back of the upper arm for at least several weeks; if the numbness remains after several months, it is probably permanent (and feels peculiar for a woman shaving under her arm).

Of more medical concern is the possibility that removing lymph nodes from the arm may affect the drainage of lymph fluid from that arm, so that the arm swells with lymphedema (see Chapter 22). Once in a great while, the axillary surgery permanently damages a nerve that regulates movement.

If removing the lymph nodes causes these problems, why do surgeons do it? A common path for breast cancer cells leaving the breast takes them through the axillary lymph channels where they can get trapped in the lymph nodes. These axillary lymph nodes are more common escape routes than the lymph channels along the breastbone or the collarbone, and are much easier to reach surgically.

Until quite recently, most surgeons reasoned that since the lymph nodes could have cancer cells trapped in them, removing them would help cure the cancer—so they removed all the lymph nodes under the arm near the cancer: a **lymph node dissection.** But, in fact, removing all the lymph nodes proved to have no effect on curing the cancer, and the side effects of the full dissection were much greater than when a smaller number were cut out. Not only was the lymph drainage system from the arm seriously injured in most cases, but the woman also lost lymph nodes (most of them cancer-free) that were an important part of her body's defense system.

However, with the coming of systemic therapies for breast cancer, the surgeons and oncologists began making treatment decisions based partly on information that currently comes only from lymph nodes. Are cancer cells present in the lymph nodes (node-positive) or not (node-negative)? How many lymph nodes are positive? Is a node positive because of a small number of cancer cells that can only be found with a microscope (**micrometastasis**), or is it obviously overrun with cancer cells? Have cancer cells made any lymph nodes stick together or become "fixed" to other tissues? Examining the lymph nodes helps stage the breast cancer and gives the doctors clues about the woman's prognosis as well as about what treatment to give her.

Many surgeons now compromise with **lymph node sampling**, removing only a few of the lymph nodes. The lymph nodes occur at three clumpy levels in the axilla. The surgeon who takes out node-containing tissue from the lower two levels nearest the breast minimizes damage, but still gets the necessary information. Later the pathologist discovers exactly how many lymph nodes have been removed (often about ten, out of a normal total of thirty to sixty).

Some surgeons still prefer to remove all the axillary lymph nodes. On the other hand, a few doctors believe most women do not need any nodes cut out. They reason that now that more women are getting chemotherapy or hormone treatment regardless of node status, removing nodes should not be necessary.

Dr. I. Craig Henderson, chief of the Oncology Center at the University of California, San Francisco, says that there are some groups of women for whom lymph node sampling is worthless, such as the 75-year-old women who will get hormone therapy no matter what their nodes show. But he stresses that for many women, information from the nodal sampling remains crucial. Most surgeons and oncologists believe that if there is a reasonable chance the node information will make a difference in treatment, lymph node sampling is worth it.

By no means is there one treatment for all women, or even all premenopausal women, regardless of their nodal status. The information about the tumor itself from the pathologist and from laboratory tests such as cell-cycle analysis is becoming

Staging System for Cancer of the Breast

Stage	TNM	Description
0	Tis N0 M0	Carcinoma in situ (Tis) with no positive axillary lymph nodes (N0) or known distant metastasis (M0)
I	T1 N0 M0	Earliest invasive cancer, with tumor smaller than 2 cm, or $\frac{3}{4}$ inches (T1) and no positive axillary nodes or known distant metastasis
IIA	T1 N1 M0	Either a tumor smaller than 2 cm with one or more positive axillary lymph nodes (N1) and no known distant metastasis
	T2 N1 M0	or a tumor 2–5 cm, or $\frac{3}{4}$–2 inches (T2), with neither positive nodes nor known distant metastasis
IIB	T2 N1 M0	Either a tumor 2–5 cm with positive axillary node(s) but no known distant metastasis
	T3 N0 M0	or a tumor larger than 5 cm or 2 inches (T3), with no positive axillary nodes or known distant metastasis
IIIA	T1-2 N2 M0	Either a tumor 5 cm or under with fixed (stuck to other tissues) axillary lymph nodes on the same side (N2) but no known distant metastasis
	T3 N1-2 M0	or a tumor larger than 5 cm. with free or fixed axillary lymph nodes but no known distant metastasis
IIIB	T(any) N3 M0	Either any size tumor with *chest* lymph node involvement (N3) but no known distant metastasis
	T4 N(any) M0	or a tumor that involves the chest wall or breaks through the skin (T4) with any number of positive axillary lymph node(s) but no known distant metastasis; this includes inflammatory carcinoma
IV	T(any) N(any) M1	Known distant metastasis (usually bone, lung, liver, brain) or to the skin or chest wall beyond the breast area

more helpful all the time, but does not yet substitute for staging how extensive the cancer is.

DECIDING ON LOCAL TREATMENT

The National Cancer Institute says in its 1990 Consensus Conference statement: "Breast conservation treatment is an appropriate method of primary therapy for the majority of women with Stage I and Stage II breast cancer and is preferable because it provides survival equivalent to total mastectomy and axillary dissection while preserving the breast." Basically, lumpectomy/radiation is worth considering for most women with Stage I or II disease—but it is not necessarily the best treatment for *every* woman. On the other hand, neither mastectomy nor lumpectomy/radiation makes sense for the woman with either Stage IIIB or Stage IV breast cancer, since her problem is not the local disease. To handle the spread beyond the breast that is causing her problems, she needs systemic therapy (see table on page 216 for descriptions of the different stages).

QUESTIONS TO ASK YOUR PHYSICIAN

Aside from any medical factors, a woman and her doctor may want to consider aesthetic, practical, and/or psychological issues:

1. How large is the tumor in comparison with the breast and where is it located? A surgeon can usually remove a one-inch tumor with a margin of surrounding tissue from a medium-sized breast and the result will look fine. However, it may be impossible to perform a lumpectomy with a large tumor in a small breast and have any kind of aesthetically pleasing results (although reconstructive surgery may be possible). When the tumor is located near the nipple, the surgeon may have to remove not only the nipple and areola but a large area around it.

2. Is there any evidence that the cancer in the breast is multicentric (has clusters of cancer cells at more than one place in the breast)?

3. Is there any problem with getting radiation therapy? Can you get to treatments reasonably easily and/or is there any problem spending the time each weekday for several weeks? Have you ever had radiation to this area before? (If this is a recurrence in a breast already treated with lumpectomy/radiation, you no longer have this option.) Do you have any medical condition, such as a connective tissue disease, that would make radiation inadvisable? Some women initially feel uncomfortable about the thought of radiation—but how do you feel about the therapy once you know more about it?

4. How easy are your breasts to "follow" over time? Not everyone agrees that this should be a factor, but the woman with breasts that are unusually difficult to examine mammographically or with the fingers may want to consider this. Do you have risk factors that might make you especially vulnerable to a second primary cancer in the breast? If you keep your breast, you want a reasonable chance that it will remain trouble-free or that any problem will be detected early.

5. How committed are you to keeping the breast—and why? How do you feel about yourself in general, and about your breasts in particular? If you undergo mastectomy, you will lose the nipple/areola sensation of that breast—how important is that to you? If you feel strongly that you want to have a breast mound of some sort, would you be comfortable with either a breast prosthesis or the risks/benefits of reconstructive surgery? Does it matter to you that after a lumpectomy, you can change your mind later and have a mastectomy, but that the reverse is not possible?

Researchers have compared several aspects of how a woman's choice of mastectomy or lumpectomy affects her later, but the results are anything but clear-cut. One study "proves" that women with mastectomies have much poorer body image a year after surgery than women with lumpectomies, while another finds little difference. One study shows "definitively" that women with mastectomies feel safer and less anxious than those with lumpectomies, but the next study refutes it.

Before deciding on a course of action, many women consult a second surgeon, a medical oncologist, and/or a "second opinion" service, such as one at a breast health center, to get varying points of view.

Whatever she chooses, it is normal for a woman to wonder occasionally if she made the right choice. But most women, most of the time—if they make a careful, thoughtful decision based on what they have heard from their doctors *and* on what they personally think and feel—will be reasonably happy with whatever they choose.

BREAST CANCER SURGERY

In some ways, breast cancer surgery is like the other cancer surgeries discussed in Chapter 7, but it has its own peculiarities.

The woman is almost always put to sleep with general anesthesia for any procedure that includes removal of axillary nodes. When she wakes up, she usually has a protective bulky bandage covering the surgical sutures or tape strips holding the outer layers of skin together. She may have an IV or heparin lock for a day or so for antibiotics. Commonly after a mastectomy and sometimes with lumpectomy/axillary surgery, she has one or more drainage tubes, each connected to a suction bulb. She does not usually have any other tubes unless she has had major breast reconstruction surgery done at the same time.

Many women undergoing either a mastectomy or a lumpectomy will be pleasantly surprised by how little pain there is in the breast area. They may be less happy with the strange sensations in the armpit area and along the back of the arm.

Some surgeons put a sling on the arm to hold it in place, but most want a woman to start using her arm fairly soon so that it does not stiffen up. As she starts moving the arm and stretching it over the next several weeks, the discomfort will become worse at first, but then will gradually subside.

Some of the sensations in the armpit may be less painful than strange: numbness, "pins and needles," or pinching/pulling feelings. Many women continue to have peculiar discomforts in the axilla once in a while for the rest of their lives. Occasionally a woman complains of sharp pains in the breast area or may report a "phantom limb" sensation where a breast has been removed.

A woman may feel more comfortable lying on her back or on the opposite side for several weeks after a mastectomy. This puts gravity to work, draining any fluid away from the area.

Depending on her surgeon, the surgery, and her response, the woman may go home the day of surgery, the next day, or several days later. The final pathology report should be ready within a few days.

If a woman has both breasts removed at the same time (bilateral mastectomy), she needs to have hospital bedside equipment placed where she can reach it easily. Until she is able to raise her arms, she will not be able to wear clothes that have to be pulled over her head; pieces that can be pulled on from below and have loose sleeves and generous armholes (a zippered housecoat perhaps) work best at first.

Many women have read results of a research study indicating that breast cancer recurred less often in premenopausal women when breast surgery was performed near the middle of a woman's menstrual cycle, possibly because of hormonal factors. Many surgeons would like to see more studies done to prove or disprove this, but at this point would not recommend postponing surgery very long for this reason.

BREAST CANCER RADIATION THERAPY

When radiation therapy is given after a lumpectomy for invasive breast cancer, it is considered the primary local treatment for the disease. It can also be used as secondary—but important—therapy along with mastectomy in certain situations. For example, when the tumor is located at the edge of the breast tissue, the surgeon may want radiation to that area as extra "insurance" (see Chapter 7 for general information about radiation).

The linear accelerator is the usual radiation machine. There should be no discomfort during the actual process. Probably the most difficult part for the woman is raising her arm, which can be uncomfortable if radiation starts soon after surgery.

If a woman is to undergo chemotherapy, breast radiation may be postponed until she finishes, or it may be given midway through; occasionally the two are given together. Otherwise, radiation begins a few weeks after a lumpectomy, when the surgical site is relatively healed.

Typically the first part of the treatment plan includes six weeks or so of radiation to the whole breast area, from collarbone to bra line and from breastbone to axilla. A total of about 4,700 rads is delivered in divided doses.

This period of radiation to the whole breast may be followed by a booster dose concentrated on the immediate area of the tumor. This is usually given as a daily "electron beam" dose for a week or so. It may be delivered by the same linear accelerator, but with the high energy field adjusted downward so the rays are not moving so fast. The radiation area is smaller and there may be more skin damage because the electron beam releases its energy at a shallow level closer to the skin. Otherwise, for the woman, it is about the same as the earlier treatments. If the tumor was deep or quite large, the booster dose sometimes involves the placement, for 30 hours or so, of tiny radioactive seeds into minute tubes threaded through the skin into the tumor area (see Chapter 7, Internal Radiation).

Radiation to the breast area after a lumpectomy for cancer is considered (ironically) quite "benign"—it does not usually cause serious side effects. Almost everyone feels some fatigue and eventually has temporary skin redness at the radiation site. The breast often is temporarily swollen and sensitive, and usually becomes permanently firmer and less droopy than it was before treatment. If there is much radiation to the axillary lymph nodes, the woman may be more vulnerable to lymphedema.

Some women develop a few lung symptoms like a mild cough during radiation; a few show radiation pneumonitis or lung inflammation, with a dry cough and slight fever, three to six months after radiation. Rib fractures can occur, but usually heal by themselves. Several months after radiation is finished, many women develop assorted arthritis-like aching or shooting pains in the breast

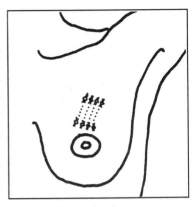

Internal radiation
(courtesy of Susan Schoen)

area, the chest wall, or the connection points between rib and breastbone. The worst part of these symptoms is that they may terrify a woman into believing her cancer has come back. What they often mean is that the body is slowly (and rather clumsily) regenerating after the treatment. A call to her doctor usually brings reassurance.

When radiation is used along with a mastectomy, the treatment field may be smaller, the number of treatments fewer, and ordinarily no booster is necessary.

SYSTEMIC TREATMENT

Many oncologists believe that cancer cells begin escaping from the breast fairly early in the course of disease, but that the body's defenses can usually demolish the occasional cell and keep the cancer in check. Systemic treatment for breast cancer—either chemotherapy or hormonal therapy—is recommended when the oncologist either knows or suspects that the body "system" outside the breast harbors more cancer cells than it can destroy without outside help.

Breast cancer is often a slow-growing and unpredictable disease, and short-term studies do not give long-term results.

This is why the statistical picture can be so muddy. Five-year survival—although it is an excellent sign—is not synonymous with cure. Thus, statistics do not talk about cures but look at or combine such factors as five-year survival, ten-year survival, death rates, and/or disease-free interval. It is the best they can do.

HORMONAL THERAPY

Since the female hormones seem to play such a major role in breast cancer, one plausible strategy for fighting the disease is to shift the body's hormonal balance in such a way as to discourage cancer growth. The first attempts to do this included removing the ovaries of some young women with fast-growing breast cancers so that the estrogen from the ovaries would no longer be available to "feed" the cancer cells; this had disappointing results.

Results with the drug tamoxifen (Nolvadex) have been much more promising. Like other hormonal manipulations, tamoxifen does not kill cancer cells directly, but instead prevents them from growing: it is a siege weapon rather than a gun or bomb. Initially, researchers thought that the drug worked as an estrogen "blocker," simply starving the cancer cells that needed estrogen to grow. Now it appears the mechanism is not so straightforward.

Tamoxifen may act as an "attenuated" (weakened) estrogen, which fools the cancer cells into accepting the "imposter," or it may act in some way researchers have not yet discovered. For instance, it sometimes appears to work on cancers that are classified as estrogen receptor-negative. (One theory is that some of the cells may have mutated to be positive.)

However, taking two tamoxifen pills every day appears to give at least postmenopausal women with breast cancer a decided survival edge. In this age group, it is statistically more effective at extending life than chemotherapy, although an individual woman may do better on chemotherapy. Postmenopausal women taking tamoxifen added an average of two years to their lives—which means that many of them added far more than two years, and some may have been cured.

Tamoxifen appears to decrease markedly both local recurrences and second unrelated cancers in the remaining breast tissue. It may also have mildly protective effects on bones and the circulatory system. There is a moderately increased risk of cancer of the endometrial lining of the uterus and possibly of the liver, but this is quite rare.

For women well past menopause, there are no known common serious side effects. Most women in this age group seem to tolerate the pills so well that even if a woman is not at especially high risk, doctors feel quite comfortable prescribing the drug. The original recommendation of two years of treatment keeps stretching to five years or even for life.

However, some premenopausal women and women not far past menopause whose hormonal balances may still fluctuate, do not tolerate the drug so easily. They may complain of hot flashes, night sweats, and similar menopausal symptoms for which hormone replacement therapy is not usually an option. Nausea, bloating, and breast tenderness and swelling for a few weeks is common, although this subsides. Some women report depression for some months—often difficult to distinguish from the emotional upheaval many women go through as they finish primary breast cancer treatment. Tamoxifen can cause birth defects if a woman becomes pregnant while taking it; it does not bar fertility.

If it does indeed increase cures and/or disease-free survival time, many women will gladly put up with these side effects. For premenopausal women, that is the unanswered question. Many thoughtful oncologists have no doubts it works, but others, including Dr. I. Craig Henderson, are still waiting for convincing scientific evidence that tamoxifen increases survival in premenopausal women. One of their concerns is that younger women, taking the drug over a longer period of time, may be more at risk for serious side effects as yet unknown.

Doctors are trying other kinds of hormonal manipulation and medications, often in women with metastatic breast cancer. One drug they would like to try is the "abortion pill" RU-486, a progesterone blocker which, if it can be studied, may someday offer hope as a new weapon against breast cancer. But as of late 1992, it is a hostage in the abortion battles.

CHEMOTHERAPY

Weighing the pros and cons of chemotherapy can be even more difficult. It is a less "benign" therapy than hormonal therapy, with more obvious side effects and toxicities; it is not something that an oncologist, in good conscience, prescribes to everyone. On the other hand, adjuvant chemotherapy (given when there is no known distant metastasis) adds an average of about three to five years to the premenopausal woman's life; that means some cures and some much-extended lives.

The woman well past menopause usually does better with tamoxifen or other hormonal therapy and does not receive chemotherapy; some oncologists contend that the reason for the relatively dismal showing for "chemo" in this age group is that doctors give gentler and much less potentially effective doses of the drugs.

For the premenopausal women with *any* positive lymph nodes, no matter how minimally positive, most oncologists will recommend a course of chemotherapy. There may be no circulating cancer cells, but few oncologists are willing to take that chance.

It is much harder for both the oncologist and the woman to decide on treatment when the woman is either premenopausal with negative nodes or in her fifties and not far past menopause (when her cancer may have premenopausal "roots"). In these cases especially, the oncologist must consider the type of tumor, its stage, and any other prognostic factors such as hormone receptor status, to make an informed recommendation, based on the statistical likelihood that there are cancer cells that need to be killed and that chemotherapy is the weapon of choice.

Many premenopausal women with node-negative tumors, especially those in certain subgroups of women, face relatively high risk that their cancer will come back: those whose cancers have a high expression of HER-2/neu oncogene, for instance, or other signs of a more aggressive tumor. It is also conceivable that a pathologist missed seeing a tiny micrometastasis. The National Cancer Institute currently advises oncologists to consider a course of chemo for any premenopausal woman with breast cancer, regardless of her lymph node status. But it is up to a woman and her oncologist to decide together.

The most common chemotherapy regimens for Stage I or II breast cancer combine three drugs: cyclophosphamide (Cytoxan), 5-fluorouracil (5-FU), and either methotrexate or doxorubicin (Adriamycin). A woman is usually on either CMF or CAF (or FAC), named after the initials of the drugs she is taking. Adriamycin is somewhat stronger and has more serious side effects than methotrexate, so it is given when the oncologist wants a more aggressive drug. But as chemo drugs and dosages go, these breast cancer chemo regimens are considered relatively tame (see Chapter 8 for general information about chemotherapy).

"Tame," however, does not mean ineffective or fun.

Ordinarily, these drugs can be given in the doctor's office so the woman does not need to be hospitalized. Cyclophosphamide can be injected into a vein or taken as pills. The other drugs are given into the vein, either "pushed" slowly with a syringe or dripped from an IV bag.

A typical course might be eight repetitions of a 3-week cycle, with intravenous injections of all three medications on day 1 and nothing else for the next 20 days. When the Cytoxan is taken as pills, a 28-day cycle is common, with injections of both methotrexate and 5-FU on days 1 and 8 in the oncologist's office. The Cytoxan pills are taken at home every day from day 1 through day 14, and then no medications are taken as the body recovers from day 15 to day 28.

The courses of adjuvant chemotherapy are getting shorter now, and usually last from four to six months (although one year is not uncommon). Chemo usually starts within a month after surgery and often before any radiation, since this seems to be a particular "window of opportunity" for destroying cancer cells. An alternative strategy, especially with a somewhat larger or more aggressive tumor, is to begin treatment with several months of chemotherapy, then perform the surgery, and finish off with more chemo: a kind of treatment "sandwich."

The common temporary side effects of the drugs are fatigue, digestive tract complaints, and hair loss (usually complete loss with Adriamycin, hair thinning with CMF). Loss of menstruation and/or menopausal symptoms often occur in premenopausal women; these changes are more likely to be permanent if the woman is over 40.

Weight gain (much more often than weight loss) happens so often with breast cancer chemo that it may be a side effect of the drug. Although it is not inevitable, it is common for a woman to gain twenty pounds or more, and the weight may take a long time to lose.

No one is quite sure why weight gain occurs. It may be that these particular chemo regimens bring about some changes in the woman's metabolism that make it easier to gain weight, harder to lose it. Possible contributing factors might be menopausal changes, frequent snacking to keep ahead of queasiness, or lack of exercise. Also, some women are taking the steroid pill prednisone as part of their chemotherapy, and that causes weight gain.

Besides general chemo side effects, there are some special cautions with the breast chemo drugs. If a woman is taking Adriamycin, her oncologist may order special heart function tests. Ordinarily, however, heart damage occurs only when the cumulative dosage of the drug exceeds a certain amount, and oncologists are careful to keep below that amount. In fact, the possibility of heart damage is the "dose-limiting" factor for Adriamycin. Many women taking Adriamycin complain of nightmares and other temporary psychological changes.

The woman taking Cytoxan will be cautioned to drink about three quarts of fluids on the days she receives the drug. The end products of Cytoxan are notoriously rough on the bladder as they pass through and can cause a severe bleeding irritation called hemorrhagic cystitis. While the woman may feel "water-logged," drinking all those fluids dilutes the Cytoxan and washes it out of the body before it can cause problems.

Treating Stage III or IV Breast Cancer

Stage IIIA breast cancer, which has no known distant metastasis but either a large tumor and positive axillary nodes or a smaller tumor and "fixed" axillary nodes, is treated with a whole smorgasbord of therapies. Typically, chemotherapy shrinks the tumor before a mastectomy is done; radiation is often part of the package.

Chemotherapy becomes the primary rather than the adjuvant treatment when inflammatory breast cancer is involved, or the chest lymph nodes, chest wall, or skin over the breast has a tumor in it, or when there is known distant metastasis (Stages IIIB or IV). Surgery and/or radiation to the breast area are not usually used. Many different drugs and combinations are being tried, sometimes in very high doses in conjunction with an **autologous bone marrow transplant** (see Chapter 14)—and sometimes with quite good results. Taxol, manufactured from the bark of a particular species of yew tree, and its chemical "cousins" have been much in the news, but there are *many* promising agents being tested. Other strategies use only one chemo agent, given either in weekly low doses or as a continuous slow drip into the vein through a small pump which the woman carries or is implanted under the skin.

Clinical trials in the community or at a comprehensive cancer center can be a major resource for this woman. Early clinical trials of biological therapies have started. One study, for instance, is testing the use of laboratory-grown clones of the body's own antibodies. If these trials prove successful, they may herald new treatment options for every stage of breast cancer.

Kerry McGinn

Chapter 14

❖

Beyond Basic Treatment for Breast Cancer

Most women have all sorts of other questions about living with breast cancer. How do I get my arm moving again after surgery? What about an external breast prosthesis or reconstructive surgery? What kind of follow-up care do I need, and what can I do for myself? What if the cancer comes back, or I have metastatic cancer? How does a bone marrow transplant work? This chapter discusses these questions and more.

REGAINING ARM MOBILITY AFTER BREAST SURGERY

After either a mastectomy or a lumpectomy with lymph node surgery, it is hard at first to move the arm on that side freely. It hurts along the upper arm when the woman tries to reach above shoulder height. If the doctor told her to restrict arm movement for a couple of weeks to protect the new surgery (a controversial precaution), she may have a stiff shoulder. The worst scenario occurs when, to avoid pain, she avoids raising the arm for several weeks and the shoulder joint becomes "frozen."

But while avoiding movement actually leads to more pain, carefully stretching those muscles and keeping the shoulder joint mobile slowly gets rid of the discomfort. Ordinarily, a woman can regain a comfortable and full "range of motion" and reasonable strength 6–8 weeks after surgery—or at least be well on her way. She begins exercising her arm and shoulder, sensibly and gradually, as soon as her surgeon gives the go-ahead, and then increases her range a little every day.

The doctor may give her a set of exercises; in some hospitals a physical therapist will routinely see patients after breast cancer surgery. A Reach to Recovery volunteer can be requested through the local ACS unit to visit her, demonstrate exercises, and leave her literature and a ball to start squeezing in her hand before she is ready for more vigorous exercise.

One standard exercise involves standing a few inches in front of a wall, bending the elbows, and placing the palms of both hands on the wall at about shoulder height. Then, moving the arms from the shoulder, the woman "walks" her hands up the wall as far as they will go, and then back down. The idea is to have the arm protest a bit, but not "scream." The woman does this several times a day, a little higher each day. (Light pencil marks on a washable wall let her appreciate her accomplishment.)

In pendulum exercises, the woman bends at the waist and swings her arm slowly from the shoulder: front to back, side to side, and/or in increasing circles in front of her. Scratching her back as high as she can reach toward the opposite shoulder blade helps the shoulder regain another kind of mobility.

Heat, such as in a shower, can make it easier to stretch; some women find an ice pack before or afterwards also helpful. A bag of frozen peas covered with a piece of cloth makes a good reusable, moldable ice pack.

Should the shoulder show any signs that it is "frozen" with adhesions because it has not been used, prompt physical therapy is essential. Freeing a shoulder is not a do-it-yourself project.

BODY IMAGE AFTER MASTECTOMY

Many women are bothered sometimes by how they see themselves after a mastectomy. For some, body image after mastectomy is persistently, overpoweringly negative. They look in the mirror and see someone ugly, "less a woman," undesirable. The focus narrows to a tiny piece of themselves; they become "the scar." Concentrating on the scar sometimes means that they have found a way to ignore the more painful reality of a cancer diagnosis.

Certainly, every woman with a mastectomy needs time to mourn the lost breast. Many begin to accept the changes by touching the scar, massaging it, making it physically part of themselves. Some dream about the lost breast; some find dance or other movement helps make them "whole" again.

The major strategy for positive self-image is broadening the focus. A woman is infinitely more than her breasts. Now is the time to look at all the rest of herself. Broadening the focus also means looking outside herself, at the world, to see what she can contribute. (If a narrow scar a few inches long looks pretty small when compared to a whole woman, it looks even smaller when compared to a whole world.) When distress is severe, counseling may be helpful.

Many women—even those with supremely healthy body images—want to minimize the physical results of a mastectomy, either by wearing an external breast form or undergoing reconstructive surgery. It is an individual preference.

When my friend Betsy had both breasts removed, for instance, she was quite happy (as was her husband) to "go bare": "My breasts weren't big to begin with. The mastectomy scars look quite nice, I'm not lopsided at all since both breasts are gone, and I just feel 'freer' this way. I don't have to worry about breast prostheses and don't have to undergo more surgery. This is just right for me."

THE BREAST PROSTHESIS

Some women feel quite happy "going bare," but many women feel lopsided and unattractive and want something to take the place of the missing breast. An external prosthesis (breast form), properly fitted, not only can make the woman's clothes fit better, but can also balance the weight of a remaining breast so that she does not get backaches.

That is what Sheila wanted—and got. "I could not face the thought of more surgery, but I had visions of some scenario like a breast form falling out of my swimsuit. With the new technology, though, I have a prosthesis that feels like a normal breast, is the same weight as my natural breast, and stays in place on my chest with special strips. It's a comfortable, easy solution for me."

For at least the first two or three months, until the surgical area is completely healed, a woman needs something lighter than a "real" weighted prosthesis. Her Reach to Recovery volunteer will bring her a temporary breast form, a simple fabric casing into which the woman can put the appropriate amount of Dacron "fluff." At first, before the woman can wear a bra, this can be pinned under her nightgown. After a few weeks, when the woman can wear a bra, a comfortable alternative against the skin is a fluff of lambswool, purchased at a drugstore or more cheaply from a dancers' supply company. A light foam rubber "sleep breast" is another option then, or it can be the permanent choice for the woman who does not need to balance a heavy breast.

The permanent prosthesis matches the remaining breast closely in both shape and weight and can look very natural under clothing. It can be an expensive investment, although if the doctor writes a prescription it is often covered by health insurance, at least in part.

But the fact that a prosthesis is relatively expensive has lured many entrepreneurs into the market, and that means that a woman can choose from many different models. Some of the newer breast forms stick securely to the breast with velcro strips and some kind of adhesive. Others are made of tiny beads so that the breast "moves" like a real breast. Often, a simpler, less expensive prosthesis may fit a woman's needs quite nicely.

Most local American Cancer Society units have a display board of different breast forms and/or a list of local merchants who provide expert and sensitive fitting. Prostheses can also be ordered by mail, although the woman loses the advantage of a personal fitting.

A woman may be able to wear most of her clothes "as is"

over her regular bra and prosthesis. Some bras and swimsuits are made with a special pocket for the breast form that does not adhere directly to the skin. Otherwise, clothing can be easily altered. Many women look for or make pretty nightwear, perhaps with Greek draping on one side, for instance, in which they feel attractive without a prosthesis.

If a bra rides up—either because one side is lighter than the other or the woman has a double mastectomy—it can be anchored with a "V" of elastic sewn to the bottom of the bra and attached (with a stitched-on garter, perhaps?) to panties or a girdle.

BREAST RECONSTRUCTION

For other women, an external prosthesis is not enough. Either before a mastectomy or at any time afterwards, these women turn to the reconstructive (plastic) surgeon for help. They want to look "normal" and "like myself" again. They find the absence of a breast or a major indentation in the breast after a lumpectomy a constant and unwelcome reminder of the cancer when they want to move on with life. Or they feel "less a woman" without breast curves, and flinch at changing at a gym or having a sexual partner see them without clothes.

Perhaps they find an external prosthesis an intrusive nuisance or uncomfortable. Or they suffer from backaches or other problems from not having a breast on one side. Virtually every woman—no matter how old she is, how long ago she had breast surgery, and how much the chest area was damaged—is a candidate for some kind of breast reconstruction if she wants it.

Anne thought that people might laugh at her for wanting breast reconstruction at age 65, "But the people I cared about thought it was a great idea. They knew it was important to me, my gift to myself. Before this, I wore a good prosthesis, but it never felt like 'me.'

"I didn't expect or want to be a beauty queen after reconstruction, so my expectations were pretty reasonable. I really like the way I look and feel now. Sure, it's not quite the same as my other breast, but I'm mighty happy with it—in clothes and even out of them."

On the other hand, many women do not want reconstructive surgery. They may be quite content without it, or even be strongly opposed on feminist grounds, and see no need for it. They may not want any more surgery, or may be concerned about possible risks. It is strictly an individual choice.

What does reconstruction offer? The first step is to create a breast mound, using one of several possible techniques. The challenge is making a breast that looks like a breast, with some droop and a normal "crease" underneath. If the woman simply wants something that looks normal under clothes, a mound may be enough for her, but many women want a nipple and areola as well. Finally, making the reconstructed breast reasonably symmetrical with the other breast may mean surgery to make the remaining breast smaller or less droopy.

How does the surgeon make a breast mound? Occasionally, if the woman has enough skin remaining after the breast is removed, the surgeon may be able to slip a breast-shaped implant filled with silicone gel or saline (salt water) into a pocket in or under the chest muscle. While it is easier initially to put an implant above the muscle, it is more prone to slippage, rupture, and other complications there. If the woman can flex her breast—an unusual talent indeed—the implant has been placed in the chest muscle. An implant can be inserted during the mastectomy surgery or in a separate surgery later. This is a relatively simple procedure.

The body normally forms a fibrous scar capsule around any implant. However, in some cases, the body is too enthusiastic about "walling off" this "intruder" and, in time, the new breast comes to feel rock-hard. This is the most common complication of implant surgery; whether or not it occurs depends on the woman's body and the type of implant product. Other risks, as with any surgery, include infection and bleeding into the site.

Many people are questioning the long-term safety of silicone implants, especially if there is a rupture or a slow silicone "bleed." Others believe that they are generally safe for women in most cases, but that safety studies need to continue. Currently, the woman who wants a silicone implant for reconstructive surgery can still get one.

When a woman does not have enough skin remaining after a mastectomy to fit over a standard implant, she may have tissue expansion. The idea behind a tissue expander is that the body will recruit more skin over a gradually expanding implant—rather like what happens to the skin of the abdomen during pregnancy.

When first inserted in a pocket in the chest muscle, the silicone tissue expander looks like a small collapsed balloon, connected to a port that rests under the skin. Over the course of several weeks, the expander is filled (two or more ounces at a time) with saline injected by syringe through the skin and into the port. Each injection, spaced every week or so, stretches the skin a little as the new breast gets bigger. (Rather like being 13 years old again, but the process is certainly faster!)

This tissue expander is often a temporary measure to prepare the chest pocket for a final silicone gel or saline implant, inserted during a second surgery. Some, however, are made so that the expander stays in place permanently while the port is removed. There are many kinds of expanders, including "double-lumen" ones with an inner empty chamber for saline, and an outer chamber filled with a small amount of silicone gel to give the breast a more natural shape.

After the expander has reached the desired size, the surgeon typically continues inflating it until it is about one-third overfilled and leaves it that way for several weeks. The theory is that this helps the breast develop a natural droop when the permanent implant is inserted or the permanent expander is deflated to its final size.

Many women complain of minor discomfort and a "tight skin" sensation for a few hours after each injection. The major complaints come during the overinflation period, when the breast can be quite uncomfortable and may look rather like a large baseball perched on the chest. The same surgical complications can occur as for the regular silicone gel implants.

How do these assorted implants compare with a "natural" breast? It very much depends not only on the surgeon's skill but

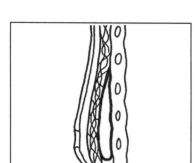

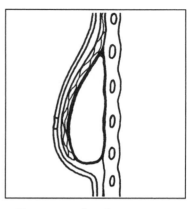

Tissue expander before expansion

Tissue expander after expansion

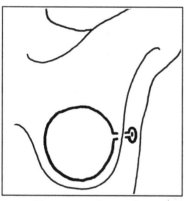

Tissue expander in place
(courtesy of Susan Schoen)

also on how a woman's individual body responds. The implanted breast rarely matches the other breast perfectly; it is typically firmer and has less of a droop—"perkier" or "more youthful" is how the surgeon might put it—but many look and feel quite natural, both in and out of clothes. It is important to know, however, that while the "real" breast may change with aging or weight gain or loss, the implanted breast stays the same. Also, current implants are not made to last a lifetime and may need replacement eventually.

There are various **muscle flap** reconstructive procedures that use a woman's own tissue, moving skin, muscle, and sometimes fat to create a new breast mound. These are lengthier surgeries that require an expert surgeon. They involve considerably more surgical pain than the implant procedures and entail relatively long periods of recuperation.

The **TRAM flap** (transverse rectus abdominus myocutaneous flap technique) is sometimes nicknamed "tummy tuck" surgery because it uses abdominal tissue to make the new breast. To be eligible for the surgery, the woman needs an ample supply of abdominal skin and fat; the surgery not only gives her a new breast (or breasts) but also flattens her abdomen somewhat.

During the operation, the surgeon prepares an island of skin and fat atop a large vertical abdominal muscle. The muscle is cut at one end while the other end remains attached to its original site and blood supply. The whole "flap" is then tunneled under the skin to the mastectomy site where the surgeon shapes it into a breast mound and stitches it in place. The abdominal wound is closed.

The surgery takes several hours. For the first few days, the woman usually requires considerable pain medication for the abdominal pain where the muscle was cut. (No matter how much they have heard, few women are prepared for just how much it hurts initially.) Also, it may be hard for her to stand up straight at first. There is a large scar on the abdomen as well as any breast scars. With such major surgery involving the abdomen and the blood supply, possible problems include infection or a flap that dies because it does not get an adequate blood supply. The woman often wears an abdominal binder for the first weeks and may never recover her full "sit-ups" capacity.

A good TRAM flap, however, looks very natural. It is soft, droops nicely, and often matches the other breast closely. The day after surgery, a woman wonders why in the world she ever sought such torture, but a few weeks later, she usually loves the results. The tissue is her own, only one surgery is needed for the breast mound, and she does not have to worry about possible complications with an implant.

Muscle flaps can come from other parts of the body besides the abdomen. The **LATS flap** (latissimus dorsi flap technique) for instance, rotates the fan-shaped latissimus muscle from the mid-back along with an attached island of tissue, tunnels it under the armpit skin and shapes it into a breast mound. The island of skin from the back fits over the mound. Since the latissimus muscle does not have fat over it, however, a silicone implant is usually necessary too. There is a back scar and per-

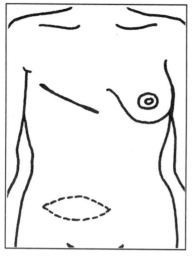

TRAM flap areas of surgery

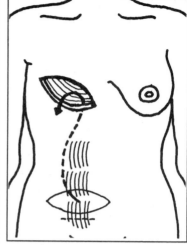

TRAM flap procedure

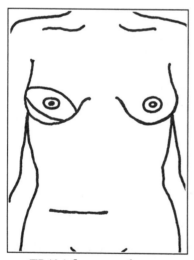

TRAM flap areas of surgery
(courtesy of Susan Schoen)

haps some decreased muscle power for some activities.

Although they require a surgeon specially trained in microsurgical procedures, the **microsurgical free flap procedures** are becoming more popular. The surgeon cuts completely free the tissue from abdomen, back, or buttocks, shapes it into a breast mound, and uses microsurgical techniques to attach the blood vessels to blood vessels on the chest wall. Because the free flap does not carry its own blood supply with it, there is an increased risk that it will not "take."

However the breast mound is made, the surgeon has a choice of techniques for making the nipple and areola later, when the breast shape has settled. The nipple can be constructed from the nipple of the other breast (one nipple makes two); sometimes it comes from a small flap of breast skin twisted on itself or from the ear lobe or somewhere else in the body. The areola can come from a doughnut of skin removed from elsewhere, often from the thigh, and/or from medical tattooing of minute dots with a dye to match the areola. Since the new nipple and areola have no nerve supply, they do not have any sensation.

There are two bodies of opinion about whether reconstruction should be done at the time of mastectomy, if possible. One point of view holds that it is safe to do it at the same time and that it saves the woman both an extra surgery and some unnecessary mourning for her lost breast. The other point of view is that, if there is a chance the woman will undergo chemotherapy, she could be at more risk for infection because of the reconstructive surgery, and that she will appreciate her new breast more if she waits.

In any case, in order to be happy with the results, a woman needs accurate information and reasonable expectations beforehand. Besides listening to the reconstructive surgeon, who is typically sincerely enthusiastic, she might want to talk to a woman or two who has undergone the same surgery. There is plenty of information readily available, both pro and con, such as Nancy Bruning's book, *Breast Implants: Everything You Need to Know* (see Resources).

FOLLOW-UP AFTER BREAST CANCER

Even if a woman is presumed cancer-free after treatment, she usually sees at least one doctor every three months or so for about two years. Then unless there is a sign of more cancer, the schedule often stretches out, perhaps to every six months for a few years, and then to every year. A regular touching-base is part of the program for life.

During her visits, the woman tells her doctor about any concerns she has. In both asking questions and doing the physical examination, the doctor pays special attention to:

— the area where the cancer occurred, including the incision site, remaining breast tissue, nearby lymph nodes, and chest wall

— the other breast (if intact)

— the organs that are especially vulnerable to breast cancer metastasis (bones, lungs, liver, and brain).

At least once a year, it is sensible for the woman to have a gynecological exam because she is at some increased risk for ovarian cancer.

How often blood work, X-rays, and other imaging studies are ordered depends on the woman, her cancer, and the doctor's individual philosophy. Blood tests might include a complete blood count, a chemistry panel and, perhaps, CA 15-3 and/or CEA tumor marker assays. In the blood count and chemistry panel, the doctor looks for any red flag values that might mean something is wrong with the bone marrow, bones, or liver. An abnormal value does not necessarily mean cancer, and may drift back into normal range as inexplicably as it left.

Mammograms of the breast with a lumpectomy and the intact breast may be scheduled every six months or every year. Many doctors order periodic chest X-rays, bone scans, and sometimes liver and/or lung CT scans. Obviously, if the woman has a specific complaint, appropriate tests need to follow it up.

Monthly breast self-examination is even more important after breast cancer than before. The procedure for examining the breasts does not change after a lumpectomy/radiation, although the radiated breast is likely to feel firmer than the other one. A palpable lump in the incision area is often scar tissue, but since this is also the prime site for a cancer recurrence, the doctor needs to evaluate *any* change.

LOCAL RECURRENCE OR METASTASIS

Breast cancer can be cured—but it is not always. Sometimes it comes back, or sometimes it is not discovered until it has spread to a distant organ.

A local recurrence means that some cancer cells in the breast were not destroyed the first time around by surgery and/or radiation. These cells seem to have stayed within the breast area, but they continue dividing until they become large enough to detect.

Recurrence is staged, as the original tumor was, by the size of the tumor, the presence or absence of positive lymph nodes, and any known distant metastasis. The oncologist often recommends systemic chemotherapy or hormonal therapy based on staging and prognostic tests as if this were the first time around. However, local treatment this time may be different because one or more of the local therapy options has already been exhausted. For example, if the initial treatment was lumpectomy/radiation, and the new local recurrence is invasive cancer, a mastectomy is the usual treatment, since radiation cannot be used in the same place again. Alternatively, if the recurrence is duct carcinoma in situ, with the cells confined within the duct and no radiation needed, a second lumpectomy can be done.

It is uncommon for cancer cells to be left in the local area after all the breast tissue has been removed in a mastectomy, but it can happen. Then there may not be any place for the cells to grow except on the chest wall or the skin, and it can be much harder to get rid of them in those places than in breast tissue. A cancer growing into the skin or the chest wall is classified as Stage IIIB. The treatment plan may include chemotherapy, radiation, and possibly surgery. Since there is no one commonly accepted protocol for treatment in this situation, the woman may want to check with a comprehensive cancer center to see what is offered.

What about distant metastasis? Whether the cancer was originally diagnosed as metastatic or its spread was discovered later, it obviously is not good news, but it is not hopeless. For one thing, wherever the cancer spreads it is still *breast* cancer; breast cancer that metastasizes to the lung is not nearly as lethal as most primary lung cancers.

The most common distant organ for breast cancer to target is bone. Bone is not an organ necessary for life, so metastasis of bone does not kill women, and the symptoms can often be relieved with radiation and/or chemotherapy.

While regular-dose chemotherapy is not considered curative with metastatic breast cancer, it can sometimes achieve long periods of control or even complete remission (where no trace of the disease can be found). Higher-dose chemotherapy may be given with support from blood transfusions or medication to stimulate the white blood cells. Autologous bone marrow transplant offers very high-dose chemotherapy with a real possibility of cure. Clinical trials are trying not only new chemotherapy agents and methods of hormonal manipulation, but also ways to jump-start the body's defenses with biologic therapy. Since women with metastatic disease statistically have less to lose, they may be eligible for studies with bigger curative payoffs.

And some women, using all sorts of methods, just thrive on beating the odds, defying the statistics. As the Wellness Community, a nationwide support network of cancer patients, would say: even if a woman has only a 1% chance of survival, she has a 100% chance of that 1%.

At some point, however, the woman with metastatic breast disease may have to decide how hard she wants to push, to fight—and the only correct answer is what *she* wants to do. She needs to know that, should pain become a problem for her, there are almost always good solutions for it, if her health professionals pursue them aggressively. Cancer pain management is evolving so quickly and creatively that it is hard for doctors to keep up with it. Even when cure is not possible, comfort always should be. The Johns Hopkins Oncology Center and the Cancer Information Service run a Cancer Pain Hotline: (800) 422-6237.

AUTOLOGOUS BONE MARROW TRANSPLANT

Since chemotherapy drugs do not have perfect aim, they destroy not only the cancer cells but also other rapidly-dividing cells in the body. Standard doses of chemotherapy drugs kill cancer cells in reasonable numbers while allowing the normal cells to bounce back readily. Achieving the maximum cancer cell kill while avoiding irreversible damage to the rest of the body is what chemotherapy is all about.

As chemotherapy dosages rise, the body system that gives out long before any other is the bone marrow, where blood cells are made. The red cells and platelets can be replaced somewhat with blood transfusions, but what cannot be replaced from the outside are the white cells that protect the body from infection. If oncologists did not have to worry about the bone marrow, they could give massive (and theoretically curative) dosages of chemotherapy drugs to women whose cancers have not been cured with lesser doses.

An **autologous bone marrow transplant (ABMT)** lets oncologists do exactly this. They keep the woman's bone marrow in reserve for a "rescue" when it is needed; then they can administer huge doses of chemotherapy that kill the bone marrow, knowing that they have more. It is a grueling, expensive, somewhat dangerous procedure, without great statistical success in breast cancer. But some women with known metastatic disease, or at very high risk for it because of many positive lymph nodes and/or a very aggressive tumor, see it as their only real chance of survival.

The first step involves several cycles of conventional doses of chemotherapy to see if the cancer is sensitive to the drugs. This is the time to assess whether any lesser treatments might work, such as relatively high-dose conventional chemotherapy followed by blood transfusions to replace platelets and red blood cells, and injections of a special medication called **granulocyte colony-stimulating factor (G-CSF)** to rebuild the white blood cells.

If ABMT is chosen, the rescue agent is either bone marrow or special "stem" blood cells from the woman's own body, harvested and then stored for later use. The procedure is "autologous" because the transplant comes from the woman's own body. This avoids problems of a donor mismatch and possible transplant rejection, which can happen when the transplant comes from another person. Because the bone marrow comes from a woman with cancer, however, it could have some stray cancer cells in it, so any marrow cells are checked carefully.

For a bone marrow harvest, the woman is put to sleep with a general anesthetic. Needles are inserted into large bones, typically the pelvic bones, and one to two pints of the marrow—a fluid—is withdrawn into syringes. Because many needle insertions are necessary, the harvest area can ache for several days. The marrow is then specially prepared so that it can be stored until needed.

Instead of using bone marrow, ABMT often uses **stem cells**, special immature blood cells from the general blood circulation that can work to repopulate the bone marrow. Using stem cells avoids the problem of possible contamination with cancer cells. **Pheresis**, the process of obtaining stem cells, is like a long and complicated blood donation. The blood is drawn off into a special machine that separates out the stem cells and then recycles the rest of the blood back into the woman. The process is repeated many times over two to four hours to get a good supply of stem cells.

As the woman learns about and prepares for the ABMT procedure, the transplant team learns about her, including her psychological readiness for a stressful procedure. If the decision is made to go ahead, the woman enters the hospital, and over the next few days is given huge doses of chemotherapy. Symptoms, such as severe nausea and mouth sores from the chemotherapy, are treated with medications.

Her blood is monitored frequently for the dramatic postchemo drop in white blood cells that indicates that the bone marrow is destroyed and the transplant is needed. At this point, the woman has no body defenses; the strategy is to keep her free from outside infection. She is placed in an isolation room; this may be a "laminar flow" room where special air flow patterns keep contaminants away from her and nurses give most of the care through heavy plastic sheets. She is also given antibiotics to protect her from her own "normal" bacteria, which could be lethal to her now.

Now the stored stem cells or bone marrow are given back to the woman like any other intravenous fluid, probably the easiest and most undramatic part of ABMT. It takes two to three weeks for the new bone marrow to "take" and start producing enough blood cells to protect her.

Until this happens, the woman is extremely vulnerable—and so the anxious waiting starts. She receives constant intravenous blood transfusions, antibiotics, nutrition, and medications to help with the symptoms of high-dose chemotherapy.

Confined to her room, she may feel isolated, bored, scared, miserable because of symptoms, and uncomfortably dependent on healthcare professionals and high technology. She may start thinking of herself as nothing but a profoundly interesting blood count, and wonder why she ever got into this.

But finally, if all goes well, her blood count shows a white cell or two, and then a few more, and then a wonderful surge as her new bone marrow becomes functional. When the white blood cell count rises enough, she can wear a mask and take a few steps outside her room. A few days later she can go home.

Hopefully she is cured and the cancer is gone forever. In fact, too often it reappears. Even if the cancer has not been vanquished, however, its progress may have been markedly slowed so that low doses of "salvage" chemotherapy can keep the disease in check.

Proponents believe that if women were treated earlier with ABMT, before they had such widespread and overwhelming disease, the success rate would be far higher. Treating only "last-ditch" patients, they point out, is scarcely a fair test of ABMT. On the other hand, it is a difficult, very expensive procedure that carries with it a possibility of death from the treatment.

Some oncologists consider ABMT "state-of-the-art" treatment for breast cancer, while others believe it is both unproven for this disease and unnecessary for most women. Many insurance companies balk at paying for what they consider experimental therapy, but some have been forced by the courts to pay for the procedure.

The woman who is interested in ABMT can get information from her doctor, an ABMT center, NCI's Cancer Information Service, and by a literature search. It also helps if she can talk to at least one woman who is a veteran of the procedure.

Kerry McGinn

PART THREE

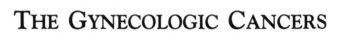

THE GYNECOLOGIC CANCERS

The word **gynecology** comes from the Greek words *gyne* and *gynaikos* which mean "woman," and *logia,* meaning "study." In the strict sense of the word, a "gynecologist" would be one who is deeply involved in the study of women. In reality, gynecology is limited to disorders of the female reproductive system. It would be wonderful if gynecologists actually were steeped in the study of women. Perhaps there would be greater understanding of what problems of the reproductive system actually mean to a woman.

THE NORMAL FEMALE REPRODUCTIVE SYSTEM

The female reproductive system includes the external genitalia—what we used to call "the private parts." The vulva consists of two folds of skin called the labia, which cover the openings of the vagina and urethra (the tube leading from the bladder to the outside of the body) and the clitoris. The vagina is a stretchy canal that extends from the vulva to the cervix, which is the opening between the vagina and the uterus (womb). The Bartholin's Glands in the lining of the vagina produce and secrete a lubricating mucous.

The two fallopian tubes (sometimes called "uterine ducts" or "oviducts") carry ova (eggs) from ovary to uterus. Usually, fertilization takes place in a Fallopian tube. The fertilized ovum, or "zygote," travels on to the uterus and is embedded in the uterine wall (endometrium), resulting in pregnancy. If the ovum is not fertilized, the uterus prepares to shed the endometrium through the menstrual cycle and the process of menstruation. This whole process is directed by hormones, some of which are produced by the ovaries.

Estrogen and **progesterone** are hormones produced by the ovaries. (The word "hormone" is derived from the Greek word *hormao,* which means "I stir up" or "I set in motion.") Estrogen is responsible for the development of sex characteristics in teens: growth of pubic hair, enlargement of breasts, and the beginning of menstruation. The main function of progesterone is to prepare the uterus to receive a fertilized ovum. Progesterone secretion stops if fertilization does not occur and starts

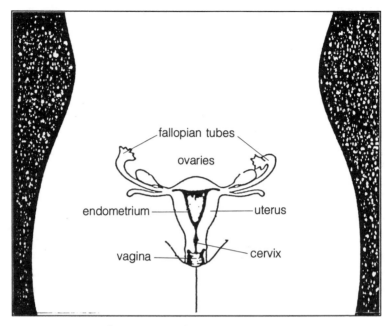

The normal female reproductive system
(*Reprinted from the NCI booklet* What You Need to Know
About Cancer of the Cervix)

again when a new ovum begins developing in the ovary. This is a regular cycle that happens about every 28 days throughout a woman's childbearing years. After menopause, hormone production in the ovaries slows down, but there is still some estrogen production there as well as in other hormone-producing organs such as the adrenal glands.

THE GYNECOLOGIC CANCERS

The gynecologic cancers affect organs of a woman's reproductive system. They account for about 13% of all cancers in women and 6% of all cancers (including men, women and children) diagnosed in the United States. Any of the female reproductive system's organs may be the site of a specific type of cancer. Cancers involving the uterus are the most common,

(32,000 new cases per year, or 6% of all cancers in women) followed by cancers of the ovary (21,000 new cases per year, or about 4% of all cancers in women) and uterine cervix (13,500 new cases per year, or 2% of all cancers in women). Many gynecologic cancers have high cure rates due to new techniques for detecting precancerous problems early, new methods of treatment, and better understanding of the usual patterns of these cancers. As a result, a woman with a gynecologic cancer has a better chance of successful treatment today than ever before.

I am almost forty-three years old. My earliest memories of learning what it meant to be female were the awkward attempts my mother and I made to talk about having periods—menstruation. The awkwardness was not my mother's fault: no one had ever told her anything. She later shared with me that when she got her first period, she thought she was bleeding to death.

I remember being introduced to female and male anatomy through a book with pictures using dogs as the anatomical models. Given my age group, and that of my mother, I know that we were not unique in the hard time we had figuring out how to talk about this subject. How *do* you talk when the parts of your body you need to discuss are called "private" parts? Children learn not to talk or think about these parts of their body, that they should not touch "down there." These are taboos that confuse children *and* adults.

My 65-year-old mother recently had her very first Pap smear. She still has not had her first mammogram. I have problems realizing that as a daughter, regardless of the fact that I can be a reasonably good cancer nurse specialist, I can only do so much to influence my mother. When I talked with her about a Pap smear or a mammogram she said, "My doctor never told me that I needed it." "But Mom," I said, "there are all kinds of ads and articles about Pap smears, mammograms, cervical, uterine, and breast cancers in newspapers and magazines. How could you not think that these messages apply to you?" She offered no answer—and I wanted to scream.

My mother is no different from millions of women—certainly no different from the millions of women in her age group. In general, women (and men too, to be fair) are not very good advocates for their own healthcare rights. Strauss and Howe in their book *Generations* referred to my mother's as the "silent generation." This silent, go-along stereotype is reflected in their attitudes toward health: "Whatever happens is meant to be and I have no control . . . " Physicians and other healthcare providers are perceived as the experts—they have advanced education and should be looked to for advice and guidance. If an action is not advised, then it is not taken. Nor is it brought up by the lesser-educated person. Not only is this level of trust misplaced and misguided, it also puts most of the responsibility on the doctors and nurses. In any modern healthcare system, the responsibility for a person's health has to lie mostly with that person. I cannot force my mother to get a mammogram or a Pap smear, and neither can her doctor. But no good doctor would refuse to allow her a mammogram or Pap if she requested it.

No woman should rely on doctors, or nurses, or anyone else to make decisions about her health and healthcare needs. Each woman has to be her own advocate—or have a friend, spouse, lover, daughter, son, who takes an advocacy role on her behalf if she cannot assume this role for herself. That is the point of this book: to help you, the reader, get an idea of what is possible and necessary; to help you take an active role in ensuring that you or someone you love gets the best care possible when the diagnosis involves cancer. You *can* separate facts from myths. You *can* make decisions. And you can feel you have made the best choice, given the available options.

The real question is, how do we convince our mothers, or our sisters, that early detection measures are worthwhile? What makes some women willingly get a mammogram or a Pap smear, or regularly do breast self-examination? What makes others avoid these self-care measures?

Are they are too busy? Can many women not afford to have medical check-ups? Do insurance policies not pay for screening tests? Do women fear that there may actually be something wrong? And, if there is something wrong, how can she pay, or take the time, to have it treated?

Or is it that women are embarrassed to have their "private parts" examined? Do they want to avoid the cold metal speculum used for gynecologic examinations or sitting in a cold, boring, exam room with nothing on but a silly-looking paper gown, waiting for a busy doctor? The reasons why women fail to get routine check-ups are probably combinations of all these things, with different reasons more important to some women than to others. But this is behavior our generation and the generation of our daughters must begin to change.

Pamela Haylock

Chapter 15

❖

Cancer of the Ovary

"Why did Gilda die?" This is the title of an article in *People Magazine* from June 1991. The article describes the problems American comedienne and actress Gilda Radner had before finding she had ovarian cancer. Her trouble started as "stomach and colon problems." At first, her symptoms were thought to be emotional—she even called herself "the Queen of Neuroses." Then she thought she had Chronic Fatigue Syndrome. After reading about Gilda's death, you might wonder if her life could have been saved by taking a simple blood test for the tumor marker CA-125. Maybe if she had been quizzed about her family history, ovarian cancer might have been considered much sooner. Gilda Radner had symptoms for over a year before she was finally correctly diagnosed.

WHAT IS CANCER OF THE OVARY?

Lifetime statistics indicate that one of every 70 newborn girls will develop ovarian cancer at some time in her life. There were about 21,000 new cases of ovarian cancer in the U.S. in 1992. Cancer of the ovary is responsible for more deaths than any other gynecologic cancer. More than 12,000 women die of this disease each year in the United States alone. The major reason so many women die from cancer of the ovary is that few women have symptoms early in the course of disease. These numbers might be misleading and cause women undue concern.

In reality, ovarian cancer is fairly rare. The gynecologist in a general OB-GYN practice sees, on the average, only one case of ovarian cancer over several years. Many experts believe we will soon be able to offer more effective treatment against ovarian cancer. New discoveries in the biology of cancer cells and information about how this cancer acts promise new approaches to treatment.

The ovary is a complex organ. The two major functions of the ovary are to release germ cells (eggs, ova) regularly and to produce steroid hormones. Each special function of the ovary is performed by certain cell types and each of these types of cells can be transformed into a cancer cell. Because of this complexity, tumors arising from the ovary are complex as well. Still, 80% of ovarian cancers develop from the surface epithelium on the outside of the ovary. These cancers are referred to as **malignant common epithelial cancers of the ovary**.

The International Federation of Gynecology and Obstetrics (FIGO) further divides ovarian epithelial tumors into three categories: **benign tumors, cancers with low malignant potential (LMP),** and **tumors with very clear malignant characteristics.** The low malignant potential tumors are usually found in younger women. They are often found at an early, more curable stage of disease, and make up about 15% of all ovarian epithelial cancers. The average age at diagnosis is about 40 years, as compared to 53 years for the other forms of epithelial ovarian cancers.

Other forms of ovarian cancer include **malignant clear cell tumors** which are found in about 5% of women with ovarian cancer.

NONEPITHELIAL CANCER OF THE OVARY

Nonepithelial cancer of the ovary usually occurs during childhood and teenage years. These cancers are diagnosed and staged in the same way as epithelial cancers. Most of these are called **germ cell** and **stromal** cancers, and account for about 15% of ovarian cancers.

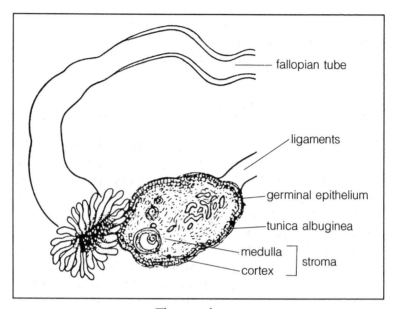

The normal ovary
(courtesy of National Cancer Institute)

Germ cells are involved in the development of the sexual organs of a fetus. Some of these cells stop developing during fetal life—they might be dormant for many years and eventually give rise to both benign and malignant tumors inside the ovary.

Stroma refers to structures that provide support for organs. In the ovary, various kinds of tissues form stroma. Stroma called **granulosa cells** and **Theca cells** surround the site on the ovary where the ovum is released each month. Granulosa cell tumors occur most often in women after menopause. The symptoms include an abdominal or pelvic mass, abdominal pain, and bloating. Most women with stromal tumors also have abnormal uterine bleeding. Treatment for women who still want to have children consists of removing the cancerous ovary and fallopian tube. Other women usually have a total hysterectomy, which includes removing both ovaries and fallopian tubes.

Sertoli and **Leydig cells** resemble cells of the male testes. Tumors involving these cells account for a very small number of ovarian cancers. Most occur in women 20–40 years of age.

These tumors produce hormones that cause a woman to take on male sex traits like facial and chest hair. Treatment consists of removing the ovary and fallopian tube.

THE NATURAL HISTORY OF OVARIAN CANCER

"Natural history" refers to the way a certain form of cancer behaves when it is allowed to go its own way, without any form of treatment. Cancer of the ovary, of course, starts with the ovary. The epithelial cancers, which are the most common, begin on the epithelial surface of an ovary. They commonly spread through direct extension: tumor cells penetrate the tissue surrounding the ovary and invade structures next to the ovary. These structures include the fallopian tubes, uterus, bladder, rectum, lower colon, and the peritoneum (the sac lining inside the abdomen). Peritoneal seeding, tumor cells in the peritoneum, is the most common route of spread. Peritoneal seeding allows cancer cells to lodge on the surfaces of the liver, diaphragm, bladder, and large and small bowel. The resulting irritation inside the peritoneum causes the formation of fluid called **ascites**, which causes the abdomen to swell.

The lymph channels and nodes around the ovaries provide another pathway for the spread of ovarian cancer cells. Lymph nodes most likely to hold cancer cells are those that surround the aorta (the body's major blood vessel that leads away from the heart) and those in the pelvis.

Blood vessels can and do carry cancer cells, but blood circulation is the least common method of spread for ovarian cancer. Cancer cells that are carried in blood vessels are likely to lodge in the liver, lung, pleura of the lung (tissue surrounding the outside of lungs), kidney, bone, adrenal glands, bladder, and spleen.

Death from untreated ovarian cancer is usually the result of large amounts of cancer cells in the abdomen. Cancer cells in the bowel and the tissues that attach abdominal organs to the abdominal wall—**the mesentary**—cause these organs to stop working. The failure of these organs to function causes

Germ Cell (Non-epithelial) Tumors of the Ovary

Type	Description
Dysgerminoma	Endodermal sinus tumor; embryonal carcinoma. Less than 5% of ovarian cancers. Usually occurs at 10–30 years of age. 25% have metastases at diagnosis. Both ovaries may be involved. hCG and AFP tests are usually negative. In early stages of disease, surgery may preserve fertility. Additional treatment may use chemotherapy or radiation therapy.
Endodermal sinus tumor	Second most common. Occurs mostly in teens and young adults. Most common symptom is abdominal pain. hCG test is usually negative, but AFP is often increased. Women who have whole tumor surgically removed have a better prognosis. After surgery, combination chemotherapy is given. Radiation therapy is not effective.
Embryonal carcinoma	4% of germ cell cancers. Occurs mostly in teens. Usually found as a mass in the abdomen or pelvis. Other symptoms include those resembling puberty (in a prepuberty girl), irregular vaginal bleeding, lack of menstrual periods, and abnormal patterns of hair growth. hCG and AFP are positive. Treatment consists of removing the cancerous fallopian tube and ovary and combination chemotherapy. Radiation therapy is not effective.
Choriocarcinoma	Mixed germ cell tumors. Occurs mostly in girls before puberty and young women. Symptoms involve unexpected signs of puberty—pubic and axillary hair, uterine bleeding. Adult women have signs of ectopic pregnancy. hCG can be found in blood and urine. Gestational choriocarcinoma is treated with surgery and combination chemotherapy. Nongestational choriocarcinoma is treated with surgery.

(continued)

(Continued)

Teratoma	Usually occurs before age 20 and often involves only one ovary. Symptoms include pelvic mass, abnormal uterine bleeding. Pain may or may not be noticed. hCG and AFP are both negative. Treatment involves surgery to remove the affected ovary and fallopian tube followed by chemotherapy. Radiation is not usually useful.
Mixed germ cell tumors	Contain at least two germ cell types. Success of treatment depends on the size of the tumor and the cell types it contains. Treatment includes surgery followed by chemotherapy.

more problems, including bowel obstruction, liver failure, and altered fluid balance. Widespread cancer can cause sepsis (infection and bacteria carried in blood), heart failure, and collapse of blood vessels. These combined problems are fatal.

WHO GETS CANCER OF THE OVARY?

The risk factors for ovarian cancer involve age, pregnancy, diet, environment, menopause, and history of another kind of cancer. Ovarian cancer is more common in industrialized Western countries such as Switzerland, the United States, and Scandinavia than anywhere else in the world. In the United States, ovarian cancer is more common among older Caucasian women with a Northern European family history. This trend probably relates to diet and environmental factors, not heredity. Some studies suggest that diets rich in vitamin A and fiber reduce the risk of ovarian cancer, while diets high in saturated fats might increase the chance of developing ovarian cancer.

The risk for nongerm cell ovarian cancer increases as women age. Most ovarian cancer happens to women 55–59 years of age; fewer than 10% occur in women younger than 35.

This increased risk relates to the number of ovulations. Pregnancy before age 25, early menopause, and use of birth control pills all reduce the number and frequency of ovulations in a woman's life and seem to offer some protection against ovarian cancer. Women with more than 40 years ovulating, those who enter menopause later in life, women who have their first pregnancy after age 30, and women over 45 who have never been pregnant are all at higher risk for ovarian cancer.

Genetic factors

Ovarian cancer is known to run in families. This may be because of inherited factors, sharing of a similar environment, or a combination of these things. A woman's chance of developing ovarian cancer is much higher if her mother, sister, or daughter has had it. In some treatment centers, women with a strong family history for ovarian cancer are offered the option of having their ovaries removed—**prophylactic oophorectomy**—when they decide not to have any more children. Some doctors believe that since the ovary is no longer "needed," removal of the ovary *before* cancer develops is a method of preventing cancer. This prophylactic or preventive surgery is not endorsed by all cancer experts. Some studies suggest that this procedure does not prevent the development of cancer and there are also questions about the value and function of ovaries after menopause.

A history of other forms of cancer

A woman who has already had breast or colon cancer has a higher risk of developing ovarian cancer. Cancer of the ovary sometimes occurs at or near the same time as cancers of the breast, colon, and uterus. This suggests that these cancers may all have a common cause. The initial workup for any of these cancers must include testing for the others.

Ovulation induction

A study reported in 1993 seems to connect the use of drugs that stimulate ovulation—the so-called "fertility drugs"— with an increased risk of ovarian cancer. So far, only one study has documented this risk, and the evidence is scanty. Still, the study has been taken so seriously that information about this risk is included in the informed consent for women who take these drugs.

PREVENTIVE MEASURES

We do not know what causes ovarian cancer, so specific preventive measures are impossible to define. While prophylactic oopherectomy is sometimes recommended for women with a strong family history, many find the side effects of removing ovaries and ovarian function—side effects like those of menopause—to be very difficult. In addition, any surgery has risks. A decision to have prophylactic oopherectomy needs to be carefully thought out, with all the pros and cons weighed.

Dietary therapies are often promoted as a preventive measure for cancers. Even though the relationship of diet—vitamins, fiber, and fat—to ovarian cancer is not clear, the benefits of a healthy diet go beyond simply reducing the risk of ovarian cancer.

EARLY DETECTION

Why isn't there a way to screen for ovarian cancer as there is for cervical cancer? So far, there is no simple test to screen women for ovarian cancer. CA-125 is an antibody developed by the body in response to some cancers and it can be detected by testing blood samples. At this time, CA-125 is either not found in early-stage ovarian cancer or the type of testing we have is just not sensitive enough. When CA-125 testing is positive, it does not always indicate ovarian cancer, so the CA-125 is a nonspecific test. After a positive test, additional testing, maybe including surgery, may be needed. Some people, most notably Gilda Radner's husband Gene Wilder, advocate use of the CA-125 as a screening tool. The argument against this position is that mass screening with CA-125 for women without symptoms does not have a valid role in a cancer that affects relatively few women.

For women who have two or more immediate family members with a history of ovarian cancer (mother, sister, daughter), a combined approach using the CA-125 along with transvaginal ultrasound and manual pelvic examinations at regular intervals can be used to detect early ovarian cancer. But even in women who may be at higher risk, the value of screening is not proven. Routine pelvic examinations done with an annual checkup will find one ovarian cancer in 10,000 women examined. The number of ovarian cancers found in this number would increase *if* the women being examined had developed symptoms. A doctor should assess further if a postmenopausal woman's ovary is large enough to be felt during the pelvic examination.

In women *without* a family history, ovarian cancer is likely to be detected at a later, more difficult to control stage. Early signs and symptoms of ovarian tumors are often vague if they exist at all. In over three out of four cases, the cancer has spread outside of the ovary at the time of diagnosis.

Signs and symptoms

The signs and symptoms of ovarian cancer are usually vague and can easily be attributed to other causes. See a doctor or nurse practitioner if you have these problems and they persist over a period of time:

- abdominal swelling or bloating
- discomfort in the lower abdomen
- feeling full after a light meal
- nausea or vomiting
- not feeling hungry
- gas, indigestion
- losing weight without dieting

- a constant need to go to the bathroom

- diarrhea or constipation

- bleeding that is not part of a normal menstrual period

Other symptoms

Ascites causes swelling of the abdomen. Jane noticed that despite *not* gaining weight, she could not zip her jeans: this was the first symptom of her ovarian cancer. Gilda Radner described abdominal swelling, fatigue, and pain in her thighs and legs. If the cancer spreads to the muscle under the lung that controls breathing (the diaphragm), fluid may build up under the lungs, causing shortness of breath.

A women absolutely *must* demand attention when she has persistent, unexplained digestive system symptoms, especially if she is over 35 and has a personal or family history of problems related to ovarian function.

Noncancerous ovarian masses

Most ovarian tumors are benign; only one of five—20%—of all neoplasms of the ovaries are cancers. After a woman notices symptoms, additional tests will determine if the neoplasm is benign or malignant. The diagnosis is made only after complete microscopic examination of the tumor mass by a pathologist. Ovarian neoplasms are either solid or cystic (fluid-filled).

Endometriosis is a condition where endometrial glands and other endometrial structures are found outside their normal place inside the uterus. The ovaries, support ligaments of the uterus, peritoneum, and the bladder are the most common sites for endometriosis. It occurs most often in women 35–45 years of age. Endometriosis can also increase CA-125 levels.

Masses in the fallopian tubes usually result from inflammation or a tubal (ectopic) pregnancy. Actual neoplasms of the fallopian tubes are rare. Other masses in this area can be tissues "left over" from fetal development.

The most common mass found in the abdomen is stool in

the lower colon. Examinations after cleaning out the bowel with enemas will confirm or rule out stool as a cause of symptoms of an abdominal mass.

Inflammatory diseases of the small and large intestine may cause symptoms like those of ovarian cancer, such as diarrhea, nausea and vomiting, lack of appetite, and sometimes passage of blood or mucus from the rectum. Abscesses may form. Pain may or may not be noticed. Diverticulitis and other forms of inflammatory bowel disease are examples of conditions that can cause these symptoms.

Tumors of the intestine and kidney might also cause symptoms that can be confused with those of ovarian cancer. Description of the symptoms and X-ray studies are used to find the correct location of the tumor.

DIAGNOSIS

The diagnostic process is likely to take several trips to the doctor's office or to the hospital for X-rays and other laboratory tests. Some lab tests require days to complete and report, while staging tests take more time. Still, all of this testing is very necessary. A complete and accurate picture of the problem, cancer or not, is crucial for planning the right treatment. All the while, the woman and those who care about her are forced to wait and wonder. Uncertainty is probably the most difficult part of the diagnostic process.

The diagnostic procedure starts with a complete "history." This is a series of questions and discussions about the woman's family, past health experience, and pregnancies—including abortion, miscarriage or stillbirth. A complete history should cover the following:

- Has any female family member ever had cancer of the ovary?

- Description of diet: vitamin supplements, fat content, fiber content

◆ Bowel habits
— frequency of bowel movements
— any diarrhea?
— any constipation?
— any gas pains?
— changes in bowel habits; when was a change noticed?

◆ Bladder habits
— number of times to pass water each day?
— color of urine
— changes in bladder habits; when was a change noticed?

◆ Menstrual history
— age when menstrual periods began (menarche)
— age when menstrual periods stopped (menopause)
— are or were periods regular?
— are menstrual cramps usual?
— has there been a change in periods? Describe these changes.

◆ Pregnancies
— number of pregnancies
— number of live births
— any difficulties becoming pregnant
— possibility of pregnancy now

After the history, a physical examination will include a Pap smear and a manual examination of the rectum and vagina. The doctor is looking for lumps or changes in the shape of the pelvic organs. A Pap test may be done, but ovarian cancer usually does not show on Pap testing; the pelvic examination is the best method for finding ovarian tumors in an early stage. It is best if the bladder is empty, and sometimes laxatives, enemas, or both are used to empty the colon and rectum before the exam. The exam reveals the size, shape, and location of a mass in the abdomen. Benign tumors usually feel smooth and are fluid-filled. They are movable, usually only involve one side, and are smaller than a tennis ball. Malignant tumors will most likely feel solid, have irregular walls, and are not movable. Ascites is usually found with malignant tumors.

Laboratory tests of blood and urine will assess liver, kidney, and other body functions. Depending upon the type of tumor suspected, levels of CA-125 and other tumor markers in the blood might be tested. Alpha-fetoprotein (AFP) and human chorionic gonadotropin (hCG) tests might be ordered if a germ cell tumor is suspected. hCG is the hormone that is detected in some pregnancy tests, but also shows up in some cancers. AFP is usually found in the human fetus, but it is also present in people who have cancers of the liver, testicle, lung, pancreas, and ovary. CA-125 is also elevated (above 35 units/ml) in 80% of women with epithelial ovarian tumors.

Usually, this part of the workup takes place in the doctor's office. Some tests require that blood or urine samples be sent to special outside laboratories.

After a complete physical exam and history, tests in the diagnostic process are likely to include:

- **uterine sounding** to outline abnormalities in the abdomen

- **intravenous pyelogram (IVP)** to outline kidneys, uterus, and bladder; also helps judge the size of a mass and adds information about kidney function

- **barium enema,** if there are symptoms involving the intestines or digestive function; rules out tumors in the rectum and lower (sigmoid) colon

- **chest X-ray** to look for fluid around the lungs and other tumors in the chest

- **pelvic ultrasound** to define the size and shape of a mass; also may be done to rule out pregnancy

- **CAT** or **CT scan** may be done during diagnosis to define the size and location of a mass

- **MRI (Magnetic Resonance Imaging)** may be used during diagnosis but is more useful to monitor effects of cancer therapy

Diagnostic Imaging Techniques Used for Ovarian Cancer

Exam	Information about the exam
Barium enema	Restrict diet beforehand to clear fluids, e.g., apple and cranberry juices, water, coffee, tea. Laxatives and enemas are given to clean out the bowel. The enema will feel cool and may cause cramps. The exam will take 30–60 minutes.
Ultrasound	There may be diet restrictions. The bladder should be full unless the doctor asks that the bladder be empty. A gel will be applied to the skin of the area being examined. A transducer, which makes sound waves is passed over the skin. The woman may feel pressure, but no pain. The exam takes about 30 minutes.
CT Scan	Be prepared to lie *very* still on a hard table for around 30–60 minutes. The body is passed through a tunnel in which X-rays are taken at precise intervals to make a computerized three-dimensional image.
MRI	Might be used to look for small tumors but is most useful in checking for the effectiveness of treatment. The body is placed in a tunnel in which X-rays are taken to make a three-dimensional image.

- ◆ **laparoscopy**

- ◆ **laparotomy:** almost always necessary in the end, this surgery can define the exact location and look of the mass and remove as much of the tumor as possible

STAGING

After a cancer diagnosis is made, staging tests are done to find out if the cancer has spread to other parts of the body. The exact definition of the stage of disease is needed so that the best treatment can be planned.

Laparoscopy permits the doctor to see directly inside the abdomen and pelvis. Usually, a laparotomy—a surgery to open the abdomen and examine the organs directly—is required to accurately stage the cancer. During the laparotomy, the surgeon looks at all the abdominal organs and does a biopsy of the tumor. Microscopic examination will reveal the presence (or absence) of cell changes that make up what we know as cancer or "malignant changes." Some laboratory techniques can be done immediately, so the rest of the surgical procedure depends on what is seen through the microscope. If an organ is found to contain cancer cells, the surgeon will either remove the whole organ, or at least as much of the cancer as is possible.

The staging surgery is also the first treatment. Since most women with epithelial cancers already have some cancer spread, more therapy is almost always needed. Adjuvant therapy decisions are based on the stage, size, and location of any tumor that was not removed, presence or absence of ascites, and tumor cells in the ascitic fluid.

Stages of ovarian cancer

The International Federation for Gynecologic Oncology (FIGO) has outlined a staging system for cancers of the ovary, which offers physicians and other healthcare providers a sort of common language for discussing ovarian cancer. In its basic form, the FIGO staging system flows from the earliest, most limited stage, Stage I, to advanced disease with involvement of other organs, Stage IV. It is different than the TNM staging system described in the discussion of breast cancer in Part Two. Some doctors use the TNM system, while others prefer to use the FIGO system (see page 267).

FIGO Staging System for Cancer of the Ovary

Stage	Description
I	Growth limited to the ovaries
IA	Growth limited to one ovary; no ascites; no tumor on the external surface; capsules intact
IB	Growth limited to both ovaries; no ascites; no tumor on the external surfaces; capsules intact
IC	Tumor either Stage IA or IB but located on the surface of one or both ovaries; or with capsule ruptured; or with ascites present containing malignant cells; or with positive peritoneal washings
II	Growth involving one or both ovaries with pelvic extension
IIA	Extension and/or metastases to the uterus and/or tubes
IIB	Extension to other pelvic tissues
IIC	Tumor either Stage IIA or IIB, but located on surface of one or both ovaries; or with capsule(s) ruptured; or with ascites present containing malignant cells; or with positive peritoneal washings
III	Tumor involving one or both ovaries with peritoneal implants outside the pelvis and/or positive retroperitoneal or inguinal nodes; superficial liver metastasis equals Stage III; tumor limited to the true pelvis but with histologically proven malignant extension to small bowel or omentum
IIIA	Tumor grossly limited to true pelvis with negative nodes but with histologically confirmed microscopic seeding of abdominal peritoneal surfaces
IIIB	Tumor of one or both ovaries with histologically confirmed implants of abdominal peritoneal surfaces, none exceeding 2 cm in diameter; nodes negative
IIIC	Abdominal implants greater than 2 cm in diameter and/or positive retroperitoneal or inguinal nodes
IV	Growth involving one or both ovaries with distant metastases; if pleural effusion present, there must be positive cytology to allot a case to Stage IV; parenchymal liver metastasis equals Stage IV

TREATMENT FOR EPITHELIAL CANCER OF THE OVARY

Stage I

Total hysterectomy—removal of the cervix, uterus, fallopian tubes, and both ovaries—is the treatment of choice for women with Stage I ovarian cancer. In this surgery, a fold of the peritoneum, the **omentum**, is also removed. During the actual operation, the surgeon will look for signs of cancer cells inside the abdomen. About one quarter of these women will have lymph nodes in the area removed also.

For women with Stage I cancer who want to become pregnant later, removal of only one ovary and fallopian tube might be possible. This decision is made based on the grade of the cancer cells (see Chapter 4).

Surgery alone does not always cure even this early stage cancer: the cancer reappears in about 20% of women. There is no common opinion about what might be the best adjuvant therapy for Stage I ovarian cancer; recommendations are based on the grade of the cancer cells. Adjuvant therapy might consist of radioactive phosphorus or chromic phosphate placed into the abdomen, systemic chemotherapy, and radiation therapy of the abdomen and pelvis. Chemotherapy often prescribed for early stage ovarian cancer includes Melphalan or chlorambucil and usually continues for one year.

After a year of chemotherapy, many women are asked to have another laparotomy—**"second-look surgery."** During this operation, the surgeon explores the abdomen looking for signs of cancer cells. If there is no evidence of cancer, therapy can be stopped. If cancer cells are found, radiation or other chemotherapy drugs are considered. Although the second-look surgery has become standard practice, the long-term benefits have to be weighed against the risks of surgery and a frank doctor-patient discussion of risks and benefits is always warranted.

In 1990, the largest clinical trial of early stage ovarian cancer treatment was reported. Results of this study showed that chemotherapy for women with well-differentiated cancers did *not* add to the success of cancer treatment. However, an 18-month program using the chemotherapy drug Melphalan helped many women with poorly-differentiated tumors survive ovarian cancer. In this study, some women received only chemotherapy, others received chemotherapy and intraperitoneal radioactive phosphorus. The success of these regimens—defined as lower rates of recurrence—depended on the grade of the cancer cells. Lower grade, more differentiated cancer cells indicate that the cancer is more likely to be cured by this treatment. Research studies are now being done to find the best treatment for Stage I ovarian cancer.

Stage II

The surgery offered for Stage I ovarian cancer is also the treatment of choice for Stage II. Some surgeons will wash the abdomen out during surgery with radioactive phosphorus. Since so few women are diagnosed at this stage, very little is really known about Stage II ovarian cancer.

Stage III and IV

These stages of ovarian cancer are not cured by surgery alone. In fact, some doctors believe that surgery should not be done for women with advanced ovarian cancer. To make matters even more confusing, no single form of treatment is recognized by doctors as the best, and there is controversy about what might be the best type of surgery. Some surgeons give women with advanced ovarian cancer one or more doses of chemotherapy before surgery, contending that the chemotherapy shrinks the tumor and makes cancer cells less likely to escape during surgery. Other surgeons prefer to delay surgery until a full course of chemotherapy is completed. Sometimes radiation therapy is given directly into the abdomen during surgery.

At this time, the NCI recommends treatment with total abdominal hysterectomy, including removal of the fallopian tubes and omentum. As much tumor as is possible should be removed. NCI also recommends that surgery be followed by either a chemotherapy program or total abdominal and pelvic radiation therapy. Chemotherapy drugs most likely to be used include cyclophosphamide, cisplatin, carboplatin, hexamethyl-melamine, and doxorubicin. Some of these drugs, particularly cisplatin or carboplatin, may be used alone in what is called "single agent therapy." Other drug treatment programs use "combination therapy," combining two, three, or four drugs in a prescribed schedule.

Specific Treatments

Second-look surgery after a chemotherapy program is completed is the most accurate way to find tumors or cancer cells that were not destroyed by chemotherapy. Even though many doctors recommend second-look surgery, its use is debatable. No study has actually shown an advantage in terms of survival for women who go through the second-look operation and NCI recommends that it be done *only* by a surgeon trained in gynecologic oncology as part of a clinical trial when a new treatment strategy is being considered.

Intraperitoneal (IP) chemotherapy—chemotherapy that is placed directly into the peritoneal cavity—is sometimes used to treat both early and advanced ovarian cancer. Since ovarian cancer usually spreads to the peritoneum, placing anticancer drugs directly into the peritoneal cavity makes sense. Levels of the drugs that spread out to the systemic circulation are kept low. Most often, women are asked to go through intraperitoneal chemotherapy *after* surgery and *after* they have completed a course of systemic chemotherapy.

Intraperitoneal (IP) chemotherapy is given through a tube or catheter that is inserted through the abdomen into the peritoneal cavity. If IP chemotherapy is recommended but only one or two doses are planned, a temporary catheter might be used instead of a port. These catheters are similar to those used for kidney dialysis. Examples include the Tenckhoff (tenk'-off) and Trocar catheters. They require quite a bit of care and attention while they are in place. For this reason, ports are preferred by many women and their doctors.

A port provides easier access to the peritoneal cavity than other types of access devices and is usually recommended when therapy is likely to involve several IP procedures. The IP port is similar to the port used for vascular access (see the chart "Access to a Central Vein," page 106). The port limits the discomfort and bother related to using temporary access devices. Once the port is in place and the surgical incision has healed, it requires little or no care. There are many kinds of ports, and their care differs according to the type used. Although the port can stay in place for several years, it will be removed when it is no longer needed. (This requires a minor operation.)

A doctor or nurse can help the woman learn the kind of care a port might entail and can discuss what sort of access device is best. She should ask questions about where it will be located and whether it will be visible, what sort of tasks will be needed to care for the skin around the port and if there are any special procedures needed to care for the catheter.

During IP chemotherapy, 1–2 quarts of fluid with anticancer drugs are allowed to flow into the peritoneal cavity and remain there for up to 24 hours. After the prescribed amount of time, the fluid is allowed to drain out. Some of it might stay in the peritoneal cavity: this will be absorbed by the body and is not a serious problem.

Women who have IP chemotherapy describe the sensations while the fluid is in place differently. Usually, pain is not a problem. If discomfort is felt it is usually compared to gas pains, feeling full or bloated, or having cramps. In practice, I have noticed two things that make a difference. First, most women report that it is more comfortable if the solution is warmed to about body temperature before it is used. The bag of solution can be placed in a microwave oven for a minute or so to take the chill off. Cramps are often the result of letting the solution flow in too fast and slowing the drip rate can help relieve this. Just changing positions in the bed—turning slightly to one side—might increase comfort also.

There are concerns about the use of IP chemotherapy. There is no guarantee that the drugs placed into the peritoneum will come into contact with cancer cells. The techniques used to access the abdomen must be absolutely sterile. Bacteria entering the body through the IP catheter can cause serious infections. And, even after IP chemotherapy has ended, bowel obstruction and bowel adhesions can occur as a late reaction. Other concerns center on the fact that no one has identified the best drug or combination of drugs to use. Of course, the biggest question of all is: can IP chemotherapy offer a woman more hope for cure, or at least control, of her cancer?

Taxol is thought by many cancer experts to be the most important cancer drug of the 1990s. It has potential for use in the treatment of cancers of the breast and ovary. Until it received FDA approval for use in ovarian cancer in January 1993, this drug was available only through clinical trials. Taxol has side effects that can be at least as dangerous as other anticancer drugs. Early reports about Taxol's anticancer effects pitted many factions against each other: women who believe Taxol is their only chance for survival, doctors, the drug industry, and environmentalists. It takes one Western yew tree (*Taxus brevifolia*) to produce two to three doses of Taxol. Bristol-Myers Squibb Company has developed a synthetic drug that has the same anticancer effects as Taxol. The NCI and a French company, Rhone–Poulenc Rorer, Inc., have signed a research agreement for the development of **taxotere**, a partly synthetic version of taxol. Currently, Taxol is used in treatment plans for women with refractory (not responding to initial treatment) ovarian cancer. In clinical trials, it is being used in combination with cisplatin, carboplatin, and cyclophosphamide.

Radiation therapy is not widely used to cure ovarian cancer in the United States. There is a British report of the use of abdominal radiation therapy to treat women with early stage disease, but it is no more effective than the chemotherapy protocols in use. Radiation therapy does have a place in combined modality protocols: it might be used before or after a chemotherapy regimen. Radioactive phosphorus and gold have been used to treat early stage ovarian cancer. Radioactive phosphorus is infused into the peritoneal cavity in a half quart of fluid in much the same way as IP chemotherapy. The woman is asked to change her position every ten to fifteen minutes to allow the fluid to distribute throughout the abdomen.

Radiation can be used to treat specific unpleasant symptoms caused by the cancer. It can reduce tumors or masses that cause pain, bleeding, or other distressing symptoms. Sometimes radiation can be used to slow down the formation of ascites. In these situations, radiation therapy might take only one or two treatments but it can provide a great deal of comfort.

WHEN OVARIAN CANCER RECURS

Any therapy for recurrent disease will be for the purposes of controlling symptoms, aiming for a remission, and/or improving the quality of life. Treatment for recurrent disease might involve cisplatin or carboplatin chemotherapy, especially if these drugs were effective in treating the woman's cancer before. Taxol's FDA approval specifies its use in the treatment of recurrent ovarian cancer. Other drugs that might be used include ifosfamide and hexamethylmelamine. Hormonal therapy with tamoxifen, megestrol acetate, and leuprolide have also resulted in remission for a few women.

THE FUTURE

Biologic therapy may soon be a fourth form of therapy for ovarian cancer. Experimental studies are being done that use interferon alone and interferon in combination with chemotherapy to treat women with small amounts of tumor left after surgery. Other studies are examining IP interferon.

Second-look surgery may be replaced by the use of antibodies combined with radioactive substances to pinpoint cancer cells. Tumor-associated antigens, such as CA-125 and CA 19-9, might eventually be more useful in finding ovarian cancers early. If these measurements are perfected, they might negate the need for second-look surgery.

Treatment for ovarian cancer is changing very quickly. The National Cancer Institute encourages all women with ovarian cancer to consider taking part in a clinical trial, available through cooperative study groups in several treatment centers. A doctor or oncology nurse should be able to help locate a clinical trial that might be appropriate. More information is available through NCI's Cancer Information Service (see Resources).

❖   ❖   ❖

Ovarian cancer is a very scary disease. Despite some progress in treatment, it is the leading cause of death from gynecologic cancers and the fifth leading cause of death for American women. Like all kinds of cancer, the best defense against ovarian cancer is to *find it early*, and this requires that every woman really know her body well. Each woman has to be watchful for symptoms that "just do not feel right." All women should have some idea of individual risk factors—especially those that relate to personal and family history. Every woman has to be open in her talks with her doctor or nurse practitioner and share her concerns and her unique history. Lastly, every woman has to be her own best friend. If ovarian cancer is a possibility, a woman's best chance for survival is her demand for the right diagnostic tests.

Pamela Haylock

Chapter 16

❖

Cancer of the Uterus (Endometrial Cancer)

The uterus—the womb—lies between the bladder and the rectum. It is usually the shape and size of an upside-down pear, but during pregnancy expands as the fetus grows.

Cancer of the uterus—endometrial cancer—is the most common gynecologic cancer in the United States. It accounts for about 7% of all new women's cancers, affecting 32,000 women a year. Even though endometrial cancer affects so many women, few die from this cancer. Early diagnosis is the major reason: most cases are discovered before the cancer spreads outside of the uterus. Most women with endometrial cancer can look forward to complete cure of their disease.

The uterus is made up of two layers of tissue: a muscular, outer layer called the **myometrium** and an inner layer called the **endometrium**. The upper portion of the uterus is the **fundus**, the central portion is the body or **corpus**, and the lower end is the **cervix**. The fallopian tubes attach to both sides of the fundus and extend to each ovary.

Like all human tissue, uterine cells normally wear out, die, and are replaced by new cells. Sometimes, abnormal growth takes place and tumors are formed, which can be benign or malignant.

Fibroid tumors or **leiomyomas** are benign and most of them do not cause serious symptoms. Some cause no symptoms at all, and require no treatment. Fibroids are seldom painful, but large fibroids can press on the bladder or rectum and be uncomfortable, and some may cause excessive bleeding during menstruation. If fibroids become painful and cause discomfort and bleeding, they can be surgically removed.

Endometrial hyperplasia is an abnormal increase in endometrial and stromal cells that can affect all women, even teens. Some experts believe endometrial hyperplasia is a precancerous condition (it can be compared to cervical intraepithelial neoplasia (CIN)). Some areas of hyperplasia can revert to normal with or without medical treatment. Sometimes hyperplasia persists; other times, if untreated, it can go through phases of increasing abnormalities until it becomes a true cancer. There is no way to predict which women will develop cancer. Most endometrial hyperplasia is thought to be caused by ongoing estrogen stimulation. The most common cause is several menstrual cycles in which an egg is *not* produced.

Heavy uterine bleeding is the major symptom of hyperplasia. Other symptoms might include a history of skipped or delayed periods, or long intervals between periods.

The development of cancer from hyperplasia seems to be fairly slow, taking five years or more.

TREATMENT FOR ENDOMETRIAL HYPERPLASIA

It is important to have a full workup because both hyperplasia and cancer can be present in a woman's uterus at the same time. Here are general treatment guidelines: actual recommendations vary according to the woman's age and the cell pattern of the tissues involved.

Teenage girls can be given hormone therapy—estrogen-progestin pills—in an attempt to stimulate menstrual cycles for at least six months. Tissue samples from the uterus will be tested three months after hormonal therapy. If the samples are normal, the teen will be followed for signs that normal menstruation and ovulation are occurring. Additional hormonal therapy is used if ovulation does not occur.

The childbearing-age woman is treated with hormone therapy for three months. Tissue sampling will be done right after she completes the hormone therapy. Hormone therapy to induce ovulation can be prescribed when the tissue samples are normal. If the woman is not interested in becoming pregnant, she can continue to use the estrogen-progestin hormones to induce normal, though artificial, menstrual cycles.

The woman nearing or in menopause may be treated with a hysterectomy or low doses of progestin. The need for hysterectomy is determined by the severity of the hyperplasia, the woman's wish for sterilization, and the presence of symptoms like severe uterine bleeding. In some cases, hysterectomy may be recommended if a uterine tumor is suspected.

For the **postmenopausal woman,** unless she is not physically able, hysterectomy is usually recommended. Women who have not had a period for at least two years and have hyperplasia very often have endometrial or ovarian cancers too. Progestin therapy might be offered to a woman whose physical condition will not allow her to go through an operation.

RISK FACTORS

Like most cancers, age is the most important risk factor for the development of uterine cancer. Most women who develop uterine cancer are 50–59 years old. Less than 25% are diagnosed before menopause.

Another risk factor for endometrial cancer is the use of estrogen replacement therapy for menopausal symptoms. The risk for developing cancer increases with the length of use and the dose of estrogens. The risk increases after 2–4 years of use and is greatest when large doses are taken. So far, it is not known if or when the risk drops to that of a "nonuser" after estrogen is stopped.

Women who are obese produce more estrogen than women who are near normal weight. Their risk for developing endometrial cancer is similar to that of women who take estrogen replacements. Women with polycystic ovaries and some ovarian tumors are also more prone to develop endometrial cancer. The combined effects of hypertension (high blood pressure), diabetes, and obesity cause more women to develop uterine cancer. It is not clear why hypertension has an effect on the uterus; it may be that it is caused by the diabetes and obesity and is not directly related to uterine cancer.

Women who began menstruation early and women who went into menopause late are more prone to develop uterine cancer. Women who have never been pregnant are at slightly higher risk than women who have been pregnant. Also, women of higher social and economic status, those who live in cities, and those of Jewish descent seem to be more at risk for uterine cancer.

Women who have had external radiation therapy to the pelvis are at higher risk to develop uterine sarcoma. A history of pelvic radiation therapy seems to be related to the development of cancer in 10–25% of women with this form of cancer. Some women might have received radiation therapy anywhere from 5–25 years before the development of uterine sarcoma.

PREVENTION

Protective Factors: as strange as it seems (and I cannot believe I have to say this) cigarette smoking has been linked to a *reduced* risk for uterine cancer—especially in women over 50 and those who are postmenopausal. The biologic effects of smoking on estrogen production may be the reason for this effect. However, *no one* should take up smoking to counteract the possibility of uterine cancer: both active and passive smoking have so many more serious—and less treatable—health hazards for women!

The use of progestins (another female hormone) with estrogen replacement therapy seems to either remove the risk or at least delay its onset. Birth control pills which combine estrogen and progesterone in the same pill used for at least 12 months seem to offer some protection with this effect lasting for at least 15 years after the pills have been stopped.

EARLY DETECTION

Endometrial cancer is unique among most women's cancers in that it produces symptoms very early. Any new onset of heavy vaginal bleeding is a warning signal—even abnormally heavy bleeding in a premenopausal woman. Although this symptom is frightening, it does cause most women to get medical care immediately. For some women, a blood-streaked, watery vaginal discharge that is either constant or seems to come and go might be a first symptom. Very rarely, low back pain is noted by women who have advanced disease.

On the other hand, vaginal bleeding is not always a sign of endometrial cancer. Other cancers, like cancer of the cervix, vulva, and vagina, might cause similar symptoms. Vaginal infection can also cause vaginal bleeding. Sometimes bleeding from inflammatory bowel disease, hemorrhoids, kidney and urinary tract problems can be confused with bleeding from the vagina.

DIAGNOSIS

Endometrial cancer is diagnosed by pretty much the same process as other gynecologic cancers. A complete history will be taken by the nurse and/or doctor. The physical examination will include an exam of the vagina and genitals. The bimanual exam helps define the size, position, and shape of the uterus. The Pap smear that is so useful in the diagnosis of cervical cancer is not as valuable in the diagnosis and workup of endometrial cancer. Still, a Pap smear is likely to be included in a full workup since it might pick up some endometrial cells as well as cells from the cervix. Endocervical curettage provides tissue samples from the endocervical canal and is done *before* samples are taken from the endometrium. Endometrial samples can be done by aspiration, biopsy, or a D&C. Any suspicious area on the cervix should also be biopsied in order to rule out cervical cancer.

Chest X-rays evaluate the status of the lungs and possible metastasis to the lungs. A **urogram** (X-ray of the urinary tract) and a barium enema are used to look for tumors blocking or pressing on the ureters or bowel. Cystoscopy and sigmoidoscopy help the doctor decide if the tumor has spread to the bladder or rectum. Ultrasound and a CT scan may be used to determine the extent of disease.

TYPES OF UTERINE CANCER

The most common form of uterine cancer, **adenocarcinoma,** starts in the gland-filled lining of the uterus. Sometimes cell types are mixed in the same tumor; this is called **adenosqua-mous carcinoma.** These two types of tumors make up almost 90% of all uterine cancers. Other less common types of adeno-carcinomas are **clear cell, undifferentiated, secretory, squamous,** and **papillary.** The clear cell and papillary types grow and spread more quickly and require more aggressive treatment.

Uterine sarcoma is very rare—it makes up less than 5% of all uterine cancers. It originates in the muscle or supporting tissues of the uterus.

TREATMENT

Cancer of the endometrium is treated with combinations of radiation, chemotherapy, surgery, and/or hormones. Surgery is the most common treatment for both adenocarcinoma and sar-coma of the uterus. Total abdominal hysterectomy that includes removal of the fallopian tubes and ovaries is most often recom-mended. During surgery, it is important that the surgeon have tissue samples sent to the pathologist for examination of proges-terone receptors.

Some doctors feel the addition of internal radiation after surgery has some benefit. If the tumor is found to have invaded deep into the myometrium (at least half the depth), post-operative external radiation therapy is added. If cancer cells have spread to the nearby lymph nodes or to more distant sites, radiation, chemotherapy, and hormones are likely to be added to the overall treatment plan.

Staging of Endometrial Carcinoma (FIGO System)

Stage	Characteristics
0	Abnormal hyperplasia or carcinoma in situ
IA	Tumor is limited to the endometrium
IB	Tumor invades less than halfway through myometrium
IC	Tumor invades to greater than halfway through myometrium
IIA	Endocervical glandular involvement only
IIB	Cervical stromal invasion
IIIA	Tumor invades serosa, adnexa, and/or positive peritoneal cytology (cells present in peritoneal fluid)
IIIB	Vaginal metastases
IIIC	Metastases to pelvic and/or lymph nodes around the aorta
IVA	Tumor invades into bladder and/or bowel
IVB	Metastases to distant organs, into the abdomen or inguinal (groin) lymph nodes

For women who are unable to have surgery because of other health conditions, treatment can consist of radiation therapy alone. In these women, cure rates are not as high as for those who have surgery.

The combination of surgery plus chemotherapy is being studied at the National Cancer Institute for both adenocarcinomas and sarcomas that have spread outside of the uterus (Stage III and above). Drugs used in clinical trials so far include ifosfamide, cisplatin, and doxorubicin.

ADVANCED OR RECURRENT DISEASE

Treatment for advanced and recurrent disease varies according to how much or how far the cancer has spread and which organs and body systems are affected.

In advanced sarcoma, clinical trials currently combine two or more chemotherapy drugs. For women with carcinoma, both internal and external radiation therapy might be of benefit if there is evidence of large tumors. If the pathologist has detected hormone receptors on the tumor cells, hormonal therapy can be useful, especially to treat metastases to the lungs. These hormonal drugs, called progesterones, include hydroxyprogesterone (Delalutin), medroxyprogesterone (Provera), and megestrol (Megace).

Recurrent sarcoma and carcinoma are not generally considered curable. Instead, therapy can offer hope for controlling the disease and managing distressing symptoms like pain, bleeding, feelings of abdominal pressure, and so on. Treatment goals are guided by the extent and location of the cancer and the symptoms. Women with recurrent sarcoma could be offered chemotherapy through several ongoing clinical trials. Sometimes, too, individual doctors adopt treatment plans from clinical trials even though the patient may not be enrolled into an actual trial. Sarcoma trials are currently underway that look at the effects of various combinations of chemotherapy drugs that are individually known to have some positive effect on sarcoma. Some sarcomas have responded to radiation therapy, and progesterone hormone therapy can be helpful for women with some recurrent sarcoma.

Recurrent endometrial carcinoma can sometimes respond to radiation therapy. When a recurrence has been limited to only the vagina, radiation has provided a cure for a few women. Women who test positive for estrogen and progesterone receptors respond better to progestin therapy. Negative receptor status usually says that a woman will not get much benefit from hormonal therapy. On the other hand, negative receptor status sometimes predicts a better response to chemotherapy. Tamoxifen, the drug often used to treat postmenopausal women with breast cancer, is sometimes useful in the treatment of endometrial carcinoma—especially with those for whom progesterone therapy did not work.

In some women, even though other organs seem to be negative for cancer cells, there is evidence that the cancer has probably spread outside of the uterus. During surgery, fluid from inside the abdomen (peritoneal fluid) is collected and examined for cancer cells. The presence of these cells might mean that the cancer is more advanced than was previously thought; treatment plans are likely to be changed in light of these findings. Clinical trials are being developed to find the most effective treatment for this situation.

FUTURE TRENDS, CLINICAL TRIALS

Treatment for early cancer of the uterus is very effective and most women with early disease can be cured. However, there is no standard treatment—no treatment that is endorsed by the majority of doctors—for metastatic cancer of the uterus. Current studies are looking at ways to manage advanced disease more effectively. Most of these studies evaluate the effects—both positive and negative—of combining drugs, hormones, surgery, and radiation. The studies might vary by the order in which each of these standard therapies are used and the doses given.

Some experts advocate the use of intraperitoneal radioactive phosphorous when cancer cells are found in the peritoneal fluid during surgery. (Radioactive material in a fluid is allowed to flow into the abdomen in much the same way as when intraperitoneal chemotherapy is given.) Other approaches include use of external radiation to the whole abdomen. Other studies are testing the effect of systemic chemotherapy versus no chemotherapy for women who have cancer cells in the peritoneal fluid.

AFTER TREATMENT

After hysterectomy and removal of the ovaries, women are at high risk for **osteoporosis** (brittle bones). These women can prevent or at least diminish the problem by increasing dietary intake of calcium to 1,500 mg/day (by taking supplements, eating dairy products, etc.). A vitamin D supplement improves the body's ability to use calcium. Weight-bearing exercises like walking, step aerobics, and swimming minimize and can even stop bone loss. Large amounts of caffeine and fiber can *reduce* the amount of calcium that is absorbed.

After treatment, a woman still needs an annual Pap smear, and a general exam of the uterus, cervix, ovaries, and/or vagina (depending on the type of treatment). Although many women forego annual gynecologic exams and/or general medical exams after hysterectomy, for some (especially older women) the lack of regular medical checkups results in the development of other problems. For example, elderly women who have had hysterectomies are found to have advanced vaginal or vulvar cancers much more frequently than women who continue to get annual or regular gynecologic checkups.

QUESTIONS TO ASK YOUR PHYSICIAN

1. Should I get a prescription for a progestin along with estrogen replacement therapy?

2. What will be the long-term side effects if these treatments are recommended?
   — surgery (see section on hysterectomy and surgical treatment for cervical cancer, Chapter 17)
   — radiation therapy
     — will there be changes in sexual function?
     — what can I do to prevent or at least decrease side effects?
   — chemotherapy
     — what are the side effects of each drug?
     — what can I do to prevent or at least decrease these side effects?
   — hormone therapy
     — the same questions as for radiation and chemotherapy

3. Will the surgeon request hormone receptor testing on surgical specimens? If not, why?

4. What is the schedule for follow-up examinations and what will be included in the exams?

ESTROGEN REPLACEMENT THERAPY

Estrogen replacement therapy (ERT) is often prescribed after a hysterectomy or menopause. However, its major risk is that estrogens are a large factor in the development of endometrial hyperplasia, which is in turn related to the development of endometrial cancer. This association is very strong for post-menopausal women—the very group in which three-fourths of all endometrial cancer is found. Estrogen from any source can cause the development of hyperplasia. The role of estrogen in the development of endometrial cancer is receiving a great deal of attention in both the scientific and lay press. **DES (Diethyl-stilbestrol),** a synthetic estrogen, has been a known carcinogen since at least 1940, but it was used to prevent miscarriages from the mid-1940s right on into the '80s and is blamed for an increased incidence in rare gynecologic cancers in the daughters born to women who took DES. However, it is still used in estrogen replacement therapy (for more on DES, see Chapter 18).

In the past, a woman with a medical history that includes uterine cancer would not have been given estrogen replacement. Recent studies have demonstrated that uterine cancer does not absolutely rule out estrogen replacement therapy.

How ERT is used

Clearly, ERT is useful in the treatment of menopausal symptoms, but its use must be weighed against the risks it brings. Before a doctor prescribes ERT, the woman must go through a complete history and physical to identify her risk factors. If she has any history of abnormal uterine bleeding, she needs a more thorough evaluation that will include getting tissue samples from her uterus. Some doctors require this sort of intensive testing even for women who have no known problems or risks. Most, however, believe that women with a normal history and normal physical findings can be safely placed on ERT. The starting dose is usually 0.625 milligrams (mg) each day. The drug of choice is a conjugated (specially created) estrogen. The more common estrogen preparations and doses vary, but the effects are the same. Common doses are:

Ethinyl estradiol	0.02 mg
Conjugated estrogens	0.625 mg
Estrone	1.25 mg

The dose is likely to be much higher for a young woman who goes into menopause early after surgery or radiation therapy removes or destroys her ovaries. Doses should be increased *only* if symptoms are very severe and intolerable. Most doctors recommend that the estrogens be given in a cycle, with 5–7 days each month off the drug. Some prefer using progestin therapy in the cycle—giving progestins the last 10 days of each monthly cycle in addition to the estrogen. This treatment schedule mimics the normal menstrual cycle and therefore might result in bleeding that resembles menstrual bleeding, even in women who are late postmenopausal. This schedule also limits endometrial growth. Some doctors prescribe estrogen and progestin doses daily—either continuously or on weekdays only with no drugs given on Saturday and Sunday. This schedule prevents bleeding.

In some situations, estrogens cannot be given. Menopausal symptoms can be relieved to some extent by daily doses of progestins such as megestrol acetate (Megace) or medroxyprogesterone (Provera). While these drugs reduce the hot flashes and sweating they may cause vaginal dryness, increased appetite, and subsequent weight gain.

Women on ERT need medical checkups every 6–12 months. This checkup should include:

— blood pressure

— breast exam

— pelvic exam

— uterine tissue sampling if there is abnormal bleeding

Pamela Haylock

Chapter 17

❖

Cancer of the Cervix and Cervical Dysplasia (CIN)

Cancer of the cervix is diagnosed in about 13,500 U.S. women each year. Before cancer cells develop, some cells of the cervix go through abnormal changes called dysplasia. The size and shape of individual cervical cells, or the structure of the tissues made up of these cells, may alter. A Pap smear can find these abnormal cells, and the right treatment during the dysplasia stage can prevent cells from going through more changes that would turn them into cancer cells. This is why an annual Pap smear is so important.

NORMAL STRUCTURE OF THE CERVIX

At the lower end of the uterus, the tissue is squeezed together to form the cervix. The cervix is about one inch long; its lower end extends into the upper part of the vagina. The **internal cervical os** is the opening on the uterine side of the cervix (os is the Latin word for "mouth"). On the vaginal end of the cervix, another small opening, the **external cervical os**, connects the inside of the uterus with the vagina.

Normally the cervix is mostly composed of mucous membrane and connective tissue. Mucous membrane, a special form of epithelium, is the same type of tissue that lines the mouth, the entire digestive system, the reproductive organs, and the urinary tract. Connective tissue gives form and shape to organs. The mucous membrane of the cervix blends with the mucous membrane that lines the vagina; the area where cells of the cervix and cells of the vagina blend is the **transformation zone**, so-called because the cells on one side are of one specialized type and the cells on the other side are another type. These normal cells are constantly being shed, just like cells from the skin are shed. The testing known as the Pap smear or Pap test (named after Doctor Papanicolaou, who discovered that cells from the cervix are shed into vaginal fluid) involves scraping some of these shed cells from the surface of the cervix and looking at them under the microscope.

DYSPLASIA OR CERVICAL INTRAEPITHELIAL NEOPLASIA (CIN)

Intraepithelial neoplasia is a premalignant (precancerous) change that can occur on the cervix, the vulva, and the vagina. Intraepithelial neoplasia involving the cervix, **Cervical Intraepithelial Neoplasia (CIN),** affects over 50,000 American women each year. For some women, CIN will progress to cancer. There is no way to predict whether CIN will or will not become cancer or the time frame in which the changes take place.

When I was 25 years old, I worked on a study that involved women with early stage cervical cancer. I was reading what seemed like volumes of books and articles about cervical cancer. After I went to my gynecologist for a routine checkup, I was shocked when the doctor's office called to tell me that my "Pap smear wasn't quite normal" and asked that I schedule a biopsy. In the time between that phone call and my appointment, I read everything I could get my hands on about cervical cancer. By the time I had the biopsy, I was convinced that I had it. But I didn't bother to read much about dysplasia. I had the colposcopy and biopsy on a Thursday, and the pathology results would not be ready until the following Tuesday. In the five days I had to wait, I drove two hundred miles to Chicago to be with a friend. I was a basket case.

To make a long story short, the pathology report was fairly good: I did not have cervical cancer. I did, however, have fairly severe dysplasia. The treatment of choice at that time was cryosurgery (destroying the abnormal cells with extreme cold), which I had without problem. There was a school of thought that birth control pills were a factor in cervical dysplasia, so I was introduced to a diaphragm. (Newer forms of birth control pills are not as likely to cause dysplasia.) It took almost two years for my Pap smear tests to revert to normal, but they did, and have been normal for the past eighteen years.

Cervical dysplasia or CIN can be scary. I knew enough to know that abnormal cells can be a sign of cancer. This experience showed me that even the slight chance of cancer is really frightening. The fact that my diagnosis was not cancer and that my Paps have remained normal is a positive comment on the value of routine checkups and early treatment for CIN. The most important message is: do not be paralyzed with fear when you find you have CIN. Go through the diagnosis process and get the right treatment as soon as possible.

Dysplasia literally means "bad molding," and refers to abnormal tissue development. The degree of dysplasia is based on the proportion of normal cells that are replaced by abnormal cells and the severity of cell changes. CIN Grade I (mild dysplasia) involves less than one-third of the thickness of the cervical epithelium; CIN II (moderate dysplasia) involves one-third to

Precancerous lesions: CIN, carcinoma in situ, invasive cancer

two-thirds of the thickness of the epithelium; CIN III (severe dysplasia and carcinoma in situ) represents two-thirds to full-thickness involvement of the cervical epithelium. Cervical Intra-epithelial Neoplasia (CIN) is classified by the proportion of normal cells that are replaced by abnormal cells.

WHO GETS CERVICAL CANCER AND CIN?

The average age for women to have CIN is around 28. Over the past few years, more women in their late teens and early 20s are found to have CIN. In one study involving 800 women with CIN, a third of the women were 20 years old or younger at the time of diagnosis.

The risk factors for CIN and cervical cancer are the same: cigarette smoking, economic status, sexual activity, and viruses. Many of these factors are related and sometimes it is not possible to identify any one specific risk. For example, African American, Hispanic, and Native American women are at a higher risk for CIN and cervical cancer. This is most likely related to economic status, not genetics or hereditary factors.

Women who do not eat enough foods containing vitamin A are at higher risk for CIN and cervical cancer.

Women who have their first sexual experience at an early age and have several sexual partners over the years are more likely to develop CIN and cervical cancer. A problem in pin-pointing any one of these risks as *the* cause of CIN is that women living in poverty often marry and have children earlier than other women.

A woman with only one sexual partner is still at risk if her sexual partner has had many other partners. A woman who is married to a man whose previous wife had cervical cancer is at higher risk to develop CIN.

CIN and cervical cancer occur less often in Jewish women. For a time it was believed that male circumcision has a protective effect. Most authorities now discount this theory, but have no better idea about why Jewish women are less likely to develop CIN and cervical cancer.

CIN seems to be a "venereal" or sexually transmitted disease (STD), but as yet no single virus or bacteria has been proven to be the main cause of CIN. For a while, herpes simplex virus type II (HSV-2) was thought to be the culprit. HSV-2 is sexually transmitted. But research has shown that HSV-2 cannot change normal cells to abnormal cells and it is no longer believed to cause CIN.

Now, the human papillomavirus (HPV)—the virus that causes genital warts—is under suspicion. HPV is found in up to 90% of all women with CIN. Women with CIN and HPV are often 7–10 years younger than women with CIN who do not have HPV. Many experts believe that HPV is a cause of CIN and that HPV makes cell changes happen over a shorter period of time. If a woman has HPV, she is 15 times more likely to develop cervical cancer. If the woman with HPV is under 21, her risk of developing cervical cancer increases by 40 *times*. There is some evidence that the herpes virus might weaken the immune system, which allows a cancer to get started.

There is some contrary evidence. In one study, Native American women with dysplasia were found to have had fewer lifetime sex partners and fewer sexually transmitted diseases than women with normal Pap tests. In another survey of women with HPV, non-Hispanic white women had cervical HPV more often than did Hispanic and Native American women.

Women who smoke and those who inhale secondhand smoke have increased cervical cancer and CIN rates. Toxic chemicals formed by cigarette smoke have been found in cervical fluid and cervical cells. These chemicals weaken the immune status of the cervix. Younger women, especially teenagers, are even more likely to develop CIN and cervical cancer when they inhale cigarette smoke. This is because the cells of the cervix go through major changes during puberty that make them more likely to be damaged by toxic chemicals. The risk also seems to increase if the young female smoker is exposed to HPV through sexual contact.

PREVENTION

There are 65 known human papillomavirus types. The HPV virus can rest on a cell's surface without causing infection or injury. If the cells are damaged with tiny cuts or scrapes found after sexual intercourse, HPV can get inside and infect them. There, the virus starts to multiply. It is thought that 20–30% of adults are infected with one of these virus types, but most have no ill effects because their immune systems stop the virus. Only 3–4% of women who have the virus develop abnormal cervical cells, and most of these revert to normal after medical treatment or by themselves. For some women, the cells turn into cancer. The most suspect types in relation to CIN and cervical cancer are HPV 16 and 18. Despite new tests for HPV, its presence has not been a good predictor of cervical cell abnormalities. So far, widespread testing for HPV is not thought to be useful for routine CIN and cervical cancer screening.

Prevention of CIN and cervical cancer involves providing information for women—especially teens—about ways to decrease the chance of exposure to HPV and other carcinogens. The use of **barrier-type contraceptives,** such as a condom, during sexual intercourse is one way to decrease exposure to cancer-causing viruses.

One study found that women who did not have CIN or cervical cancer had a higher rate of male sexual partners who had had a **vasectomy.** Many researchers think that vasectomies done at an early enough age could be a protective factor.

There are some indications that **vitamin A, vitamin C,** and **beta carotene** offer some protection against the development of CIN and cervical cancer.

The risk of exposure goes up with the number of sexual partners a woman has. Women should have regular pelvic exams and Pap smear screening. These should begin *before* a woman becomes sexually active. In several studies, teens who are sexually active before age 17 have been found to be more likely to develop CIN.

Based on knowledge of how HPV works to cause cancer,

researchers believe the development of a vaccine against the virus is possible and that this could prevent CIN.

DIAGNOSIS

Finding CIN and cancer of the cervix usually starts with an abnormal **Pap test**. No single test can determine absence of cancer cells in all women, but several tests used together reduce the chances of missing cancer. Accurate diagnosis involves a step-by-step process that includes colposcopy, colposcopy-directed biopsy, endocervical curettage (ECC) or Loop Electrocautery Excision Procedure (LEEP), and pelvic examination.

The colposcopy is done using a simple process. After a Pap test, the cervix is rinsed with acetic acid solution (similar to vinegar). The rinse removes mucous and excess cells. The acetic acid also accents the difference between normal and abnormal tissues. The most abnormal-looking part is then selected for biopsy.

Some respected authorities recommend that all women having colposcopy, unless they are pregnant, should also have **endocervical curettage (ECC)**. In ECC, a large speculum is inserted into the vagina to gain access to the space between the internal os and the external os (cervical canal). The whole surface of the cervical canal is scraped or cut away with a cu-rette, a knife-like tool. This is done twice. Women feel some discomfort during ECC, but the discomfort is usually minimal. After ECC, punch biopsies of the cervix can be done, using the colposcopy findings as a guide. All of the tissue removed is collected and examined by a pathologist. ECC gives proof of the absence of cancer cells inside the cervical canal.

During **loop electrocautery excision procedure (LEEP)**, the suspicious area is excised and the remaining tissue is cauter-ized. LEEP is both a diagnostic test and a treatment. Some diagnostic centers routinely use LEEP with ECC; others use either one alone. Tissues removed during LEEP are examined by the pathologist.

Sometimes **conization** is needed to rule out invasive, more advanced cancer. Women with positive ECCs need conization.

It involves removal of a part of the cervix with a scalpel or a laser for examination by a pathologist. Conization is important in finding the extent of the cancer cells' invasion, which in turn determines the best treatment plan (see the figure on page 53).

Postmenopausal women with abnormal Pap smears most often need conization because the cancer cells are usually located inside the cervical canal. Some doctors ask women to put estrogen creams into the vagina for several days before colposcopy and biopsy to further highlight cervical tissue changes.

Conization is an outpatient surgery that is done under general anesthesia. After the woman wakes up from the anesthesia, she can expect to go home on the same day if bleeding is not severe. After four weeks, the woman is examined to check the healing process.

In general, use of the laser instead of a scalpel results in fewer problems with bleeding and infection. The laser also reduces the chance of cervical stenosis after healing. **Stenosis** is a narrowing of the cervical opening that occurs as a result of scar tissue on the cervix. A narrow cervical opening can block the

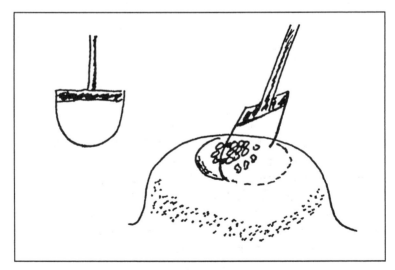

Loop Electrocautery Excision Procedure (LEEP): the excision loop is used to remove affected area with CIN

path of sperm traveling from the vagina to the uterus, causing fertility problems.

For women who have abnormal Pap testing during pregnancy, colposcopy allows the doctor to see the cervix as well as possible. Conization is not often used during pregnancy *except* when the biopsy results suggest cancer. The cervix is filled with blood vessels during pregnancy, so avoiding the larger cone biopsy is in the pregnant woman's (and her baby's) best interests. A pregnant woman with a diagnosis of very early cervical cancer can be allowed to deliver her baby vaginally, and more complete therapy can be given after delivery.

TREATMENT FOR CIN

Treatment options for CIN are observation, local excision, electrocautery, cryosurgery, laser vaporization, conization (laser or knife), and hysterectomy. The best treatment depends on the woman's age, her desire to have children in the future, the precise location of the abnormal cells, and the results of the colposcopy. Very simply, treatment involves destroying or removing abnormal cells. In a few instances, if the involved area is small and the abnormal cells are low grade, no immediate treatment is needed. If this is the case, the woman must be reliable: she must return to her doctor for follow-up exams with Pap smear and colposcopy at the doctor's discretion. This recommendation is most often made for pregnant women or women who are at high risk for infection (immunosuppressed).

Repeat exams at three and six months are sometimes recommended for women with CIN I. If a biopsy is done, the area removed may be the only area affected and biopsy alone might be the cure. For CIN II, the Pap smear should be repeated in two weeks. Suspected infections can be treated during the two-week interval. If the abnormal cells are still found, the woman should have a Pap smear every six months. Some doctors include colposcopy in the follow-up exams for CIN II.

Excision (cutting out the abnormal cells) is used when the results of the colposcopy are not certain, if ECC is positive, and/or CIN is all or partly in the endocervix (the cervical canal). Excised tissue can be examined under the microscope so that an accurate diagnosis can be made.

Electrocautery is a method of "local destruction" of abnormal cells, and has been used to treat CIN for many years. During electrocautery, electric current in passed through a metal rod that touches, burns, and destroys abnormal cells. It has been especially useful in the treatment of CIN I and II and is less effective in the treatment of CIN III. Although electrocautery is effective treatment for mild to moderate CIN, it does have some disadvantages. Some women have slight to moderate pain during and after electrocautery. It also causes scar tissue to form on the cervix, which reduces the ability of the cervix to stretch as it must during the delivery of a baby. For these reasons, electrocautery has gone out of favor with many doctors and fewer women choose this treatment option.

Cryosurgery is another form of local destruction that is as effective as electrocautery. Cryosurgery involves freezing the abnormal cells and tissue with carbon dioxide or nitrous oxide, which are applied using a probe called a "cryoprobe." As the "frozen" cells die off, they are replaced by normal cells. Cryosurgery can be done in the doctor's office or at an outpatient clinic. Most women report cramps during the procedure, but have few problems afterward. Women have a water-like vaginal discharge for several weeks after cryosurgery. They should not use tampons, douche, or have sexual intercourse for four weeks after cryosurgery; this "pelvic rest" period is needed to reduce the chance of infection. Pap smear and colposcopy will be repeated in four months. (Pap smears done before four months would still show evidence of the damage from freezing.) After the first four-month test, Pap smear and colposcopy will need to be done every six months. It is not unusual for Pap smears to remain slightly abnormal for 1–2 years after cryosurgery.

The major advantage of cryosurgery is that it does not cause as much scarring as electrocautery. On the negative side, the cryoprobe may be either too large or too small for the area to be treated. Therefore, some women may be "overtreated" and others "undertreated." The doctor's ability to detect recurrent or remaining disease is affected by the location of the abnormal area. Detection is more difficult if the abnormal area is located within the internal os—abnormalities outside the external os are easier to find and follow. Separate studies report failure to cure rates for cryosurgery of 5%, 7%, and 12% for CIN I, II, and III, respectively.

Laser vaporization is a popular and effective treatment for CIN. The word "laser" is an acronym for "Light Amplification of Stimulated Emission of Radiation." Laser can destroy most CIN of all grades; the procedure can be done in the doctor's office and does not require sedation or anesthesia. Women say they feel cramps while the procedure is being done. Vaginal discharge and bleeding usually last for about two weeks. Like electrocautery and cryosurgery, four weeks of "pelvic rest" is advised. A Pap smear and colposcopy should be done after four months and then every six months.

Laser vaporization is as effective as electrocautery and cryosurgery for treatment of CIN, but it is usually more expensive. Vaginal discharge continues for a shorter period of time, compared to electrocautery and cryosurgery. Bleeding and pain are more common with laser vaporization than with cryosurgery. Laser vaporization offers precise destruction of small areas and does *not* damage normal tissue. It can also reach and treat areas of the cervix that cannot be reached by cryosurgery and electrocautery. For these reasons, it may prevent the development of cancer. Some doctors reserve laser treatment for cases in which CIN involves a larger area and/or extends into the external os. Laser might also be used if cryosurgery or electrocautery have failed to destroy the CIN.

Conization is used as a treatment for CIN as well as a diagnostic procedure.

Hysterectomy, removal of the cervix and uterus, was once the most common treatment for CIN. Even today women who are beyond childbearing years may be offered hysterectomy. Of course, the choice of hysterectomy should be left up to the woman. She should know about other treatment alternatives, the risks involved with hysterectomy, and have a clear idea of the benefits of hysterectomy as an option. Follow-up of hysterectomy is the same as for the other, more local forms of treatment. Because of a history of CIN, this woman has a higher chance of developing CIN of the vulva and vagina.

CARCINOMA IN SITU

Carcinoma in situ is a preinvasive cancer. Carcinoma in situ of the cervix is also called CIN III and Stage 0 carcinoma. Without treatment, carcinoma in situ usually turns into invasive carcinoma. It can be treated with the methods described for CIN, including vaginal hysterectomy (removing the cervix, the uterus, and part of the vagina). CIN treatments such as electrocautery, laser, and cryosurgery can be used for CIN III as long as the woman knows that there is a higher risk of treatment failure. During hysterectomy, removal of the upper part of the vagina is not necessary when there is no sign of cancer in the vagina. (Cervical carcinoma in situ extends into the vagina in fewer than 5% of all cases.) In the United States, hysterectomy (removal of the entire uterus and cervix) has been the treatment of choice for women whose childbearing years are over or women who are interested in permanent sterilization. It is very important for all women, even the woman who has had her uterus and cervix removed, to continue to have regular pelvic examinations that include Pap smears.

CANCER OF THE CERVIX

Most cancers of the cervix start in the transformation zone. **Squamous carcinoma** is the most common and usually occurs in older women. **Adenocarcinoma** occurs in younger women. Adenocarcinoma is often more aggressive and does not respond as well to treatment. The natural history of cervical cancer— the course it would take if left untreated—involves other pelvic structures first, then spread to lymph nodes. Eventually the cancer metastasizes to the lungs, liver, and bones.

Early-stage cervical cancer, like CIN and carcinoma in

situ, may not cause symptoms. As the cancer continues to grow without treatment, the first symptom might be a watery, blood-tinged vaginal discharge that the woman might not even notice. The woman may notice some painless bleeding that occurs at times other than during her normal period. She may notice spotting after sexual intercourse or douching. As the cancer grows, the bleeding might get heavier, more frequent, and might last longer. Some women notice that their periods also last longer and/or that the blood flow is heavier than normal. Eventually, the bleeding is constant. Women who have passed menopause are likely to notice these changes, since for them bleeding is more likely to be thought of as abnormal.

Symptoms of more advanced disease include pain in the flank or leg. This pain is related to pressure from the tumor on the ureters, the pelvic wall, and nerves. Many women with advanced disease describe pain on urination and notice blood in their urine. Advanced disease may block the urinary tract or the bowel. Blocked lymph channels and blood vessels can result in swelling of one or both legs.

Because of the use of routine Pap smears, most women with cervical cancer are diagnosed at earlier, more treatable stages of disease. Usually these early stages of disease have no symptoms. After an abnormal Pap smear, a woman must go through additional tests to define the problem—CIN versus actual cancer—and the extent of the disease.

STAGING

The extent of the cancer is determined through several tests. The bladder is assessed by cystoscopy, done under general anesthesia or local anesthesia with sedation. If there are suspicious areas, biopsy can be done during cystoscopy. Intravenous pyelogram (IVP) is a special imaging study to measure the size of the kidneys, detect blockages, and evaluate suspicious masses. The large intestine (colon) and the rectum are assessed through sigmoidoscopy, proctoscopy, or barium enema examinations. Other imaging studies that might be used to evaluate the extent of the cancer include a chest X-ray, CT scan, ultrasound, or MRI. Blood tests check the function of the liver and kidneys, the presence or absence of anemia or blood loss, and the likelihood of an inflammatory reaction or infection.

As with all kinds of cancer, a classification system gives doctors and the healthcare team a common language for discussion of cervical cancer. This is outlined in the chart on page 301.

TREATMENTS

Treatment options for invasive cancer depend on the woman's age, her general physical condition (including any unintended weight loss), the amount of cancer present, and her wish to save ovarian function. *The extent of the disease is the most important clue to the chance of cure.* The cure rate is nearly 100% in Stages 0 and IA and goes down to 5% in Stage IV. Staging also determines the choice of treatment. Treatment is most likely to include surgery, radiation therapy, or both. Chemotherapy has not been very useful in the treatment of cervical cancer.

In early cervical cancer, cure rates are exactly the same with either radical hysterectomy or radiation therapy. The choice of treatment is based on the size of the tumor on the cervix and evidence of the tumor extending into the vagina. Surgery can effectively remove small tumors. If a tumor is larger, radiation will probably be selected because it offers fewer problems than a big surgical procedure. In general women under 70 are more likely to have surgery, though this is not a hard and fast rule. Many older women are in good health and are able to tolerate surgery. The woman who has surgery needs to be in generally good condition. If she has other medical problems—for example, lung or heart problems—radiation therapy may be easier for her. If the woman has distorted pelvic anatomy, maybe from other earlier surgery, she may be better served by surgery since the success of radiation depends upon the even and predictable dispersal of radiation through tissues. A past history of pelvic inflammatory disease or inflammatory bowel disease increases

FIGO Staging and Classification of Cancer of the Cervix

Stage 0	Carcinoma in situ
Stage I	Carcinoma confined to the cervix
Stage IA	Carcinomas not visible to the eye but seen with microscope
Stage IA1	Minimal microscopic evidence of stromal invasion
Stage IA2	Carcinoma detected microscopically that can be measured, is not deeper than 5 mm and not larger horizontally than 7 mm
Stage IB	Lesions larger than in IA2
Stage II	Involves the upper vagina, but not the lower third of the vagina, or some invasion into the parametria—the outer layer of the uterus
Stage IIA	Involves the vagina but not the parametria
Stage IIB	Involves the inner layer parametria
Stage III	Involves the lower third of the vagina or extends to the pelvic walls; obstruction of one or both ureters without involvement of the vagina or parametria
Stage IIIA	Involves the lower third of the vagina but does not extend to the pelvic walls
Stage IIIB	Involves one or both parametria and extends to the pelvic walls
Stage IV	Extends outside of the reproductive tract
Stage IVA	Involves the bladder or rectum
Stage IVB	Cancer spread outside of the pelvis—for example, to lungs, bones, or liver

the risks of bowel problems with radiation therapy.

The advantages of radical hysterectomy over radiation therapy are:

- ♦ young women can keep ovarian function
- ♦ reproductive capacity and fertility can be maintained:

surgical techniques can move ovaries to a higher location outside a pelvic radiation therapy field.

♦ sexual function is less affected by surgical techniques
(though some might debate this)

♦ there is less chance of bowel complications

On the other hand, during surgery the vagina may be
shortened. Some of the most common complications of surgery
include bladder problems and formation of fistulas, or open pas-
sages in the tissue. The choice of surgery may not rule out the
need for radiation. During surgery, if lymph nodes are found to
contain cancer cells, postoperative radiation therapy will be
recommended.

Delayed complications of surgery do happen, though rarely.
For example, 3% of all women who have radical hysterectomies experience bladder problems. These include problems beginning urination, increased need to urinate, and decreased
bladder capacity. Most women do describe some decrease in
sensations related to the need to urinate that lasts up to six
months after surgery. Because of these problems, women are
more prone to urinary tract infections during the immediate
postoperative period.

In general, surgery is used for all cervical cancers Stage 0
through IIA. Women with Stage IIB and III are more likely to
be treated with radiation therapy.

Early stage cervical cancer includes cancers that have not
invaded the cervix deeper than 3 millimeters (3 mm is a little
less than ⅛ inch). Some experts call this "microinvasive carcinoma" or "microcarcinoma." Under a microscope, the pathologist needs to decide if the cancer cells have spread beyond the
3 mm limit and/or if there are cancer cells in nearby lymph
channels or blood vessels. Early stage disease also includes the
category called "early stromal invasion," in which a few isolated
cancer cells are seen with early signs of spread.

The woman with early stage disease can be treated with
conization (for women who may not be able to endure surgery
or those women who wish to preserve fertility) or simple hyster-

ectomy. If there is evidence of deeper spread, the woman might have a **radical hysterectomy**—removal of the uterus, upper third of the vagina, the parametrium on each side, and pelvic lymph nodes. Removal of the ovaries and fallopian tubes (**salpingo-oophorectomy**) might also be recommended, particularly if the woman is over 40 and is postmenopausal. Keep in mind that the cure rates are exactly the same for women who have hysterectomy and those who have other forms of treatment with radiation therapy.

In invasive carcinoma, the treatment will be much more aggressive. In Stage I and II, surgical removal of the cancer is possible. The surgery should include removal of the lymph nodes for any woman with cancer staged greater than IA1. Some surgeons prefer to do a vaginal hysterectomy and remove lymph nodes. Stage IB and IIA cancers can be treated with radical hysterectomy and one or two intracavitary radiation treatments. Lymph nodes removed during surgery are examined under a microscope to look for cancer cells. The presence or absence of tumor cells is an important predictor of the chance of cure. Women who have "positive" lymph nodes will usually need external radiation therapy to the entire pelvis after surgery. Radical surgery is indicated only for women who are considered healthy enough to go through surgery.

Women with disease staged at IIB and beyond are usually treated with high doses of external pelvic radiation and intracavitary radiation.

Radiation therapy

Early and advanced stage disease can be treated with radiation. Sometimes radiation will be used alone as the major treatment; other times, it will be used in combination with surgery. Radiation can be from an external radioactive source (a machine) or given internally by inserting radioactive substances directly into the area affected by cancer (brachytherapy). Brachytherapy, as discussed in Chapter 7, allows a high dose of radiation to target known cancer cells while sparing normal tissues that surround the cancer. Protection of the normal tissue reduces overall dam-

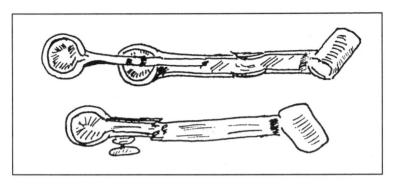

This pair of stainless steel **ovoids** is placed into the top of the vagina while a woman is under general anesthesia. The oval cylinders at the ends are hollow and hold a radioactive source. The ovoids rest against the cervix. After the applicators are in place, the vagina can be packed with gauze to prevent the applicators from being dislodged during the implant procedure.

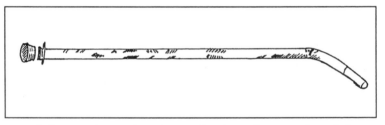

A hollow stainless steel **tandem** is placed into the uterus through the vagina. It is sometimes used with ovoids in the treatment of cervical, vaginal, and uterine cancers. A radioactive source like radium or cesium is placed inside the tandem during an afterloading procedure and left in place for a prescribed time period—usually 48–72 hours. The tandem is about 8–10 inches long and ¼ inch in diameter.

age, side effects, and complications. Intracavitary implants can be used before or after external radiation therapy.

Brachytherapy can be done either with a vaginal applicator or by placing small steel needles into the parametrium; these are "afterloaded" with seed-shaped bits of radioactive material. This interstitial (meaning "between tissues") method might be used when the cancer is advanced. Advanced cancer may have changed the vagina's size and shape, making the use of the applicators difficult or impossible. Interstitial implants do cause more problems and complications than other applicators. Still, interstitial therapy is being used more often and is under study in many cancer research centers.

Specific information about the implant procedure needs to be provided by the radiation oncologist and/or the radiation oncology nurse. Radiation therapy affects organs that lie in the path of the beam: side effects that occur soon after radiation therapy ends—and maybe even while treatment is in process— can include skin reactions, inflammation of the bladder, bowel, and rectum. Side effects that do not reveal themselves for 6–24 months after treatment has ended include vaginal changes (dryness, fibrosis, loss of ability to stretch), vaginal shrinkage (stenosis), and discomfort or pain with sexual intercourse.

The effects of radiation on sexual function depend on the body area included in the radiation field and the total dose of radiation used. Most sexual changes caused by radiation relate to the effects on ovaries and the vagina. When the ovaries are in the radiation treatment field in a premenopausal woman, ovarian function stops permanently and the woman will go into menopause. The symptoms and sexual changes in this woman will be similar to those of older women who go through menopause. She might experience hot flashes, mood swings, decreased lubrication of the vagina, and thinning of the vaginal tissues. Any of these symptoms can interfere with sexual function.

If the vagina is included in the radiation field, the vaginal canal shrinks and becomes rigid. The woman will have a loss of lubrication and vaginal sensation. To prevent these changes, a woman can take several actions, such as resuming sexual activity as soon as possible, and using a vaginal dilator with a water-soluble lubricant (more about these in Chapter 18).

Short-term side effects from radiation to the pelvic area can include diarrhea, nausea, vomiting, bladder irritation, weight loss, and fatigue. Any of these side effects can affect a woman's desire or physical ability to have sex.

ADVANCED AND RECURRENT CERVICAL CANCER

Cancer will recur or return in about one-third of all women with invasive cervical cancer. Most cervical cancers recur within the first two years after therapy. The exact location where the cancer recurs relates to the type of therapy initially used. After hysterectomy, about one-fourth of these cancers recur in the upper part of the vagina or the area where the cervix was located. After primary treatment with radiation therapy, recurrent cancers are most likely found in the cervix, the uterus, the upper vagina, and the pelvic wall. The most common signs and symptoms of recurrent disease include:

— weight loss

— leg swelling, often involving only one leg

— pain in the thigh or buttock area

— bloody vaginal discharge

— signs of blocked urinary tract

— cough

— chest pain

The prognosis for women with recurrent or advanced cervical cancer depends on where the cancer is found. The most favorable prognosis is for women with what is called "central" recurrence: cancer found in the pelvic area. The outlook is not so hopeful for women whose cancer is found in bone, lungs, liver, or other areas outside of the pelvis.

Radiation therapy for advanced cancer

When cancer comes back in areas outside the pelvis, radiation therapy can offer relief of symptoms, but not cure. Pain from bone metastases can be controlled by radiation. In some cancer treatment centers, external radiation is used when cancer recurs in the cervical area. These women are treated with a second full course of external radiation.

Chemotherapy for advanced cervical cancer

So far, chemotherapy for cervical cancer that has spread outside the pelvis has not been very effective. Some studies have reported a "good response" to some chemotherapy agents (mitomycin C, vincristine, bleomycin, doxorubicin, methyl CCNU, cisplatin), but a good response is not a lasting response: the cancer is not completely destroyed. Although some women did live longer, these studies usually do not report on the quality of life these women experienced during this "good response" time.

Surgery for advanced cervical cancer

For women with *only* central recurrence—no cancer found in areas outside of the pelvis—a major surgical procedure called **pelvic exenteration** may offer hope for cure.

The pelvic exenteration is a very extensive operation. It involves removing most or all the major organs in the pelvis in addition to those removed in the radical hysterectomy: the bladder, or rectum, or both, are also removed. Urine and stool then need to be "rerouted" to openings on the abdomen so that body wastes can still leave the body. The results of this type of surgery can have huge psychological affects. The woman who opts for this surgery must be emotionally stable and prepared to go through a long, difficult recovery process.

Nearly 10% of women who have pelvic exenteration die during or soon after the operation. Complications immediately after surgery are mostly caused by heart and lung problems. Infections affecting the pelvic wall cause severe problems too. Bowel complications can occur for a period of time starting right after surgery to as long as 18 months later. Urinary tract and kidney problems are likely to be lifelong issues. The surgery itself is lengthy: in one study, each woman's operation took over seven hours. Most women stayed in an intensive care unit for one to two weeks, and were in the hospital for between five and six weeks. Of these women, over one-third can be expected to live longer than five years after surgery. Despite all of the hardships and risks of pelvic exenteration, this radical and risky surgery may hold the only chance for cure. If pelvic exenteration is suggested, a woman must weigh her risks and what she hopes to achieve by having the surgery. She must have a very clear idea of what body changes will be involved with a urinary or bowel diversion—changes that will affect her for the rest of her life.

Hysterectomy

Hysterectomy is controversial. In the United States alone, nearly a million hysterectomies are performed each year, yet there are only a few *real* reasons to have a hysterectomy. Over 1,000 women die each year from complications after hysterectomy, and serious thought has to go into the choice. After a hysterectomy, many women describe drastic changes in their sexual response. For many women, removal of the uterus or womb is disturbing. These issues should be considered before a woman signs the consent form.

One reason hysterectomy has lost some favor of late is that younger women who still want to have children are being diagnosed more often with CIN. This increases the need for treatment that preserves a woman's childbearing capacity.

What kind of hysterectomy?

There are two ways to remove the uterus. In an **abdominal hysterectomy** the uterus is removed through an incision in the abdomen. In a **vaginal hysterectomy** the uterus is removed through the vagina. A surgeon *should* recommend an approach based on the reason for the operation and the easiest and safest approach. A vaginal hysterectomy leaves no visible scar and is recommended when there is no risk that the uterus is abnormally attached to the intestine or other structures, and when the uterus is small enough to be removed safely through the vagina. The abdominal approach should be used when there are more risks associated with a vaginal approach or when the surgeon needs to look closely at the other abdominal organs. Surgeons suggest that the vaginal hysterectomy requires more effort and more skill.

Hysterectomy operations are also categorized by what organs and structures are removed during the surgery. In a **radical hysterectomy**, the uterus, cervix, supporting ligaments and tissues, upper part of the vagina, and pelvic lymph nodes are removed. The ovaries and fallopian tubes might also be removed, but this is not part of the standard operation. A **simple hysterectomy** removes the uterus, and possibly the ovaries, fallopian tubes, and cervix. The doctor should explain the variations in hysterectomy: the exact details have much to do with the woman's future healthcare plans.

In his book *Women and Doctors*, which is highly critical of his peers, John M. Smith, M.D. outlines the following indications for hysterectomy:

1. Cancer of the uterus, fallopian tubes, or ovaries

2. Menstrual bleeding that does not respond to treatment and causes the woman to be anemic

3. Large, benign tumors of the uterus that block or will soon block the urinary tract, cause severe pain or uncontrollable bleeding, *and* cannot be treated or removed while leaving the uterus in place

4. Chronic pelvic inflammatory disease that causes pain and is not treatable by any other means

Noted surgical gynecologists Philip DiSaia, M.D. and William T. Creasman, M.D. have numerous medical journal papers and gynecologic oncology textbooks to their credit. In the most recent edition of their textbook, *Clinical Gynecologic Oncology* they advocate vaginal hysterectomy, for the most part, for women who have carcinoma in situ. They indicate that hysterectomy might be the treatment of choice for CIN in women who have completed childbearing and want permanent sterilization. They warn that removing the upper part of the vagina is *not* indicated in either CIN or carcinoma in situ.

Dr. Smith warns that "*any* other situation requires that you get some specific answers to a few questions, weigh the risk versus the benefits, and decide for yourself." Dr. Smith suggests that women facing a decision about hysterectomy should get the following information in order to make a good decision:

1. What *exactly* is wrong and what are all the possible treatment approaches?

2. What are the possible effects of doing nothing?

3. What complications and/or problems are connected with all possible treatments, including hysterectomy?

4. What are *all* the effects that any treatment, including hysterectomy, might have?

5. Is it necessary or recommended that the ovaries be removed?

If hysterectomy is a woman's choice, the bad effects—barring surgical complications—should not be serious. Menstrual periods will stop. Hormonal cycles will continue if ovaries are left in place, but there is no uterine lining to shed and bleed. There is no risk of pregnancy and no need for birth control measures. There will be no further risk of uterine or cervical cancer if all uterine and cervical tissues are removed. Estrogen replacement after menopause can be used without increasing the risk of uterine cancer.

Removing the ovaries, however, is another issue. Many surgeons recommend removing the ovaries, especially if the woman is close to or past menopause. Unless a premenopausal woman has a family history of ovarian cancer, most experts recommend that her normal ovaries *not* be removed. Removal of functioning ovaries puts a woman into "instant" menopause. Without the estrogen produced by ovaries, the woman is likely to have symptoms associated with menopause: hot flashes, mood swings, and decreased vaginal moisture. There is also evidence to suggest that small amounts of estrogen are produced by ovaries even after menopause and experts are not quite sure what function this estrogen has. All in all, the general advice is to avoid removing normal tissue.

Complications of hysterectomy

As with any major surgery, hysterectomy is not without risks, which must be weighed against its benefits. These risks can occur even when the surgeon performs the operation with great skill. Some relate to any surgery while others are specific to the area directly affected by the operation. For example, blood clots can form in the veins of the pelvis or legs when anyone is immobile for an extended period of time. These clots can break free and move to the lungs, causing sudden death. After surgery, hemorrhage or abnormal bleeding can occur which, if not dealt with quickly and successfully, can also result in death. Other general risks that can result in death include infection, anesthetic complications, reaction to drugs used, surgical mistakes, and administration of a wrong medication.

There are other risks that are not fatal but still cause serious problems. Fistulas—abnormal connections between organs —occur only rarely, but can be the result of surgical error, nutritional deficits, and previous radiation therapy to the abdomen. The most common fistula related to hysterectomy is a "vesico-vaginal" fistula (connecting the bladder and the vagina), resulting in passage of urine into the vagina. A fistula repair surgery is difficult and may not be successful. During hysterectomy, a ureter (the tube that carries urine from the kidney to the bladder) might be accidentally tied off or blocked. If this is not corrected, it can cause the loss of a kidney.

After surgery, a woman can expect some discomfort and tiredness. It is important that she knows what is normal and what is not. Very often, nurses offer preoperative teaching. They might work with the surgeon in an office setting, in a hospital, or surgery or gynecology clinic. The more a woman knows about what to expect during and after the surgery, the less anxious she is likely to be. Knowledge is a real source of power—one that every woman facing surgery can use. Information needed includes that related to any surgery, including information about what will be expected of the "patient" immediately after she awakens from the anesthetic. Many women are surprised at how much seems to be expected of them and are not prepared to take an active role in the healing process— at least not quite so soon. For these women, the surgical nurse seems almost like a villain, ready to inflict all kinds of torture! Indeed, women are often surprised that they will be up sitting in a bedside chair within a few hours of surgery. The routine coughing and deep breathing exercises might be painful or at least uncomfortable. To most women, it is hard to believe that they could be expected to go home after a mere three to five days!

Right after any operation, the major priorities for surgical nurses include the effective function of their patient's lungs, keeping the incision free of infection, keeping the normal skin in good condition, allowing the intestines and urinary system to return to normal, and helping the patient to be reasonably comfortable. Each of these nursing priorities, involves the active cooperation of the woman. These activities need to be discussed *before* the operation (see Questions to Ask Your Physician later in this chapter).

Overall, the death rate from hysterectomy is about 12 out of 10,000 operations. This might not seem a huge risk—unless you or the woman you care for is one of those 12. There is no accurate predictor of any of these complications. In some cases, a hysterectomy may be the best answer for a woman's gynecologic problem. The horror is that at least a few of these 12 women did not need to have a hysterectomy. The bottom line is that each woman needs to make sure she fully understands the risks and benefits of whatever treatment option she selects.

Sexuality issues after hysterectomy

Changes in sexual behavior after hysterectomy have not been well-documented. Sexual behavior includes both sexual function and sexual desire. Of all the phases of sexual activity, sexual desire is the least understood. In women who have had cervical cancer, almost half describe some degree of disruption in what had been their normal sexual behavior. In one study, one in three reported changes in desire, excitement, and orgasm.

One in three women also reported pain or discomfort with sexual intercourse. It is known that the uterus plays an important role in the stages of the female sexual response, so it is likely that a woman can expect some changes following hysterectomy. Exact changes have not been fully described but almost half of women who have hysterectomy in which the ovaries are also removed describe a decreased sexual response, and a reduced desire for and frequency of intercourse. On the other hand, some women became sexually active, or resumed sexual activity after treatment. A decrease in sexual response might be caused by changes in hormone production (when ovarian hormones are no longer present) and removal of the cervix and uterus that trigger orgasm for some women. Many woman describe their orgasm as "different"—not better or worse—than it was before hysterectomy. Most women describe a temporary loss of sexual desire for anywhere up to six months after treatment, and report that desire returns during the first year.

Many women report that pain with intercourse is a problem. Removing the upper part of the vagina and vaginal shortening causes pain for some women.

Both body image and self-esteem are greatly affected by diagnosis and treatment for a gynecologic cancer. Often, women fear rejection, isolation, and unacceptability. Women with a new diagnosis of gynecologic cancer describe a decrease in both sexual activity and sexual satisfaction. Sometimes the woman's sexual partner has fears or misconceptions about the cancer and its treatment.

Many women who believe their sexual adjustment after surgery is good credit their success to supportive sexual partners. A second major factor in successful adjustment is the ability to get accurate information about what to expect after surgery. A woman and her partner can better adjust to changes by exploring their feelings about sexual expression and satisfaction. It is important that the woman (and her partner) have a clear understanding of what her sexual functioning can be during and after therapy. Many women find that counseling that includes sexual information is a crucial part of successful adjustment.

QUESTIONS TO ASK YOUR PHYSICIAN

1. How long will I need to stay in the hospital or clinic?

2. How long can I expect to be off work?

3. What activities should I do and which activities should I avoid?

4. Should I expect bowel function changes, for how long, and what treatment is needed?

5. Should I expect urinary function changes, for how long, and what treatment is needed?

6. Regarding follow-up care:
   — How often do I need pelvic exams and Pap smears?
   — What is the plan and schedule for follow-up appointments?
   — Are there self-care activities to help prevent complications? (For example: signs and symptoms of infection, who to call, how to avoid infection, etc.)
   — What medications will be needed, on what schedule, and what are the side effects?
   — Will I need other treatment modalities after surgery? (for example, radiation therapy)
   — What are signs and symptoms of recurrent disease that must be reported to the doctor or nurse?

7. What changes in sexual function can I expect?

8. Are there other lifestyle changes I need to know about?
   — Use of barrier-type birth control devices (diaphragm or condom)
   — Quitting smoking

9. What and where are the community resources to help meet the demands of treatment and survivorship?

It is most important that each woman facing treatment—whether it is a hysterectomy or another treatment option—have a very clear understanding about what is expected of her:

what her "job" is in the treatment process versus what is the job of the surgeon, the nurse, and any other member of the healthcare team.

❖   ❖   ❖

Hope for the future includes the creation of treatment programs that combine surgery, radiation, and chemotherapy. Drugs being tested include hydroxyurea and cisplatin used with radiation therapy. Early research results hold promise for more successful treatment.

Pamela Haylock

Chapter 18

❖

Cancer of the Vagina

The vagina connects the cervix and the vulva. It is the passage-way for fluid to leave the body during menstrual periods, the entry for sperm to reach an egg to create a baby, and the birth canal through which a baby travels during a normal vaginal delivery.

Cancer of the vagina is one of the rarest cancers in the human body. It is strange, but cancers affect the tissues on either side of the vagina—the cervix and the vulva—much more often than the vaginal tissues. It is more common for cancers to start in the cervix and spread down to the upper part of the vagina. Sometimes cancers that started in the uterus, urethra, ovary, bladder, and rectum spread to the vagina. Primary cancer of the vagina accounts for only about 2% of all gynecologic cancers.

Most vaginal cancers occur in women 50–70 years of age. The exception is for the even more rare clear cell adenocarci-noma, which usually occurs in women under 20.

Most (95%) of vaginal cancers develop from the epithelial or skinlike tissues and are squamous cell carcinoma. Other cells in the vagina can develop other types of cancer—melanoma, sarcoma, and adenocarcinoma.

RISK FACTORS

The cause of squamous cell carcinoma of the vagina is not known. Some experts suspect that fluids collect in the upper part of the vagina and cause irritation that eventually leads to cancer. Other factors that might make a woman more likely to develop squamous cell carcinoma of the vagina include a past history of syphilis, use of a vaginal pessary, prolapse of the vaginal wall, and other factors that irritate the vaginal wall.

Clear cell adenocarcinoma of the vagina is linked to *in utero* exposure to the hormone diethylstilbestrol (DES). Cancers related to DES exposure make up about 6–7% of all primary vaginal cancers. About 1 in 1,000 women exposed to DES *in utero* go on to develop vaginal adenocarcinoma (discussed later in this chapter).

It is guessed that some factors that cause cancer of the cervix might also cause cancer of the vagina, including the human papillomavirus (HPV). Women who have had radiation therapy for a previous cervical cancer may be at higher risk to develop a second gynecologic cancer. After hysterectomy, many women fail to have regular gynecologic exams, which allows a vaginal cancer to go undetected. Because this disease is so rare, proving these theories will be difficult.

PREVENTION

Without knowing the true cause of primary vaginal cancer, preventive care is geared toward finding abnormalities early. The Pap smear is the most effective method of finding vaginal cancers before symptoms develop. For this reason, it should still be used for the woman who has had a hysterectomy. Vaginal cancer seems to grow slowly, so most experts suggest that adequate screening consists of Pap smears every 2–3 three years. If there are other risk factors, she should be screened more frequently.

BENIGN VAGINAL DISEASE

Carcinoma in situ, also called **Vaginal Intraepithelial Neoplasia (VAIN),** is less common than cervical and vulvar intraepithelial neoplasia and accounts for only 0.4% of all gynecologic cancers, but its incidence is increasing. VAIN is thought to be a precancerous condition.

Most of the time, a woman with VAIN will not have symptoms; occasionally she may have spotting after sexual intercourse. Routine Pap smears are crucial to finding VAIN early. After a Pap smear, vaginal colposcopy and biopsy establish the diagnosis. In ½–⅔ of women with VAIN, precancerous cells or actual cancer cells can be found in another part of the lower genital tract (cervix or vulva). Additional tests need to be done to look for other abnormalities.

Treatment for benign vaginal disease

Surgical removal of the affected area has been the standard treatment for VAIN. For many women, curative treatment can be done during the biopsy. If there are several areas affected, partial or total removal of the vagina might be needed. Some surgeons try to create a new vagina during this surgery, but this has mixed reviews. Many women describe uncomfortable or painful sexual intercourse and other problems with sexual function after surgery.

Radiation has been used, but the structure of the vagina makes even distribution of the radiation difficult. Radiation can cause vaginal fibrosis—thickening and loss of ability to stretch—and sometimes the formation of fistulae between the vagina, rectum, and/or urethra.

Chemotherapy has been used directly in the vagina with 5-fluorouracil (5-FU). It seems to yield high cure rates with few side effects. Intravaginal chemotherapy can cause burning and shedding of the vaginal lining that is serious enough to keep this treatment from getting widespread approval. There has been no agreement on the optimal dose, length of treatment, or method of application.

The use of the laser is gaining acceptance in the treatment of VAIN. Pain and bleeding are the major problems associated with laser therapy, but these seem to be minimal. Healing is good and sexual function is not altered.

Radiation therapy through intravaginal applicators is used

in some treatment centers, but some experts do not advocate this treatment and warn that its use results in recurrence more often than other treatment methods. The vaginal fibrosis and stenosis that can result from the treatment may make follow-up examination difficult.

VAGINAL CANCER

Most vaginal cancers do not cause symptoms. However, signs of vaginal cancer include feeling the need to strain during urination or bowel movements (tenesmus), feelings of having to urinate often, pain with urination, bladder pain, vaginal discharge, or painless bleeding, especially after sexual intercourse. Some women might have a foul-smelling vaginal discharge.

Diagnosis and staging

After initial diagnosis is made through Pap smear, colposcopy, biopsy, and other diagnostic tests are needed to determine the extent of the cancer. The tests, in addition to the history and physical, include chest X-ray, intravenous pyelogram (IVP), cystoscopy, and proctosigmoidoscopy. Some doctors will also perform a lymphangiogram, in which the pelvic lymph system is injected with a dye and x-rayed, but this is commonly replaced by MRIs. A barium enema is especially needed if the woman has had a recent episode of diverticulitis, since that will be a factor in planning for radiation therapy. The chart on page 320 outlines the FIGO stages of vaginal cancer.

TREATMENT

Like all cancer treatment decisions, treatment recommendations will be based on the stage, size, and location of the cancer. Other specific factors include the presence or absence of the uterus and whether or not the woman has had radiation therapy to the pelvis.

FIGO Staging System for Vaginal Cancer

Stage	Characteristics
Stage 0	Intraepithelial carcinoma
Stage I	Cancer limited to the vaginal lining
Stage II	Cancer involves the tissue beneath the lining but does not extend to the pelvic wall
Stage III	Cancer extends onto the pelvic wall or pubic symphysis (pubic bone)
Stage IV	Cancer extends beyond the pelvis and involves the bladder or rectum

Historically, surgery has been the major treatment offered to women with vaginal cancer. Surgical choices vary from limited, local procedures to extensive, complicated operations:

♦ **Laser surgery:** uses laser to destroy cancer cells in Stage 0

♦ **Wide local excision:** removes the cancer and some of the tissue around it. Skin grafts may be needed to repair the vagina.

♦ **Vaginectomy:** removes the entire vagina. It is used when the cancer has spread outside the vagina. It can be combined with radical hysterectomy. Lymph nodes in the pelvis are also likely to be removed.

♦ **Pelvic Exenteration:** if the cancer has spread to other pelvic organs—the bladder and/or rectum—the lower colon, rectum, bladder, cervix, uterus, and vagina can be removed.

In many of these surgical procedures, skin grafts can be used to make an artificial vagina.

More and more often, radiation therapy is the treatment of choice for most vaginal cancers. Cancers of the upper part of the vagina in a woman who has a uterus can be treated with external radiation therapy. After external radiation is completed, a "boost" or extra dosage directed at the tumor with an intravaginal applicator is sometimes recommended. The intravaginal radiation can be done in two separate procedures spaced about two weeks apart.

If the woman has had her uterus removed, treatment plans can consist of intravaginal radiation therapy, external pelvic radiation therapy, and interstitial implants. A combined surgical procedure and radiation therapy called an "open implant" is used in some cancer centers. During a laparotomy—abdominal incision to provide access to the inside of the pelvis—radioactive needles are placed into the affected area. Other treatment plans combine both external and interstitial radiation therapy.

Treatment for adenocarcinoma

Treatment recommendations for adenocarcinoma are different than those for squamous cell carcinoma. The differences are based on what is known about the natural history of the disease. Even for early Stage I cancer, surgery is fairly extensive, involving total radical vaginectomy, hysterectomy, and lymph node

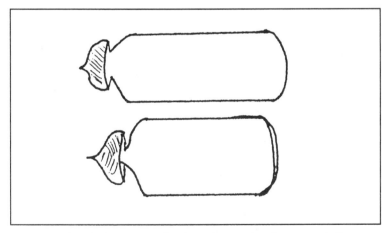

Vaginal cylinders *are made of stainless steel or lucite, are hollow, and hold a radioactive source. Some vaginal cylinders have lead shielding that protects certain parts of the vagina from radiation exposure. They are made in different shapes and sizes to conform to different vaginal contours.*

dissection. Some women may opt for combined intracavitary, interstitial, and external radiation instead. For other women, a combination of surgery (wide local excision), lymph node dissection and sampling, and interstitial therapy is possible. For later, more advanced stages, combinations of surgery and/or interstitial, intracavitary, and external radiation are given.

RECURRENT VAGINAL CANCER

If vaginal cancer does recur, it is most likely to reappear in the pelvic area and will do so within two years of initial therapy. Pelvic exenteration is the treatment of choice in recurrent disease, but it occurs so infrequently that not much is written about the surgery or its outcomes. Radiation therapy may also be used. Chemotherapy has not been effective in the treatment of vaginal cancer, or at least, there is not enough data to make clear recommendations for its use.

AFTER TREATMENT

Treatment can have side effects. Fistulae and damage to the normal vaginal tissues can be late side effects of radiation therapy. Vaginal fibrosis is also an effect of radiation therapy. Just as in other procedures that surgically disrupt lymph and blood flow, lymphedema can be a serious complication following surgery. Obviously, the extensive surgical procedures, hysterectomy and pelvic exenteration, will have long-lasting and in some cases, permanent consequences.

Vaginal reconstruction—creation of a new vagina—is done with skin and muscle flaps. Whole sections of skin and underlying muscle, usually from the inner thigh, are cut away and swung upward to create a new vagina. A tube is constructed and inverted into the pelvic cavity to replace the original vagina. Right after surgery, the new vagina will be packed with sterile gauze. Vaginal molds and special supporters called "stents" may be worn for several weeks during the healing process. Vaginal dilators may be used as soon as the incisions have healed. Estrogen cream inserted into the vagina is used to increase blood vessel formation and increase the flexibility of the vagina. Skin grafts need special care and the newly created vagina may require daily vinegar douching. Sexual intercourse can resume in about 6–8 weeks, and a water-soluble lubricant should be used. Most women report that it takes up to a year or longer to achieve somewhat normal vaginal function, but that sexual satisfaction and orgasm are possible with vaginal grafts.

The sexuality issues, body image problems, and emotional responses to treatment are similar to those discussed in the previous chapter on cervical cancer, and the following chapter on vulvar cancer.

Post-treatment follow-up consists of regular Pap smears, pelvic examinations with colposcopy, and other exams as needed.

QUESTIONS TO ASK YOUR PHYSICIAN

1. What surgical procedure will be used in treatment and what will be the short-term effects? What are the risks? What are the alternatives? Will there be skin grafts? What activities can I do and what are my limits? What wound care will I need to do for myself? How long should healing take? What can I do to speed healing?

2. Should I plan for outside help when I get home? What resources are available to me? (home care nurses, home aides, physical therapy, etc.)

3. What surgical procedure will be used and what are the expected long-term effects? Should I expect changes in urinary function? Should I expect changes in sensations from my genitals? Will my clitoris be preserved? What about other aspects of sexual function—when can I resume sexual activity? Should I use vaginal dilators? How do I use vaginal dilators? Where can I get one?

4. What is my chance for developing lymphedema? Will I have lymph node dissection? What can the surgeon do to lessen my chance of developing lymphedema? What can I do to decrease my chances?

5. What are the local resources for counseling for me and my husband or lover?

6. Will I have radiation therapy? Will it be external, intracavitary, or interstitial? When will this be scheduled and how many treatments will I have? If I have intracavitary or interstitial radiation, how long will I stay in the hospital?

7. What side effects can I expect from the radiation therapy? Are there things I can do to decrease the chances of side effects or at least minimize the side effects?

8. What is the plan for after-treatment checkups and follow-up appointments for each specialist involved?

9. Will I need referrals to physical therapy or other rehabilitation services? If not, why?

DES (DIETHYLSTILBESTROL)

Diethylstilbestrol was the first synthetic estrogen, developed in England in 1938. Many women who were exposed to diethylstilbestrol in the womb during the 1940s and 1950s have been found to have a rare kind of cancer twenty years later. The Eli Lilly drug company produced and marketed DES as a drug with effects similar to those of naturally occurring feminine hormones. When the drug was first used for women, there had been no studies of its long-term effects. Historically, it has been prescribed:

1. As hormone replacement therapy for women in menopause or women whose ovaries had been removed or never developed

2. For prevention of postpartum breast engorgement in mothers who did not want to breastfeed their infants

3. For the treatment of prostate cancer in men

4. For the treatment of breast cancer

5. For prevention of miscarriage

The 1993 *Physicians' Desk Reference* lists only two current indications for the use of diethylstilbestrol:

1. Treatment of advanced breast cancer (palliation only)

2. Treatment of prostate cancer (palliation only)

A report published in the *American Journal of Obstetrics and Gynecology* in 1948 indicated that DES might prevent miscarriage. It was based on a study of hundreds of pregnancies dating back to 1943 in which mothers thought to be in danger of miscarriage were given DES. From there, more studies led researchers to believe that normal pregnancies could be made "more normal" and could produce healthier, more "rugged" babies. As a result, even women who were not necessarily at risk for miscarriage were given DES. Prescription of DES continued unchecked until 1971, when the FDA issued a warning that DES was contraindicated in pregnancy. Even after the FDA warning, many doctors continued to prescribe DES during pregnancy and *it is still not banned*. A *Wall Street Journal* report (December 23, 1975) documented 11,000 prescriptions written in 1974 for pregnant women. Use of DES continued until 1975 in England and the Netherlands, 1977 in France, 1981 in Spain and Italy, and 1983 in Hungary. The FDA finally acknowledged that DES could cause cancer in 1975, when other hormones were linked to cancer.

The DES Cancer Network estimates that approximately 4.8 million American children born between 1943 and 1970 were exposed to DES *in utero*. And keep in mind, 4.8 million mothers were exposed as well.

In 1966, a 15-year-old girl was found to have a rare cancer of the vagina. This type of cancer, called "clear cell adenocarcinoma" was so rare that only a few cases were ever reported in all of the medical literature, and never in one so young. Over the next few years, more young women were found to have this same type of cancer. The common thread in each case was that the mothers of the girls had all taken DES during pregnancy.

The rest of the DES story is a testament to government foul-ups and misguided medical research. Despite the fact that DES had been a known carcinogen since 1940, it was promoted as a useful drug. Despite the reported relationship between DES and clear cell adenocarcinoma, it continued to be prescribed for pregnant women. Despite studies showing that DES caused more stillbirths, doctors continued to give the drug to pregnant women. Despite the fact that the FDA had received information about the harmful effects of DES by 1971, the drug was not restricted. Recommendations to doctors to discontinue use of DES during pregnancy and to notify all women who had used the drug were finally published in 1974. *And still, despite these recommendations, many doctors continued to prescribe DES during pregnancy.*

DES has also been used as a "morning-after pill"—a pill designed to prevent a pregnancy after unprotected sex. The only problem is the "morning-after pill" did not always work, and many women who took it became and remained pregnant while using high doses of DES during crucial fetal development.

For a period of 20–30 years, nearly every American woman who chose not to breastfeed was given DES (or other types of hormones) for several days after birth to "dry up" her breast milk. This use declined after 1978 following an FDA recommendation.

It is impossible to know exactly how many women took DES, how much DES they were given, and the exact timeframe of the exposure. The worst time to have been exposed to DES (in terms of *in utero* exposure) was during the first three months of a pregnancy. It is during this time, the first trimester, that the fetus's reproductive system is forming. Total dose ranges varied widely. Many women were not provided information about drugs they were given during pregnancy. Many were told they were being given vitamins. For others, dose determinations cannot be made because old medical records are not available or have been destroyed. Some doctors fear legal action and are not willing to come forth with information about patients for whom DES was prescribed.

The DES-exposed population includes:

◆ DES mothers

◆ DES daughters

◆ DES sons

◆ DES daughters who have had clear cell cancer

◆ Third generation children (children of DES-exposed offspring)   (Braun, 1991)

The women who took DES—the DES mothers—have a higher risk for breast cancer than women who have not taken DES.

Clear cell cancer is still being diagnosed in women whose mothers took DES. In 1991, there were at least five new cases—one in a 41-year-old woman. In the United States, over 600 women have been diagnosed with clear cell cancer to date. The youngest was 7, but most clear cell cancers occur between midteens and mid-20s. The upper age limit for the development of this cancer is not known. DES daughters have a higher rate of cervical and vaginal dysplasia, and carcinoma in situ (at least double the rate) than nonexposed women.

In utero exposure to DES causes birth defects, usually involving the reproductive tract. These defects can be cell abnormalities and malformations, resulting in changes in uterine tissue, blocked fallopian tubes, malformed uterus, incompetent cervix, and inability to ovulate. DES daughters who do become pregnant have a greater risk for tubal pregnancy, miscarriage or stillbirth, and premature labor and delivery. Premature babies are at risk for any of the problems encountered in premature delivery. In babies born to these mothers, the effects of DES extend to a third generation.

The limited research that has been conducted on DES sons has shown relatively few problems. Still, DES sons do have more reproductive tract abnormalities than sons who were not exposed. Abnormalities vary in severity, but can include malfunction of the genitals, benign cysts inside the scrotal sacs, malformation of the penis, sterility due to low sperm count, and testicular problems.

Everyone who has been exposed to DES is likely to have profound emotional effects. DES mothers live with tremendous guilt. DES sons and daughters live with the need for frequent medical examinations, knowledge of abnormalities and deformities, fear of developing cancer, and concerns about having a child who might be another victim of DES exposure.

By now, most DES daughters (and sons) in the United States are between 20 and 45 years old, with the majority in their mid-30s. It is estimated that 1 in every 1,000 DES daughters will develop a clear cell adenocarcinoma. The good news is that the annual increase in the occurrence of DES-related clear cell adenocarcinoma that started 20 years ago began decreasing in the late 1980s. Also, the survival rate is actually better than the survival rates for some other gynecologic cancers, probably a result of the close observation of women known to have been exposed.

So, in the 1990s and beyond, how can women best meet their healthcare needs? First, women need to know if they have been exposed to DES. Ask your mother, if you can, if she was given DES during her pregnancy with you. If she does not know, but perhaps was thought to be at risk for miscarriage, did she take any medication to prevent the miscarriage? If there is any suspicion, it should be discussed with a gynecologist who can include this information with a complete history and physical examination as well as follow-up exams.

The DES daughter should have a gynecologic examination yearly starting at age 14 *or* when she starts to menstruate, whichever comes first. The purpose of early and regular exams is to detect abnormalities and cancer at earlier stages. Exams before puberty are not usually recommended, but might be needed if a young girl develops abnormal bleeding or discharge. In this case, the doctor might wish to perform the examination while the girl is under anesthesia or at least heavily sedated.

Mothers can teach their daughters to use tampons during their periods which will stretch the vagina and make examinations easier for both the doctor and the young girl. The annual exams should include:

♦ visual inspection of the cervix and vagina

♦ digital examination of the vagina

♦ colposcopic examination on the first examination

♦ Pap smear from the cervical os and the walls of the upper part of the vagina

♦ colposcopy exam of suspicious areas

♦ biopsy of suspicious areas

♦ bimanual examination of the vagina and rectum

♦ breast examination and mammography

(DiSaia and Creasman, 1989)

Treatment for abnormal, noncancerous findings are varied and there is no standard recommendation. Some doctors prescribe contraceptive jellies and foams that will lower the vaginal pH and promote normal growth of the mucous membrane. Progesterone has also been used in the vagina for therapy. Neither of these approaches is supported by published studies. In most cases, the abnormalities disappear on their own and no therapy is needed.

The DES Registry in the United States collects information about exposed daughters who have gotten clear cell carcinoma. Studies were conducted at the University of Chicago beginning in 1951 and follow-up on these women is still being done. There is no registry in the United States that collects data on exposed mothers or their healthy sons and daughters. Registries do exist to some extent in The Netherlands, France, and Australia. However, there is a real possibility that funding for DES-related research will dry up. DES Action, a consumer group, and The Herbst Registry advocate continued research into the effects of DES exposure. During 1991 hearings before the National Institutes of Health Office of Research on Women's Health, the spokeswoman for the DES Cancer Network and DES Action USA stressed the continued research needs relating to DES. Further research is imperative to resolve lingering questions:

- ◆ What is the effect of the dose of DES given? (There were wide geographic variations in dosage given to pregnant women.)

- ◆ What other long-term effects will occur?

- ◆ What is the best way to treat people who get cancers associated with DES exposure?

- ◆ What effect will menopause have on exposed mothers and daughters?

An April 1992 consensus conference was sponsored by the National Cancer Institute that included representatives from several National Institute of Health divisions as well as DES Action. The purpose of the conference was to review data and encourage further research. Funding for new research was promised, but will depend on national budget priorities. Representative Louise Slaughter (D-NY) introduced federal legislation directing NIH to study health problems relating to DES exposure and to authorize appropriate funding. The NIH plans to issue a full report of the workshop in late 1992.

Meanwhile, DES Action continues to advocate on behalf of people affected by DES exposure. It offers information and referral services, as well as both informational publications and a quarterly newsletter. DES Action is affiliated with the DES Cancer Network, a support group that offers meetings, telephone counseling, and a newsletter, and these organizations have affiliates in 22 states. For more information contact:

DES Action   (510) 465-4011
1615 Broadway, Suite 510, Oakland CA 94612

DES Cancer Network   (716) 473-6119
Box 10185, Rochester NY 14610

Laboratory studies demonstrate that the effects of DES continue throughout the life span of those exposed. Since most of the DES daughters and sons are not yet middle-aged, it is entirely possible that the age with the greatest health hazards has not yet arrived.

Pamela Haylock

Chapter 19

❖

Cancer of the Vulva

The vulva is the outside skin or external part of a woman's vagina. It extends from the pubic mound to the rectal opening and surrounds the urethra, clitoris, and vaginal opening.

Cancer of the vulva is rare and accounts for only 4% of all gynecologic cancers and 1% of all cancers in women. Vulvar cancer occurs most often in women after menopause (85%), though it is becoming a little more common in women under 40. It appears most often in women during their mid-60s. In most Western countries, about half of all vulvar cancers are found when they are quite small (less than about ¾ inch or 2 cm in diameter) and are very curable. Routine self-examination of the vulva can increase a woman's chance of finding a cancer early.

RISK FACTORS

Little is known for certain about potential risk factors for vulvar cancer, though there are some factors that are at least suspect. It is possible that cancer of the vulva is related to sexually transmitted diseases, including condyloma and human papillomavirus (HPV). A history of other gynecologic cancers places a woman at an increased risk for vulvar cancer. Nearly a third of all women who are diagnosed with vulvar cancer had in situ or squamous cancer of the cervix at least five years earlier. A history of inflammation of the vulva with itching and burning sensations and shrinkage and thickening of vulvar tissues (leuk-oplakia) increases the chance of developing vulvar cancer.

Smoking and drinking more than two cups of coffee a day are also risk factors. Women who work as maids or in laundries, cleaning, or other garment services also have an increased risk for vulvar cancer, as do very overweight women. Some experts guess that in obese women, moisture and warmth in the genital area may relate to the development of this cancer.

Personal hygiene involving the genital area has been thought to be related to vulvitis and vulvar cancer for some time, but this has not been scientifically proven.

PREVENTION

The lack of a clear cause-and-effect relationship between any of the risk factors and the development of vulvar cancer makes hard and fast recommendations for preventive care impossible. Infection with HPV is the most seriously considered factor, so preventing infection with the virus by using condoms or limiting the number of sexual partners is one preventive action any woman could consider. Using coffee in moderation and quitting smoking should be considered too. Other preventive measures involve good hygiene of the vulva including the following suggestions:

- ◆ wipe from front to back after urination or a bowel movement

- ◆ Use white, unscented toilet tissue

- ◆ wear white panties or pantyhose with 100% cotton crotch; avoid girdles

- ◆ avoid wearing tight jeans or slacks

- ◆ use mild detergent to wash clothes and rinse clothing well; avoid excessive bleach

- ◆ sleep without panties to allow air to reach vulva

- ◆ use mild unscented soap for bathing

- ◆ avoid using "feminine hygiene products"—sprays, wipes, deodorizers

- ◆ avoid scented tampons, sanitary pads, and panty liners

(Sendella, 1987)

Other than these preventive measures, the best action a woman can take is to know early warning signs and use regular vulvar self-examination so that early diagnosis gives her the best chance for cure.

A woman should perform vulvar self-examination once each month. During the self-exam, she grows familiar with the appearance of her vulva and can watch for changes and warning signs. Then she can consult her doctor or nurse practitioner if she notices a change.

BENIGN VULVAR DISEASE

Several noncancerous conditions can affect the vulva. They include **lichen sclerosis, squamous cell hyperplasia** (formerly called hyperplastic dystrophy), **Paget's disease** of the vulva, and **vulvar intraepithelia neoplasia.**

Vulvar intraepithelial neoplasia (VIN), formerly known as Bowen's Disease, may be a precancerous problem. Like cervical intraepithelial neoplasia, VIN is also classified as carcinoma in situ. Herpes simplex virus type II and HPV are viruses suspected of starting the mutation process that leads to cancer. When the immune system is compromised, women are thought to be more susceptible to the carcinogenic effects of viral infections.

Careful visual examination of the vulva during a routine gynecologic exam is a good screening method for VIN. If abnormal areas are noted, a biopsy with or without colposcopy is needed. A biopsy that removes enough tissue must be done and will most likely require local anesthesia. A Pap smear and

VULVAR SELF-EXAMINATION

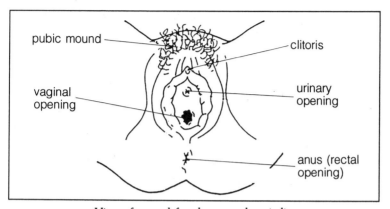

View of normal female external genitalia

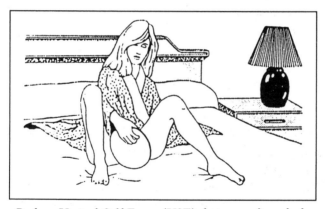

Perform **Vaginal Self-Exam (VSE)** *during or after a bath: use a mirror to make viewing easier; a flashlight can help you see a certain area more clearly*

(this series of illustrations—on pages 335, 336, and 337—reprinted from the Oncology Nursing Forum with permission from the Oncology Nursing Press, Inc. Sandella, Judy. Vulvar Self Examination (VSE). Oncology Nursing Forum 14(6):71–73, 1987.

examination of the cervix and vagina with colposcopy are important to include in the exam because of the increased chances of other gynecologic cancers with VIN.

VULVAR SELF-EXAMINATION (Continued)

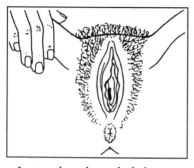

Inspect the vulva to look for any warning signs: are both sides alike?

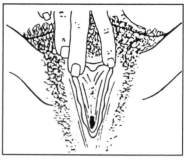

Push back the cover of the clitoris

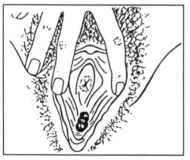

Separate the lips of the labia with your fingers and examine the inner parts: the urinary opening, the vagina, and the skin between the vagina and the anus

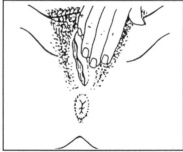

Feel the vulva for lumps or thickening; press all the areas of the vulva with the flat part of your fingers

Treatment for vulvar intraepithelial neoplasia

Treatment recommendations for vulvar intraepithelial neoplasia are based on the extent and location of the disease. If the VIN is seen in only one area and is thought to be minimal, surgical removal of the abnormal area is the likely treatment. It allows all the abnormal tissues to be assessed under the microscope. Surgical excision performed by a competent surgeon will result in a fast, complete return to normal vulvar function and appearance. Topical chemotherapy using 5-fluorouracil (5-FU)

VULVAR SELF-EXAMINATION (Contiued)

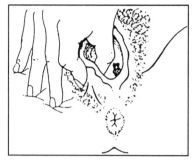

Circle the vaginal opening with your thumb and index finger

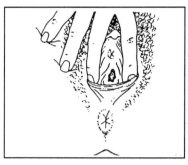

Compress the tissue; it should be soft, slightly moist, and not tender

used to be a common treatment for VIN, but it is no longer used because it causes large, painful, skin sores.

Cryosurgery has been used, but has mostly been replaced by laser surgery. Healing after cryosurgery on the vulva is slow and the woman goes through severe pain. Laser surgery has high cure rates, can be done under general anesthesia, and requires only a short hospital stay. The pain is most severe 4–5 days after laser surgery. Warm, soaking, cleansing baths (Sitz baths), oral pain pills, and complete pelvic rest (no douches, no sex, no tampons) will increase comfort and help the healing processes.

Follow-up for the first two years after therapy consists of colposcopy and a Pap smear after 3–4 months, then at least every six months if the examination is normal.

For VIN that involves several areas of the vulva, vulvectomy used to be the treatment of choice. In 1968 surgeons started using a procedure called the "skinning vulvectomy," which offers high cure rates and a more normal postoperative appearance. This procedure involves the surgical removal of vulvar skin and replacement with a skin graft. The procedure can be done so that the clitoris is saved. Clearly, a skilled surgeon is needed to perform this operation. The woman needs to understand that she will be confined to bed rest for some time after surgery to allow the skin grafts to heal.

Today a surgeon might recommend laser vulvectomy instead of the skinning vulvectomy. The laser vulvectomy does the vulvectomy without the need for skin grafts, and it can be an outpatient procedure. The cure rate and the appearance are similar to the skinning vulvectomy with fewer postoperative problems.

Interferon is being used in several experimental treatments for VIN. It seems to be especially useful in treating VIN that is associated with HPV infection.

VULVAR CANCER

Signs and symptoms of vulvar cancer include:

- ◆ constant itching of the vulva

- ◆ change of color in the skin of the vulva

- ◆ burning sensation in the vulva during urination

- ◆ change in a mole or birthmark on the vagina

- ◆ a lump or mass on the vulva—could be a wartlike lump, or fleshy, white patches

In many cases of vulvar cancer a woman has delayed getting medical attention or has been treated for vulvar problems not properly diagnosed as cancer. For these women it is lucky that vulvar cancer grows slowly and usually does not spread until the disease is quite advanced. Without any treatment, cancer of the vulva usually spreads to nearby organs (vagina, urethra, and anus) or through the lymph channels to lymph nodes in the groin and pelvis.

DIAGNOSIS

Diagnosis of vulvar cancer is made after examination of biopsied tissues. Cystoscopy, proctoscopy, intravenous urography, and X-rays of the lungs and bones are used for staging purposes. Biopsy can confirm presence of bladder or rectal involvement.

Half of all vulvar cancers are found on the labia majora, though they can appear on the labia minora (15–20%), clitoris, Bartholin's glands, and perineum—the space between the vagina and the rectum. The most common cell type (nearly 90%) is squamous cell carcinoma, but melanoma, sarcoma, and basal cell cancers can also occur.

TREATMENT OF VULVAR CANCER

The small or early vulvar cancers that make up 50% of all vulvar cancers are usually treated with surgery. More advanced cancer is most often treated with a combination of surgery and external radiation therapy. Surgery is the most common treatment used in all stages of cancer of the vulva. It can be a relatively mild operation in which only the tumor and the area immediately surrounding it are removed or it can be extensive and remove the vulva and other organs that have become involved with cancer. The surgical procedures used for vulvar cancer are:

- ◆ Wide local excision: removes the cancer and some of the normal tissue around it; can be done in a doctor's office or outpatient surgery department

- ◆ Radical local excision: removes the cancer and a larger area of normal tissue around the tumor, lymph nodes may also be removed

- ◆ Skinning vulvectomy: removes the skin of the vulva that contains the cancer

- ◆ Simple vulvectomy: removes the entire vulva, but no lymph nodes

- ◆ Partial vulvectomy: removes some but not all of the vulva

- ◆ Radical vulvectomy: removes the entire vulva and surrounding lymph nodes

Stage 0 or carcinoma in situ, also called VIN, can be treated by local excision, laser beam therapy, or skinning vulvectomy (with or without skin grafts). The cure rate is essentially 100%.

Women with Stage I vulvar carcinoma have a great chance for cure. There is no "standard" procedure that is right for every woman with this stage of disease. The three most important factors to be considered are:

1. The woman's age

2. The condition of the noncancerous part of the vulva

3. The presence or absence of lymph node involvement by tumor

If the cancer involves one tumor on an otherwise normal vulva, and lymph nodes *are not* thought to be involved, radical local excision is the treatment of choice no matter what the woman's age. This procedure usually includes exploring the lymph nodes.

If the cancer involves a vulva that also has VIN or other abnormalities, the treatment choice could depend on the woman's age. Elderly women who have had longstanding, uncomfortable symptoms and are not sexually active might prefer a radical vulvectomy. For younger women, the primary tumor can be removed by radical local excision and the remainder of the vulva treated by more conservative surgical or medical treatment. For example, topical steroids might be used to treat vulvar dystrophy, with local excision or laser therapy used to treat the VIN. In any local excision, the lymph nodes in the groin and upper thigh should be explored. Radiation therapy can be used to treat women who have health problems that would make surgery more risky.

Vulvar cancer that involves the clitoris can present a special problem. Surgical removal of the clitoris can have major emotional and sexual effects. Physically, surgery in this area can interfere with the lymph channels that supply the genital areas and can cause uncomfortable and serious swelling. Radiation therapy can be used to treat tumors involving the clitoris; it

FIGO Staging for Cancer of the Vulva

Stage	Characteristics
0	Carcinoma in situ, intraepithelial carcinoma
I	Tumor confined to vulva and/or perineum, and is less than 2 cm in diameter
II	Tumor confined to the vulva and/or perineum, more than 2 cm in diameter
IIII	Tumor of any size with spread to the lower urethra and/or vagina, or anus, and/or lymph nodes on one side
IVA	Tumor of any size with involvement of lymph nodes on both sides or tumor spreading to the bowel or bladder
IVB	Same as IVA but with metastasis to distant organs and/or pelvic lymph nodes

causes a quick, skin reaction that may require treatments to be stopped for a week or two before completing therapy.

Radical local excision is used for vulvar tumors where preservation of the clitoris is possible. If there is a large perineal wound after surgery, skin and muscle flaps might be surgically created to close the wound.

Women with Stage II cancers will usually be treated with radical vulvectomy and lymph node dissection. Radiation therapy might be used in cases where the tumor extends close to the edge of the tissues removed, if the tumor is more than 5 mm thick, and/or if lymph nodes are found to contain cancer cells. The five-year survival rates for women without lymph node involvement ranges from 70–90%; the rates drop to 40% if nodes contain cancer cells. Again, radiation therapy can be used as a first-line treatment if the woman is physically unable to withstand surgery.

Stage III vulvar cancer is treated in much the same way as Stage II. If area lymph nodes are found to contain cancer cells, external radiation therapy will be recommended after surgical wounds have healed. Some women might be given radiation therapy before surgery. The rationale for preoperative radiation therapy is that it can decrease the tumor size and thus the extent of surgery required. As might be expected, the chances for cure are reduced with more advanced cancer. The most important predictor of chances for cure is the absence or presence of cancer cells in the lymph nodes.

Recent clinical trials are testing the effects of chemotherapy (cisplatin and 5-FU) combined with radiation therapy. A small trial found a complete response (total disappearance of tumor) in six of eight women studied.

Treatment of Stage IV vulvar cancer can involve radical vulvectomy combined with pelvic exenteration. Other options might involve surgery followed by external radiation. Preoperative radiation might increase the surgeon's ability to remove large tumors. Radiation combined with chemotherapy (5-FU) is sometimes suggested.

Radiation therapy can be used to treat women who are physically unable to go through surgery. In this case, radiation might be combined with chemotherapy (5-FU). In one clinical trial, cisplatin and 5-FU chemotherapy, and radiation therapy have had some effect in two of four women treated.

RECURRENT VULVAR CANCER

Regular post-treatment follow-up is done so that recurrent disease will be spotted as early as possible. Eighty percent of all recurrences come back during the first two years after initial treatment, either in the vulva or another place. A woman's treatment options will depend on the site and extent of the recurrence. Radical excision is used to remove a recurrent tumor that has not spread. Radiation can be curative too, for women whose recurrent tumor is small and has not spread. When the tumor comes back more than two years after it was first treated, a combination of radiation and surgery is the most likely treatment option. Other surgical options include radical vulvectomy and pelvic exenteration. So far, no standard chemotherapy plan has been effective in the treatment of women with widespread or metastatic vulvar cancer.

AFTER TREATMENT

In addition to general post-treatment examinations, Pap smears, and colposcopy, cancer of the vulva and its treatment have both physical and emotional long-term effects. Immediately after surgery, most care strategies relate to preventing infection, maintaining blood and lymphatic circulation in the operative area, and adding to the body's own healing ability. Good nutrition is especially important to promote healing. Discomfort and pain can be controlled with medications.

One of the most distressing problems that can occur after lymph node dissection and removal is **lymphedema**. It happens when lymph vessels or blood vessels are injured or disrupted, the flow of lymph fluid is blocked, and as a result an abnormal amount of lymph fluid collects in the tissues of the arms or legs. Lymphedema increases the woman's susceptibility to infections. It occurs as a result of any lymph node dissection in vulvar cancer and affects nearly 60% of all women who have node dissection in varying degrees. Treatment of lymphedema is discussed in Chapter 22.

If surgery involves the loss of fat tissues around the perineum, long periods of sitting can be uncomfortable. Surgery can also create changes in the urinary system. For example, the urinary stream direction might change, or urine may "spray" instead of leaving the body in a stream. One nurse advises women with these problems to use a cone-shaped urinal that is made for women to use outdoors while camping. This product can be found in camping supply stores or mail-order magazines.

Probably the most longlasting serious consequence of vulvar cancer is the psychological stress resulting from treatment. Sexual satisfaction is very low in women after vulvectomy. External pelvic radiation can cause loss of the vagina's ability to stretch during intercourse, and scarring. If the clitoris is removed during vulvectomy, the woman loses the organ that may be most important to her sexual response and satisfaction. Genital numbness can be a problem, or sexual intercourse may be painful after surgery. And a woman may fear rejection by her sexual partner. If a woman's self- and body image are equally disturbed, it can also lower her sexual desire and pleasure. As in other cancer diagnoses, the fear of recurrence or metastasis is always a concern. Surgeons are looking for less radical forms of treatment—perhaps combinations of surgery, radiation, chemotherapy—that improve emotional and sexual outcomes.

Some women feel that allowing a sexual partner to help in postoperative wound care was partly to blame for ending or changing their sexual relations. The choice to use a husband or lover as care-giver should be carefully considered by each couple.

Vulvar cancer does leave obvious effects. Some degree of disfigurement and change in function will be a part of the woman's life forever. Husbands and partners are affected too, and both the woman and her partner will need to make adjustments throughout the years. Using vaginal dilators and/or having regular sexual intercourse can stretch the vaginal tissues; dilators are available by prescription. Using water-soluble lubricants and changes in sexual positions (for example, to a side-lying position) can also reduce discomfort during intercourse. Some women find comfort through counseling to help couples explore alternatives to vaginal intercourse and being allowed to express feelings of grief over the loss of their normal sexual function.

Vulvar self-examination is critically important after initial therapy because recurrent vulvar cancer is always a possibility. But there is effective treatment for recurrent disease that is found early. Other gynecologic cancers can affect women after treatment for vulvar cancer, and early detection is always the key to long-term survival or cure.

QUESTIONS TO ASK YOUR PHYSICIAN

1. What surgical procedure will be used in treatment and what will be the short-term effects? What are the risks? What are the alternatives? Will there be skin grafts? What activities can I do? What wound care will I need to do for myself? How long should healing take? What can I do to speed healing? Should I plan for outside help when I get home?

2. What will be the long-term effects of this surgical procedure? For example, should I expect changes in urination? Will there be numbness in my genital organs? Will my clitoris be preserved? What about other aspects of sexual function—when can I resume sexual activity? Should I use vaginal dilators?

3. What is my chance for developing lymphedema? Will I have lymph node dissection? Are special surgical precautions being used to prevent lymphedema? What can I do to decrease my chances of developing lymphedema?

4. What are the local resources for counseling for myself and my husband or lover?

5. What additional treatment will I need after initial therapy? Will I need radiation or chemotherapy? When will this adjuvant therapy start? How do I select a doctor? (Or how does the doctor decide who becomes my other doctors?)

6. What is the plan for follow-up appointments with the surgeon? With the gynecologist? With the radiation oncologist?

7. Will I need referrals to physical therapy or other rehabilitation services?

Pamela Haylock

Chapter 20

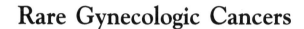

Rare Gynecologic Cancers

CANCER OF THE FALLOPIAN TUBE

Cancer starting in the fallopian tube is one of the rarest forms—less than 1%—of all gynecologic cancers. Only about 1,200 cases have ever been reported, and most are single case reports. Therefore, experience with this form of cancer is very limited and as a result, diagnosis usually happens as a result of exploratory surgery.

Who gets cancer of the fallopian tube?

Because experience with this disease is limited, hard evidence for risk factors is not available. Still, cancer of the fallopian tube seems to be found more often in women who have had several tubal infections and pelvic inflammatory disease. Most women found to have this cancer are in their 50s, although there is one reported case in a teenager.

Signs and symptoms

Most women who have cancer of the fallopian tube have symptoms including vaginal bleeding and/or clear discharge, colic-type pain, distension, and feelings of pressure in the abdomen. Each type of symptom can occur by itself or in combination with one or two others. For example, pain along with bloody vaginal discharge is common.

During physical examination, particularly if performed at the time of the symptoms, the doctor may be able to feel a pelvic mass. This is likely to be fluid-filled; if it ruptures, the discharge will increase. As the mass decreases, so does the pain, but the cancer grows. Of all patients diagnosed, very few are totally without symptoms.

Diagnosis

Diagnosis before surgery is rare. Women are examined for symptoms—which usually mimic other gynecologic or intestinal problems. Some women may have a dilation and curettage (D&C). If the D&C is negative and symptoms continue, cancer of the fallopian tube is a major suspect.

X-rays, ultrasound, and CT scans of the pelvis may or may not confirm the presence of a tumor. Even after surgery in which a mass is found, it is difficult to tell benign from malignant cells. If the mass is near or includes the ovary, it may be hard to determine if the tumor started in the tube or in the ovary. This is a very important "call" for the pathologist to make, since treatment and the prognosis for each situation is so very different.

Of the limited cases available for study, it seems that most women with this cancer have early stage, curable, disease.

Treatment

The minimum treatment for cancer of the fallopian tube is a total abdominal hysterectomy that includes removal of both ovaries and both fallopian tubes. During surgery, it is important that samples of the fluid from the abdomen be examined for cancer cells. The presence or absence of cancer cells in this fluid is an important indication of prognosis and a guideline for selecting therapy.

Post-operative therapy is indicated regardless of the extent of the cancer found during surgery. It may include the instillation of radioactive fluid directly into the abdomen (intra-peritoneal radioactive chromic phosphate). External radiation therapy has been used for more women than most other kinds of therapy. The use of chemotherapy and hormones are not well-defined at this time.

Survival statistics for fallopian tube cancers mimic those of ovarian cancer. The five year survival rate of women with early stage cancer is 60–90%, depending on the exact stage of disease, adjuvant therapy, success of surgical removal, and other factors.

GESTATIONAL TROPHOBLASTIC NEOPLASIA

Gestational trophoblastic neoplasia (GTN) (also called **gestational trophoblastic tumors** or **GTT**) is a relatively new term for a group of related tumors. In 4 B.C. Hippocrates described one form of GTN, the hydatidiform mole, as dropsy of the uterus and blamed its formation on unhealthy water. Before the mid-1950s, the prognoses for these diseases were dismal. Today, GTN is recognized as the most curable gynecologic cancer.

Gestational trophoblastic tumors involve several classes of tumors. They include hydatidiform moles (which can be complete or partial), chorioadenoma destruens (or invasive mole), choriocarcinoma, and placental-site trophoblastic tumors.

A **hydatidiform mole** is formed when a sperm and ovum join in the uterus but there is no fetal development. The cystic tissue that forms resembles a clump of grapes. The hydatidiform mole does not spread to other parts of the body.

In the United States, the hydatidiform mole occurs in about 1 of every 1,200 pregnancies. In other parts of the world, it occurs much more often. In the Far East, it is reported in 1 of 120 pregnancies.

Who develops hydatidiform mole?

Most women who experience hydatidiform mole are 50 years old or older. The risk is lowest for women 20–29. Women 15 or younger and 40 and older have an increased risk. Nutritional factors may play a role in the development of this form of neoplasia; animal fat and carotene (vitamin A) deficiency seem to be linked to higher rates of hydatidiform mole.

Women who develop hydatidiform mole during one pregnancy are more likely to develop it in subsequent pregnancies.

Symptoms

Most if not all women with hydatidiform mole notice a delay in menstrual periods for several cycles; most are thought to be pregnant. Vaginal bleeding occurs, most often during the first three months of pregnancy. About a third of these women report nausea and vomiting. Because of abnormal hormonal production, particularly human chorionic gonatropin (hCG), the woman might have symptoms of over-stimulation and function of the thyroid gland or hyperthyroidism.

Nearly half of all women with hydatidiform mole have an increase in uterine size that is excessive for the believed length of the pregnancy or gestational age. On the other hand, a third are found to have a smaller than expected uterus compared to gestational age.

Diagnosis

The diagnostic process includes a pelvic exam, ultrasound, and blood test for the hormone beta hCG. Although this hormone is expected to be present during a normal pregnancy, higher than normal levels, especially on repeated testings, might indicate hydatidiform mole. **Amniography** can be used to make a definite diagnosis. During amniography, a needle is inserted into the uterus. Dye is injected through the needle and X-rays, which highlight the distribution of the dye, reveal little amniotic fluid and a characteristic pattern of the mole.

Treatment

The hydatidiform mole is removed either by D & C and suction evacuation, or hysterectomy. The choice of therapy depends on the woman's desire for future pregnancy.

After surgery, the woman's blood and urine will be monitored at one to two-week intervals for levels of beta hCG until it reaches normal levels for two successive tests. The length of time varies for each woman, but usually lasts for at least 8–9 weeks after removing the mole. After that the hCG levels are tested every other month for a year. The woman should use contraceptives for one year after treatment.

If the hCG level does not revert to normal or actually increases during the follow-up period, remaining or recurrent hydatidiform mole is suspected. At this time, the woman goes through added evaluation and is most likely started on chemotherapy.

Choriocarcinoma

Most experts prefer to use the general term "GTN" and eliminate use of the old term "choriocarcinoma." GTN may have started as a hydatidiform mole or from tissue that remains in the uterus after an abortion or normal delivery of a baby. Malignant GTN can spread to other parts of the body, including the bowel and urinary systems, the liver, lung, and brain. Placental-site trophoblastic disease, an even more rare form of GTN, starts in the uterus where the placenta was attached.

Diagnosis

The symptoms and diagnostic workup are much the same as for hydatidiform mole. A positive beta hCG is diagnostic, but a negative test does not rule out the disease. A D&C might be useful and can provide tissue for microscopic exam and diagnosis. In some cases, a woman with GTN may have no disease in the uterus but have metastatic disease.

The prognosis for metastatic GTN is generally poor. This is especially true if any of these five factors are part of the woman's history or current status:

- ◆ the last pregnancy was more than 4 months ago

- ◆ the beta hCG blood level is high

- ◆ the cancer has spread to the liver or brain

- ◆ the woman has had chemotherapy and the cancer did not disappear

- ◆ the tumor started after the completion of a normal pregnancy

Treatment

Treatment decisions are based on the cell type, the stage of disease, the levels of beta hCG, the amount of time the disease has persisted, the sites of metastasis, and the type and extent of previous treatment.

As in the case of hydatidiform mole, treatment will most likely use surgery and radiation. The tumor is removed by D&C or hysterectomy. If disease has not spread outside the uterus, the woman is likely to be treated with chemotherapy. In this case one drug, usually methotrexate, is used for single-agent chemotherapy. Other drugs studied for use in non-metastatic GTN include 5-fluorouracil (5-FU) and dactinomycin. Treatment with this type of regimen can be curative.

Even when the disease has spread to the brain or liver, some women still have a fairly good chance for long-term survival. Treatment can be the same as for non-metastatic GTN; methotrexate is considered the drug of choice. Some women are placed on a multi-drug program that includes methotrexate, dactinomycin, and chlorambucil. Etoposide, vincristine, and cyclophosphamide might be used in other plans for combination chemotherapy. Radiation therapy seems to have a limited role in the treatment of malignant GTN.

❖   ❖   ❖

Some of the cancers that affect women are so rare that very few doctors have much experience or expertise in their management. There is also not much information available in the medical literature that could give a doctor really good guidance. For these reasons, women might want to consider requesting information about participation in a clinical trial sponsored by the National Cancer Institute or one of NCI's sponsored coop-erative clinical group trials. NCI clinical trial information is available directly through their information line. A woman can also ask her doctor for this information. At the very least, she should be able to consult with a gynecologic oncologist who can provide information about available clinical trials that are exploring her type of cancer.

Pamela Hayock

PART IV

LIFE AFTER CANCER

Chapter 21

Feelings After Treatment Ends

I swallowed my final three chemo pills with three glasses of water. Pills #250, 251, and 252. (I counted!) For months I had mentally checked off each injection and pill and wondered if this day would *ever* come.

An hour later, my husband and I packed up my cold cap and the empty pill container and headed for the county dump. There we ritually crushed the container (driving back and forth over it several times) and tossed the cold cap into the deepest garbage pit. An exhilarating moment . . .

So why did I feel more terrified than exhilarated? Why this jolt of anxiety? What in the world was the matter with me?

Nothing. I had just learned the hard way that the after-treatment road is not all rainbows and bluebirds (although there are plenty of those).

At any point after she finishes cancer treatment, a woman may struggle with

- her feelings (including fear, anger, sadness, guilt)

- her self-image and body image

- her relationships

- her goals

Some of these may be more of the same old problems that came up during treatment. Others may be new, or may be more pressing now.

Ending cancer treatment is a predictable emotional "pothole" on the cancer survivorship journey. Many people feel anxious, vulnerable, uncertain, ambivalent. It is common, normal—and temporary.

In sharing stories of life after treatment, cancer survivors have discovered that almost everyone goes through certain emotional bad patches along the way. The timing of some is predictable: however many years or decades it may be after treatment, no breast cancer patient ever undergoes mammography again without trembling a little inside.

The timing of others is less predictable, but just about everyone with cancer eventually experiences a painful range of feelings about the disease: fear that cancer will come back, grief at the losses she has had, uncertainties about her self-image.

One woman may grieve most intensely right after diagnosis or during treatment. (Of course, one never tidily "finishes" a feeling and then puts it behind forever.) Another woman, conserving all her emotional energy just to get through treatment, may not face that first excruciating blast of sorrow until after treatment ends.

What has been postponed, however, cannot be put off indefinitely. Thus, when treatment ends, some women find themselves struggling not only with the common after-treatment feelings but also with the postponed or "holdover" ones. They may doubt their ability to survive, let alone thrive. They feel wobbly and unsure, both physically and emotionally; the journey ahead looks like one rock, rut, and jolt after another.

But it gets better—and knowing what to expect and when makes it easier to get through. Techniques that other cancer survivors have found helpful may prove useful. But, whether it is the day therapy ends or decades later, simply getting through the rough spots as easily as possible is part of the challenge of living well after cancer treatment.

But not the only part.

Like other major crises, cancer provides a "window of opportunity" for change and growth. Eventually, many women —no matter how much they hate the disease—become aware of positive changes in themselves that would not have happened without cancer. Whether or not they feel "transformed," they may become conscious of a new sense of clarity, of fresh eyes for the world and the people around them. Many just enjoy and appreciate life more. Some gain a better idea of who they really are and what they truly want out of life.

Sometimes women have learned through cancer to be kinder to themselves, or have been astonished at their own strength and resilience. Whatever the good changes, many women want to hold on to them, build on them.

As time passes, however, and the immediacy of the cancer experience fades, it is all too easy to slip back into old ways. If a woman wants to live better than ever after cancer treatment, her second challenge is to keep alive the good changes that have happened because of her response to cancer.

GENERAL STRATEGIES

The general strategies for coping with feelings after treatment are similar to those that can be used during treatment. Whatever the difficult feeling, acknowledging and naming it take away some of its power.

A woman can examine what she is feeling by herself, in a group, or with a mentor, therapist, or close friend. Like women at earlier stages of the cancer journey, some women make the unspoken spoken by keeping journals or diaries. A woman can also draw her feelings, sculpt them, dance them, write poetry about them, using the creative process not only to express her emotions but to begin "resolving" them. Many women find it useful and safe to read about feelings.

For the woman who belongs to a cancer support group, the immediate post-treatment period is not the time to leave. Some localities offer after-treatment groups (often listed with the local American Cancer Society unit). Cancervive, Inc., specializes in groups for people who have completed cancer treatment.

Any mentor should be a woman who has navigated the post-treatment period successfully. The breast cancer patient who had a helpful Reach-to-Recovery volunteer earlier might contact her again, for instance. If necessary, a mentorship can be by long-distance telephone or letter; Y-ME (breast cancer), DES Action, and the National Coalition for Cancer Survivorship are possible resources (see Resources).

A psychotherapist or counselor may be able to help a woman integrate what she has experienced with cancer into the rest of her life. Many women look to a special friend who does not have cancer or to a noncancer-related group for techniques and support in identifying and coping with strong emotions: cancer patients have no monopoly on feelings of anger or vulnerability. Such groups include general women's support groups, 12-Step groups, or simply an informal gathering of women friends talking about what bothers them.

After some time passes, many women begin serving as mentors for other women or as cancer volunteers, and discover that they are helped as much as they help. As she works with the cancer "novice," the woman reexamines her own feelings, but in a new context. Being a mentor or a cancer volunteer does not require that a woman know all the answers: it simply means that she has passed this way before and is willing to listen and share her experiences.

Many women invest some of their feelings and energy in cancer political action groups or the national survivorship movement. On the other hand, the woman who finds she is spending every waking moment on cancer-related activities may need to create more balance in her life.

AFTER-TREATMENT FEARS

The "what ifs"—what if cancer comes back? what if I need more treatment? what if I die?—bedevil most cancer survivors at least once in a while. Most admit they never completely get over the fear that cancer will return. Living with a cancer diagnosis means living with a certain degree of uncertainty forever. For most of us, however, the fear eventually recedes into the background of our everyday lives. The fear and uncertainty are just *there*, rather like emotional background music.

But there are the "high-decibel" times. One, as unexpected as it is unwelcome, often comes at the completion of basic cancer treatment (surgery, chemotherapy, radiation).

A woman expects to feel jubilant, relieved. Instead, what she experiences is so at odds with what she thought she would feel, thought she *should* feel, that it staggers her.

"I just can't believe how terrified I feel—and how weird it is," confided one woman right after she finished chemotherapy. "For months, I've been trying to reach this day, cheering myself on. At the doctors' office, the nurses even gave me flowers and a big certificate to congratulate me on finishing treatment. My family and friends are all geared up to celebrate with me at this big party I was planning.

"Instead, here I am so scared I can barely function. I haven't been this frightened since I got my diagnosis. What if it comes back? How do the doctors know I'm okay? Sometimes I even feel like asking the doctor if I can have more chemo. I hated it—but it was my powerful weapon, keeping me safe. Is it always going to be like this?"

Her panic is common, and it doesn't seem to matter whether treatment involves a single surgery or months of treatment. At the end, many cancer survivors feel "as if I've been thrown out of the nest and don't know if I even have wings."

Some women on long-term hormonal therapy for cancer, such as Tamoxifen for breast cancer, continue to feel "protected"; others do not. The end of hormonal therapy can also be an anxious time.

As treatment ends, a woman may be physically weak, severely fatigued, hard-pressed to believe that she will ever feel healthy again. Whatever cancer therapy she has undergone, it takes weeks, months, or even longer for the body to recover fully—and it is difficult to wait with patience and confidence.

In addition, as a woman's treatment ends, much of her support may vanish. During treatment a woman yearns for the day when she can measure her life by something other than doctors' appointments, but right after therapy finishes, she may ache for that reassuring surveillance. And family and friends may be less "there" for her after therapy ends. They have been grappling (often with little help) with their own feelings of helplessness, anger, and sadness. Like her, they've been focusing on that magical end-of-treatment day. Now they may be so ready to get back to "normal" that they do not want to listen to her fears. No matter how much they care, they just "can't take any more."

DEALING WITH "WHAT-IFS"

We fear what *might* happen in the future. But, as oncologist William M. Buchholz, M.D., writes in *Surviving* newsletter (July/August 1989), "You become tense in anticipation of being powerless some time from now.... The antidote for fear is returning to the present."

When I am pondering "what ifs" I keep reminding myself that, *whatever* happens to me, I will never, *ever*, have to face more than one day at a time. While the prospect of "the future" may sometimes overwhelm me, I can manage 24 hours.

Sometimes I turn and face my fear, remembering the Bene Gessent creed from Frank Herbert's science fiction adventure *Dune:* "I will face my fear. I will permit it to pass over me and through me. And when it has gone past I will turn the inner eye to see its path. Where the fear has gone there will be nothing. Only I will remain."

If we feel overwhelmed by the "what ifs," relaxation techniques can bring us back to the moment and serve as first aid for fear. Slow breathing makes us pay attention to what is happening *now*. In progressive relaxation, we experience each part of the body as it tenses and then releases. We can "soften the belly," or *feel* our feet solidly connected to the ground.

Taking concrete action lets a woman feel more in control. She might draft a will or fashion a fall-back plan for the care of her young children, for instance; this practical planning (appropriate for everyone, with or without cancer) is prudent rather than morbid and allows her to relax and get on with life.

And sometimes we have to remind ourselves that the body's own strong immune system is still the state-of-the-art mechanism for destroying cancer cells. After a cancer diagnosis, we forget how long and well the body's defenses have protected us. We may blame our bodies for "betraying" us; we have to relearn to trust them.

After treatment ends, energy returns in bits and spurts. Many of us tend to overdo one day, suffer for it the next, and then wonder if we will ever feel really healthy again. But if we give them a fair chance, our bodies work diligently to get healthy again—and then to stay healthy.

Some women swear by improving their nutrition: "I've really decreased the amount of fat in my diet. When I cook a delicious low-fat, high-fiber meal for myself and my family, I know I am doing something special for all of us. It gives me back a sense of control, too, in a situation in which I felt little control: I can do something to make me healthier."

Other women start an exercise program, perhaps a post-mastectomy class. Our bodies, made to fight or flee anything that causes distress, crave physical activity. (Taking it slowly at first is better here. Rushing into vigorous exercise with a not-so-vigorous body invites discouragement as well as sore muscles.)

Some women meditate, stop smoking, sip special herbal teas, or listen to relaxation tapes. Some just try to be kinder to themselves, becoming readier to say "yes" to themselves and "no" to others. One way of being kinder involves setting realistic health expectations, ones that allow for the occasional chocolate bar or missed exercise class.

Many women, having put together for themselves a "healing package" during treatment (a combination of chemotherapy, walking, visualization exercises, and herbal teas, perhaps) continue everything but the medical therapy, and perhaps add other techniques that make them feel healthier, stronger, and more at peace. It helps many women to think of their cancer diagnosis and treatment as a kind of "midcourse correction" in life's journey, an opportunity to see what is wrong and make it better.

Yes, it is important to celebrate the end of treatment, and to mark closure of a difficult phase. A woman *deserves* to congratulate herself and to bask in the love and good wishes of others. But she also needs to know that fear and ambivalence commonly appear as unwelcome guests at the celebration—and to realize that she has some effective strategies for throwing them out.

OTHER PREDICTABLE DIFFICULT TIMES

As time passes, we recover more confidence in our ability to survive and thrive. But there are other predictable scary moments.

Any symptom, whether a twinge, a cough, or a phone number we cannot recall, can trip our internal alarm system. It doesn't take much, especially at first. Most symptoms have nothing to do with cancer, of course, and go away on their own, but sometimes it is hard to believe that.

It makes sense to get information from the doctor about follow-up care, prognosis, common symptoms that don't mean anything, and problems that need to be reported. Knowing what is important and what can be safely ignored lets a woman adjust her emotional alarm system. However, if a woman is seriously concerned about *any* symptom, it is reasonable to check with the doctor.

Are there skills she needs to know in order to monitor her continuing health? One woman reports that she felt much better after breast cancer treatment when she visited a hospital-based Breast Health Center and learned the most effective way to examine her own breasts.

Routine checkups and tests, even when there are no symptoms, can be times of predictable anxiety. Many women felt perfectly healthy when their cancers were diagnosed. Taken by surprise once, they worry that feeling fine now is no guarantee of health.

"Before my regular mammograms, I still can't sleep," admits a woman treated for breast cancer several years ago. "I thought that after a year or two, I would face checkups with total calm and equanimity, but I don't. I don't get *quite* as worked up now though!"

People who survive cancer sometimes experience the

"post-traumatic stress syndrome" (complete with sudden distressing flashbacks) common to soldiers after a war. For instance, on a cancer-related anniversary, a woman may find herself reliving the scene in the doctor's office, struggling with the excruciating fear she felt then.

Or it is a common experience to develop symptoms right before a checkup or test. Many women have learned from experience that symptoms that develop right before check-ups have more to do with anxiety than with any physical problem. Relaxation techniques, talk with a support group sister, and positive "self-talk" all can help.

Sometimes I "fast-forward" myself a few days mentally so that I am looking *back* at the event, savoring my relief. I hunt for distractions and promise myself that I will not do this again (until the next time).

Mentally "reframing" checkups and anniversaries into reassuring milestones helps many women. Focusing on the champagne afterward makes the temporary anxiety more tolerable. It is cause for celebration to check off another bone scan, another year!

Other predictable occasions of anxiety include hearing about the death of a woman from a similar cancer. In the case of a personal friend, the fear is overshadowed by grief but still exists. The death of a public figure may feel almost like the loss of a friend. (Many women report finding the autobiographies of Gilda Radner or Jill Ireland, for instance, painful and anxiety-raising—but also cleansing and cathartic.) News stories or obituaries may make us pause and worry; movies, TV dramas or novels may tap into an undercurrent of anxiety.

FEAR THAT COMES FROM NOWHERE

Sometimes a woman has a sudden, fierce anxiety, seemingly from nowhere. I use these as an emotional barometer: what have I been ignoring? I may find that the painful feelings have little to do with cancer per se, more to do with vulnerability or fear of making a choice or something else. Once I know what I am really dealing with and begin to take some action, the fear passes.

Some women, often those who "sailed through" treatment and the immediate post-treatment period, encounter an unexpected and totally unsettling period of acute anxiety several months (or even years) later. This often comes at just about the time the woman is congratulating herself on how well she has coped with the whole experience. This happens to be her individual timetable for integrating cancer into her life and the techniques are the same: acknowledging and naming the fear, shedding some tears, talking about it, and so on.

With most cancer-related fear, the common remedies are sufficient. If fear hangs on, causes severe and continuing distress, or immobilizes a woman, however, it is definitely time for professional help. This might include psychotherapy (often brief) and/or the short-term use of antianxiety medication.

ANGER AND SADNESS

Cancer wounds us with visible and invisible scars. We grieve and feel angry—and that is how it should be.

Aside from any "holdover" feelings of sadness that she may have postponed until after treatment, a woman may face specific post-therapy losses. What appeared to be a temporary loss, for instance, may prove permanent. A woman may suffer what turns out to be permanent major damage from chemotherapy, radiation, or surgery. A woman in her 30s who underwent chemotherapy for breast cancer may discover, perhaps, that her periods do not return and that she cannot give birth to the baby she longs for. Or she may mourn an accumulation of "little" physical losses: a scar that has healed "well" according to the surgeon, but is still there; a continuing numbness under her arm that always feels strange when she shaves; lessened vaginal lubrication during intercourse. Almost everyone treated for a women's cancer faces a few long-term "reminders" that she has had cancer. Admitting that these sometimes bother her in no way means that she is ungrateful that she is alive.

As treatment ends, a woman may *know* intellectually that she no longer needs the close attention from her doctors that she was getting, but that may not keep her from *feeling* a sense of loss. Women, far more than men, tend to see a relationship with the doctor as a personal one and to want to be "liked" by their health professionals. Especially when therapy has been protracted, it is not uncommon for a woman to have a sense of being rejected and abandoned when she is sent on her way after treatment ends.

If she stifled any anger or resentment toward her doctor during treatment in order to be a "good, lovable" patient, a woman still has those feelings simmering within. In addition, many patients feel angry that their health professionals did not prepare them for the difficult transition after treatment.

There are other kinds of scars. The process of renegotiating relationships may be painful. The friends who could not tolerate any part of cancer and dropped from view during the woman's treatment may be gone forever. Other people may continue to treat her differently than they once did. If a support group "sister" dies of cancer, a woman grieves the loss. Uninsured medical bills may come due, imperiling a woman's financial security.

Guilt enters the scene when what she thinks or does or feels does not match her expectations, usually internalized from our culture. Some of this is a holdover from the period right after diagnosis when the woman was trying to make sense of why she got cancer. That the cause is not knowable in most cases, with the current state of medical information, does not deter her from blaming herself: "I didn't eat right. I didn't manage stress right."

After treatment, she can feel even more culpable. Now she "knows better"—and *still* may not eat right or do her relaxation exercises! Or, expecting a "transformation" in herself because of cancer—and seeing few changes—she wonders where she has gone wrong. It is usually the expectation at fault, not the woman.

Many women are hard on themselves at the best of times. They struggle to meet the expectations of a society that keeps changing what it wants of them. Cancer can give a woman the opportunity to look at what she expects of herself and those around her. Changing the expectations to something more realistic reduces the guilt.

Although, amazingly enough, women cancer survivors do not appear to be *more* at risk for severe depression (and other acute psychiatric ills) than the general populace, they are not immune. The woman who feels immobilized by sadness for more than two weeks (major sleeping or eating problems; persistent severe "empty," guilty, hopeless feelings; a "slowed down" or very restless feeling; continuing thoughts of suicide) urgently needs professional help and perhaps antidepressant medication.

HOW WE FEEL ABOUT OURSELVES

All through her life, a woman's internal "computer" keeps adding to her mental picture of herself, her self-image (including her body image). Words women use to describe themselves during and after treatment include victim, ugly, weak, stupid, dependent—and strong, survivor, sensitive, magnificent, focused.

Crises in self-image can occur anytime during the cancer experience. Reentering "normal" life after treatment ends can make a woman question again just who and what she is, but the process is the same as earlier.

Body image concerns, however, often reach critical mass about the time treatment ends. No matter that she is an ardent feminist, no matter that she is truly convinced that what's inside is far more important than what's on the surface, a woman may still be shaken by what she sees. In fact, many of these changes improve rapidly after their low point as treatment ends. Scars fade over time, though this depends on the individual woman's body. Hair regrows, often thick, lustrous and curly, after chemotherapy ends. Her complexion gradually returns to normal.

A woman may choose breast reconstruction to replace a missing breast, use a secure prosthesis, or simply enjoy her Amazon-woman chest (the ancient Amazons removed a breast

so they could shoot their arrows better). I love the striking
poster that shows a woman, her arms stretched wide as she
embraces life, with a delicate tracing of flowers tattooed over
her mastectomy scar.

Many women find that the hardest body image change
they have to cope with is weight gain during chemotherapy.
Weight losses may reverse relatively quickly as a woman feels
healthy again, but the extra pounds common after breast cancer
chemo hang on tenaciously. If she wants to lose weight, a slow,
steady pace of about 1–2 pounds a month through healthy eating and exercise seems to work best.

Women who have undergone radical pelvic surgeries may
now have one or more openings on the abdomen, new exit(s)
for the digestive tract and/or urinary tract. A plastic pouch is
worn over the ostomy to collect stool and/or urine. Specially-
trained health professionals called enterostomal therapy nurses
can help the woman with both the practical and psychological
adjustments to these changes.

RELATIONSHIPS

During treatment many relationships enter a holding pattern.
Nobody wants to rock the boat much, and the woman undergoing therapy may lack the energy and will to make changes.

As treatment ends, exhausted family and friends may
crave an emotional break from the intensity of diagnosis and
treatment. Although this is usually temporary, it conflicts with
the woman's need for support during this difficult transition.
Everyone is upset and resentful and no one quite understands
why. Information and direct communication are key: if the
woman, her family, and friends all know that this is normally a
trying time that passes, they can relax more and help each
other while protecting themselves.

A woman may feel angry at family and friends who want
to "get back to normal" and expect her to do the same. She
knows intuitively that she is not physically or emotionally
ready for "normal" yet.

Or she may realize, consciously or not, that normal as defined by other people is not where she wants to be. During cancer treatment, many women begin paying attention to their own legitimate needs and desires, often for the first time. Reluctant to return to the precancer status quo, a woman may seek new rules for the relationship. But making these kinds of changes (and then making them stick) takes more emotional energy than she is likely to have now; the attempt may leave her feeling angry, frustrated, and powerless. Time, returning energy, and some negotiating skills can bring about a more successful outcome later.

At the same time, the other person in the relationship has been changing. Thus the relationship must be renegotiated gradually between two individuals who are in some ways new and different from what they were.

Partners

Some cancer doctors recommend that, if a woman has a partner, they plan an official getaway alone for a few days about a month or so after treatment ends, a sort of second honeymoon. This is one way to mark the end of one phase of their lives and start on a new life together. It is only a start, however, since this is an ongoing process.

It helps if neither the woman nor her partner expects too much yet: the physical and emotional wounds of cancer and its therapies are still relatively fresh and unhealed. Recognizing that this can be a difficult period is half the battle. But if they can talk about their separate and mutual uncertainties and hopes, they can use these to forge new and stronger connections.

Psychotherapist Diane W. Scott, R.N., Ph.D, in her work with women with cancer, says that in a close relationship there is not only the woman's ego and the partner's ego, but a separate something which she calls the "couple ego." As they struggle together through the crisis of cancer, the process may strengthen not only each one of the pair, but also their shared sense of what they have together. The woman may feel grateful for what her partner has done to make life easier during treatment;

many a woman finds wonderful and unexpected depths in her mate. The partner may experience with awe the courage and lovability of the woman. Knowing that they could lose each other lends a sweet and urgent edge to their journey of mutual discovery.

But, with or without cancer, most relationships do not run like Swiss watches all the time. Cancer may make some good relationships idyllic, but it may also show clearly that some are poisonous and unsalvageable. Like most people, however, most relationships are neither perfect nor dreadful; they repay the time and effort spent making them better.

It is a temptation for some women to want to change their lives drastically after cancer or to hold a flawed relationship accountable for causing the disease. Often, it makes sense to consider the first months after treatment a "sit back and take a deep breath" time. This gives both partners a chance to heal and the relationship space to settle a bit before a woman makes any radical decisions.

It is not uncommon for one or both partners to blame the cancer for all their problems. Sometimes that is an excuse, a camouflage for bigger unacknowledged problems and feelings. The idea now is to admit and accept these feelings, communicate them, and begin working together to resolve them.

If the situation does not improve after some time and effort, both partners have to decide if their relationship is worth saving. Counseling may be able to help them sort out tangled feelings and perhaps learn better ways of being together.

What if a woman does her part to build the relationship and the other person still rejects her, giving cancer as the reason? Obviously, it can be devastating. As hard as it is to keep the situation in perspective, the woman must remind herself over and over again of all the wonderful things she is and can do. Cancer has changed her, perhaps, but has not diminished her. It is the partner's loss: some people, because of their own fears and conflicts, cannot tolerate the reality of cancer in someone close to them. This is not in any way the woman's fault, but that does not mean that she will not feel outraged and shed many tears before beginning a new phase of her life.

Other family members

What about her children? They can be told that Mom's treatment is finished and (if appropriate) that she will start feeling better again. How children respond depends on the individual child, the age, and the situation. Again, children need to know clearly that they are *in no way to blame* for the illness and that there will always be someone to care for them.

Older children (including teenagers) who may have taken on more family responsibility during the treatment phase may keep some of it, or may happily or very reluctantly relinquish it. Getting back to "being a kid" can be a tricky transition, another relationship change to renegotiate. As always, talking openly means that children can get their questions answered and their fears resolved. Teenagers and parents sometimes benefit from using a "buffer" adult to help with communication, perhaps a school counselor or a trusted family friend.

Just being older doesn't save adult children from their own terrors when a mother has cancer, and they need to be included in the communication loop. When family history increases the risk of this cancer, the end of treatment period is a natural time to open the issue of how a daughter can protect herself.

This can be a difficult subject to broach. The woman may feel guilty for "handing down" a vulnerability to the cancer to her child or may not know how to raise the subject. Some daughters react by denying the danger, others by becoming panicky about their risk. If the woman can admit her feelings to herself and perhaps rehearse what to say—by herself or with a mentor or support group—it is easier to begin. Then, of course, she needs accurate information to pass along. A caring doctor, a medical geneticist, a women's health center may be able to guide the daughter to take appropriate measures to protect herself.

If the woman's parents and siblings have been part of her support team during cancer treatment, this relationship too may need to be renegotiated when treatment is over. Sometimes a woman does not know *what* she wants now (being "babied" may have been rather pleasant) and may feel like a touchy, ambivalent adolescent all over again.

Friends and others

Each woman decides how open she wants to be about the can-cer with friends, acquaintances, and coworkers. There is no one right solution, but many women handle the subject after treat-ment more or less the way they handled it earlier.

After treatment, however, the changes made because of cancer are less obvious. The wig is gone, and the lunch date does not have to be postponed because of the radiation therapy appointment. As cancer comes less often to mind, it is natural to speak of it less often. If the woman finds herself sharing her cancer experiences nonstop with everyone long after treatment ends, she may need to remind herself that there are plenty of other fascinating topics of conversation.

It is a woman's decision what to do about any friends who drifted away after the diagnosis because they couldn't handle it. If they drift back and she is interested in being friends again, she may overlook the earlier defection and consider their be-havior now a reaffirmation of her current healthiness.

What about a new friendship after treatment ends? Does this person need to know about the cancer? If the relationship is becoming a close one (certainly if the person is a potential "significant other"), it is not fair to either party to withhold the information.

SETTING GOALS

"Enjoy the moment . . . Live for today!" Yes—and no.

As she is going through cancer treatment, a woman's goal often is "getting through this." After treatment, she may want simply to get back to normal. Many women, however, feel a need to make something fresh and special of their lives, perhaps to set out in a new direction entirely. They feel a sense of rebirth, of second chance. They do not want to spin their wheels going nowhere. But, physically and emotionally drained, they do not know where to begin.

On the other hand, a woman may be scared to set goals

for fear that cancer will disrupt them again; she has been through that once already. Sometimes there may be a deep-down "don't tempt the fates" feeling: could planning far beyond today *trigger* a return of the cancer? Knowing this is superstition may not protect her from this common feeling.

Many women alternate between the two, one moment eager to brave new worlds and the next moment fearing to stick a toe in the water. They do not feel transformed, but sense some changes in themselves and wonder where they will all lead.

Energy to set goals usually requires some physical energy, and that will come in time as the woman's body recovers. During this time she takes baby steps: what can she do to make her life better in the next week? This means setting a reachable concrete goal for the near future ("I will walk half a mile tomorrow and increase the distance a little bit every day until I am walking three-quarters of a mile a day after one week").

The more concrete the goals are, the more achievable. "Getting in shape" is less helpful than "I will take this ballet class three times a week." Concentrating on one or two goals at a time seems to be more effective than reaching out in all directions at once. The woman also needs to include some intermittent monitoring: is this, in fact, a helpful goal for her?

Many women set goals for themselves, fail to meet them, and then not only give up on the goal completely but feel bad about themselves. It helps if the woman rehearses in her mind beforehand what she will do if she stumbles. This gives her a plan so that she can pick up where she left off, rather than becoming bogged down in self-loathing.

When she becomes more comfortable with short-term goals, the woman can set ones a little bigger and a little longer term. And eventually . . . .

Kerry McGinn

Chapter 22

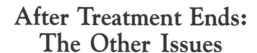

After Treatment Ends:
The Other Issues

In black moments, I sometimes think, "You mean I went through everything I went through and now there's this too? That's the *last straw!*"

Indeed, after treatment ends, a woman may discover that cancer and its therapy have affected many areas of her life besides her feelings, including

- sexual concerns

- pregnancy

- lymphedema

- early menopause

- employment and insurance

Sometimes I get downright furious. It's not fair and there is no way to pretend it is. I keep trying to remember the Serenity Prayer—although I do not always get serene.

Indeed, some things cannot be changed, and a woman simply exhausts herself trying to make them go away. But others are challenges, opportunities to make life better (or at least more interesting). By looking at a problem squarely, getting information about it, talking about it, and finding out strategies other people have used to deal with it, a woman learns what reasonable action she can take. Who knows? She may be able to take that "last straw" and weave it into something beautiful.

SEXUALITY

No cancer makes it impossible for a woman to give and receive pleasure from touching. If this is important to her, there is always a way.

However, some of the women's cancers and their treatment put hurdles in the path of a woman's sexuality. She and her partner may need to keep open minds about ways to feel sexual pleasure. Changing their techniques and expectations can broaden their lovemaking horizons.

During treatment, women may find that they have less interest in sex, simply because mind and body are so involved in getting through this phase. Then treatment ends and the woman and her partner wonder, "What now?" She may fear possible rejection at the same time her partner is concerned about appearing overeager and insensitive.

What happens now depends on what is happening in the woman's mind, in her body, and in the relationship. Whatever happens, it is likely to take some time for recovery and renegotiation. The woman and her partner need to remind themselves of this before immediately worrying that things are not "back to normal."

It helps to realize that the first experiences with lovemaking after surgery (or after a period without much sexual touching) are sometimes awkward and disappointing. The woman tries to protect new scars and her partner worries about hurting her. This can improve dramatically as the woman continues her recovery and they both relax.

The mind

The most important sex organ is not the clitoris or the vagina, but the brain. Many sexual difficulties start there—but that is also where they can be solved.

How a woman thinks of herself and her body (self-image, including body image) plays a crucial role in how she responds sexually. She needs to like herself, to think she is "worth it," desirable, and deserving of sexual pleasure. In addition, she has to be sufficiently free from fear and other overpowering negative emotions to muster the energy for lovemaking. Depression is one of the major inhibitors of sexual response: it tamps down all the feelings and vanquishes joy, spontaneity, and pleasure.

Since the period immediately after treatment ends is often full of negative feelings (as well as fears about pain), it is a tricky one for lovemaking. If a woman engages in intercourse before she is emotionally ready, her body may not respond— and she may feel worse about herself and resentful toward her partner. The more tense she gets, the more painful it is. That means her body is even less likely to respond the next time. It can be a vicious cycle.

On the other hand, satisfying lovemaking helps both mind and body to recover. Aside from the pleasure, it makes a woman feel good about herself, and that she is no less a woman because of what she has gone through. It can distract her from fear and draw her back to "normal" again. It can bond partners tightly at a time when they may especially need this closeness.

Satisfying lovemaking depends less on bedroom acrobatics than on *communication*. If a woman and her partner can say to each other directly, "That feels good," or "I'm scared that touching that spot will hurt," and can trust that the other will listen, then both can relax. Expecting a partner to be able to read one's mind simply does not work.

Thinking of lovemaking itself as a special communication, as a way of giving and receiving pleasure in many ways, takes the pressure off and lets both partners enjoy the journey. They can caress, stroke, touch, laugh, and cuddle to their hearts' content. The woman who masturbates can explore her body, listening to its old and new messages of what feels right.

The body

Many women feel violated, both physically and emotionally, by the treatments for women's cancers. To get through therapy, they begin considering their body a *thing* unrelated to them, and it takes time to move back into their altered bodies.

Possible physical changes include scars, missing organs or parts of organs, different sensations in sensitive areas, and altered hormonal balance. Obvious scars ordinarily fade in time; as long as they are healing normally, they do not need any special physical coddling during lovemaking—just some tender loving emotional care for these badges of courage.

With no uterus after a hysterectomy, a woman can continue to have orgasms, but they may feel a little different because the spasm no longer includes the uterus contracting; on the other hand, she may be more free to respond because she no longer experiences bleeding or fear of pregnancy.

If the vagina is all or partially removed, it may be rebuilt with reconstructive surgery. To keep the vaginal channel open, the woman can use either a vaginal dilator or have regular intercourse.

The woman who has lost her clitoris in surgery for cancer of the vulva may have the most difficult sexual road to travel, because the clitoris is where the most intense sexual sensations occur. For her, recovering or retaining her sexuality means becoming sensitive to the pleasures available from the rest of her body (breasts, thighs, etc.).

Many women experience areas of altered sensation, such as numbness, a pins and needles feeling, or increased sensitivity. Some are shocked by bizarre sensations in the armpit and along the arm after a breast lumpectomy and lymph node surgery; they thought that only women who had mastectomies felt those sensations. While many women are tempted to avoid these areas, consistent touching and stroking during lovemaking and at other times may actually reeducate the nerve endings and reduce the negative sensations.

When both ovaries are removed with surgery or are made nonfunctional with treatment, the premenopausal woman catapults into menopause. If she cannot (or does not) take hormone replacement therapy, she will experience physical changes in the vagina (see Menopause—Without Hormone Replacement, in this chapter).

Even in the best of relationships and with a healthy vagina, some women experience very decreased sexual desire or difficulty with arousal because of hormonal changes from chemotherapy and/or Tamoxifen. These women can ask their doctors for a blood test to measure their testosterone level. Testosterone, a hormone associated with sexual desire, is considered a male hormone—but it normally occurs in smaller amounts in women too. If the testosterone level is very low, some women are choosing to replace the deficiency with pills or injections of the hormone. (Helen Singer Kaplan, M.D., Ph.D., the Director of the Human Sexuality Program of the New York Hospital–Cornell Medical Center, is investigating this treatment.)

Any major physical change requires adjustments in lovemaking: more comfortable positions, lubricating jelly, more attention to other sensitive areas, use of fantasy, and so on. In many cases, including vaginal surgery and menopausal changes in the vagina, fairly frequent intercourse helps keeps the vagina in good condition (a clear case of "use it or lose it").

The woman needs clear information from her doctor, a nurse, a sex therapist, or a good reference book about the changes that occur. This is a legitimate part of cancer therapy for women *of any age* who are interested in continuing or beginning a sexual relationship. But many women feel reluctant to ask—and too many health professionals, raised in the same atmosphere of "things we do not talk about," either do not know the answers or feel uncomfortable telling women what they need to know.

The booklet, *Sexuality & Cancer: For the Woman Who Has Cancer, and Her Partner,* available on request from the local American Cancer Society unit, contains information about both the physical and emotional aspects of sexuality after a cancer diagnosis. Also, many a woman finds, in talking with friends or opening up in a support group, that she is not alone —that her questions and problems are all too common. (This does not mean she has to tell other people every detail of her sex life, of course. She might ask a simple question, such as, "Is anyone having trouble getting interested in sex?")

The relationship

Anyone eavesdropping on Cinderella and her Prince Charming a few years after "happily ever after" would doubtless hear a few spats and misunderstandings. Even the most long-term relationships experience some sexual difficulties at one time or another. These go with the territory when two imperfect human beings try to communicate (including sexually) over time.

Because people can use a sexual relationship to express many different aspects of themselves, sexual problems may mask all sorts of personal or relationship difficulties, big and small. Sometimes the partners themselves can disentangle the threads and work to make the situation better, but it may take a counselor to step in and take an impartial look.

After cancer diagnosis and treatment, some women in a reasonably good established relationship feel a need for a new relationship—perhaps an affair—to affirm that they are still desirable women. The thinking may go, "Of course, my regular partner will act as if I'm desirable, but that does not *prove* that I really am." It makes sense to think long and hard before acting on this kind of impulse.

BEGINNING A NEW RELATIONSHIP

When a woman and her partner have been together for some time before her cancer diagnosis, they have a shared history, good or bad. A woman interested in beginning a new close relationship does not have that—but she does have a fresh slate.

At the best of times, however, it can be scary to reach out for a new friendship. A woman may feel vulnerable, unsure of herself and of how much she can trust the partner. Cancer and the changes it has brought may make her question her desirability as a partner: who would want someone with one breast or a missing uterus or a cancer diagnosis?

She focuses so much on the negative changes that have occurred that she cannot remember the exciting positive changes, as well as the wonderful things about herself that have not changed. Cancer scars can become a convenient "cover" for more basic feelings of inadequacy: a reason not to reach for the relationship at all or a scapegoat if she is rejected.

Cynthia, for instance, was a most attractive single woman who underwent mastectomy surgery with reconstruction using a breast implant. The tissue around the implant hardened somewhat, and she became acutely self-conscious about it. She began seeing herself (as she admitted later) as a horrible rock-like breast, which just happened to have a walking, talking person attached. She was convinced that everyone else was just as aware of her breast as she was. If she ever went on a date, she spent the whole time "protecting" herself from "discovery," maneuvering herself away from even a hug. No date had a chance to discover the warm, intelligent, funny Cynthia underneath—and no date ever came back twice.

It took some months of therapy before Cynthia realized how much she had been using her "different" breast as a scapegoat for all the doubts she'd had about herself long before surgery. When she began liking herself more, she no longer had to spend all her energy protecting herself. Now she had more interesting tasks: listening to her date, talking, having fun. She learned that a woman who sincerely likes herself is profoundly desirable.

To her astonishment, she found that when she did engage in sexual relations, her partner barely noticed the scars or the "different" breast, just as she did not pay much attention to the reddened appendectomy scar which made her partner self-conscious. Each had the same reaction to the other's "disfigurement": "Is that all? What's the problem?"

After cancer, there is another scenario: the woman who collects sexual "scalps" in order to prove that she is still desirable. Aside from the dangers in a time of deadly sexually-transmitted diseases, this woman is not coming any closer to liking herself as a real person.

How does a woman tell a prospective partner and when?

Neither Miss Manners nor Emily Post has given guidelines. Some people tell casual dates; some do not. But before committing to a long-term relationship, certainly a potential lifetime partner has the right to know of a previous cancer diagnosis. And some people feel so much more at ease after they tell that they explain fairly early in any possibly serious relationship.

Explanations can be simple, honest—and honestly optimistic: "A few years ago I was diagnosed with cancer of the uterus. I had a hysterectomy and, as you can see, I'm doing very well!" (She can also enlist her doctor's help to talk to a potential mate.)

One of my favorite "how to tell" strategies was a friend who took her date to a "Survivors' Day" picnic sponsored by the National Coalition for Cancer Survivorship. Surrounded by other obviously healthy, thriving people who had been through a cancer diagnosis, she felt comfortable broaching the subject.

Occasionally, a partner cannot deal with the cancer—or gives that as an excuse to discontinue the relationship. This is not easy, but it is still better to discover the problem before wasting too much time on a fruitless relationship.

While it is specifically geared to the post-mastectomy woman, Linda Dackman's book, *Up Front: Sex and the Post-Mastectomy Woman*, can help all women with cancer diagnoses.

PREGNANCY

Saving the woman's life is the first priority in treating any cancer. Considerations of becoming and staying pregnant take second place. Some cancers and their treatments make pregnancy afterwards impossible, highly unlikely, or inadvisable.

However, some women do become pregnant and deliver healthy babies after treatment for a women's cancer. These are among the women who cheered when actress Ann Jillian gave birth to a beautiful, healthy boy a few years after a double mastectomy and chemotherapy for breast cancer.

Childbearing is an individual question, and it makes sense for the woman who truly wants to have a baby after treatment to ask questions beforehand. Occasionally, there are two equally effective treatment options and the doctor and the woman can choose the one less likely to hurt her chances of having a baby.

After treatment, a woman should consider any limiting physical factors. Have any parts of her reproductive tract been removed or severely damaged? This could be from surgery, such as removal of both ovaries so that the woman can no longer provide ova (eggs) necessary for a pregnancy. Radiation can cause similar local damage. Or a woman could have such heavy scarring after conization of the cervix that she has difficulty carrying a pregnancy to term. It is worth consulting a gynecologist who specializes in fertility issues.

During chemotherapy for breast cancer, especially with the drug cyclophosphamide (Cytoxan), many premenopausal women stop menstruating. The younger the woman is, the more likely it is that her ovarian function will resume after she finishes treatment; however, the woman over 40 or so may be close enough to normal menopause that this tips the balance permanently.

Tamoxifen (Nolvadex), a common long-term treatment after a breast cancer diagnosis, blocks the hormone estrogen in the breast but actually acts as a weak estrogen elsewhere in the body. It does not make a women infertile, but it can cause severe damage to the fetus in the uterus. Thus a premenopausal woman who uses the drug needs to use effective birth control at the same time. Removing both ovaries or destroying them with radiation so that they do not produce hormones to "feed" a breast cancer used to be more common. Now, tamoxifen does the job.

Even if she remains physically capable of becoming pregnant, a woman wants to know if she can have a healthy baby and whether pregnancy poses any special risk to her continuing health. For several reasons, many doctors advise the woman to wait two years or so after treatment ends before trying to become pregnant. The first two years are the most common time for cancer to reappear. This waiting period also allows the woman time to recover her health and energy before coping with pregnancy and the challenges of new motherhood. It is especially important after chemotherapy to protect the baby from residual effects of the powerful drugs, and that means taking time for them to leave the body. Of course, this also means that if there is any chance a woman could be fertile, she needs to use an effective method of contraception during this time. Not having menstrual periods is no guarantee of infertility.

There are many questions and few answers about pregnancy as a risk to a woman's continued health. Especially after diagnosis of a hormone-nourished cancer, both doctors and women worry that any stray cancer cells lingering in the body will thrive on all those pregnancy hormones. In truth, there is little evidence one way or the other, and more research is long overdue.

Many women argue that for them the benefits of having a baby outweigh the risks from cancer cells that may or may not be there. Still, it makes sense for any woman contemplating pregnancy to sit down with her cancer doctor first so that she can make her decision based on both head and heart. Adoption may be a good option if a woman has a positive bill-of-health from her doctor, but cannot or does not want to become pregnant.

One of the unspoken questions for many cancer-survivor women is, "What are my chances of living to bring up this baby?" It needs to be spoken. In a sense, it is an appropriate question for *any* woman who wants to become pregnant or adopt, but the woman with a cancer diagnosis is more intimately acquainted than most with uncertainty and her own mortality. Each woman's answer must be her own, but it is prudent (for every woman) to consider who will raise her child if she cannot.

LYMPHEDEMA

After cancer treatment, many women are at risk for *lymphedema*: edema, or swelling, of an arm or leg that occurs from the buildup of lymph fluid that cannot drain out freely. This can happen because a tumor is pressing on the lymph nodes in the armpit or the groin. More often, it occurs as a complication of cancer treatment: the lymph nodes have been removed to check for the presence of cancer or have been purposely destroyed with radiation therapy to the area. Lymphedema does *not* mean that the treatment itself was unsuccessful or poorly done.

Lymph is a sticky, protein-rich fluid. If it cannot drain normally, it builds up like water before a dam. If it pools long enough, it begins to stick to the linings of the lymph channels in the arm or leg, forming protein plaques which harden and make the channels even narrower and less elastic; that makes the drainage even worse and means that less oxygen reaches the tissues. In addition, since bacteria thrive in any quiet pool of protein-rich fluid, the arm or leg with lymphedema is prone to infection which can further damage the lymph vessels.

Right after surgery, many women develop some temporary tissue swelling in an arm or leg. This goes away by itself and usually does not indicate the chronic high-protein swelling of lymphedema, which tends to develop later.

Lymphedema is unsightly, and finding attractive clothing to fit over a grossly swollen limb may be next to impossible. It can also be very difficult to use a swollen arm or leg. The limb may be quite uncomfortable and heavy although, surprisingly, pain is rare unless there is infection or another problem.

Preventing lymphedema is the first goal. A lymph system damaged by surgery or radiation may still be able to function well unless an infection or other "insult" tips the delicate balance into lymphedema. That is the idea behind the common sense do's and don'ts after surgery or radiation to either armpit or groin.

A woman avoids infection by keeping the arm or leg clean and taking reasonable care to prevent any break in the skin: wearing gloves for household or garden work after breast cancer surgery, for instance, and not allowing the arm to be used for injections or blood drawing. To prevent nicks, she shaves with an electric razor rather than a safety razor and does not cut her cuticles. She cleans and cares for any tiny cut or injury thoroughly and seeks medical help at the first sign of infection.

Also she avoids constriction of the limb or pressure on

any lymph nodes in the area because that makes it harder for the lymph to circulate normally. This means no tight bands or jewelry and no blood pressure readings in the arm after breast surgery. Too, the woman protects the lymph nodes along the collar bone by not wearing over-the-shoulder handbags on that side or a very heavy breast prosthesis.

She also uses gravity to help keep the lymph from pooling in the limb. If the arm is at risk, for instance, she does not carry things with a straight arm hanging at her side, and periodically she raises the arm so that the hand is above her heart. She exercises the limb. This maintains or increases the muscle tone to help move lymph fluid out of the arm or leg.

These precautions mean being reasonably careful. They do not mean that a woman should become so petrified of the possibility of lymphedema that she wraps herself in lambswool and refuses to budge. Most women never develop lymphedema.

If the arm or leg does become swollen, a woman should seek help as soon as possible. Expert care from a health professional who specializes in lymphedema care can make the difference between a condition that is a "mild nuisance" and one that makes a woman chronically miserable. A lymphedema clinic, a physical therapist who treats the condition frequently, or a cancer center may be possible resources.

Early mild lymphedema is usually relatively easy to treat: any threatening factor is removed (an infection is cured with antibiotics, for instance). Swelling can be reduced by elevating the limb; after the swelling is gone, the woman may use compression sleeves or stockings (like support hose but heavy duty) to help lymph fluid leave the area before it can build up protein plaques along the lymph channels. These compression garments may encourage the body to form new "collateral" lymph drainage channels.

Treatment for more severe or advanced lymphedema includes use of pressure pumps, lymph drainage massage, a low-salt diet, and special bandaging techniques. The specialist also teaches the woman how to prevent more injury and prescribes antibiotics at the first hint of possible infection. Some surgeons, primarily in Europe, are working on microsurgery techniques to increase lymph drainage. Drugs to reduce the development of the protein plaques that often occurs with lymphedema and to control the amount of protein in the lymph are also being studied.

The pressure pump blows air into an inflatable "sleeve" that fits over the whole limb. Effective pumps use a "sequential" pattern of inflation. Thus, the sleeve is divided into several channels circling the limb and these channels inflate and deflate in turn to provide deep massage, increase circulation, and push the lymphedema fluid out of the arm or leg. The safest pumps use a system of "gradient" pressures which means that they compress most firmly at the wrist or ankle (high "grade" of pressure), less firmly as they move up the arm or leg.

Manual lymph drainage massage helps open existing lymph channels. The gentle pumping motions focus on the connective tissue rather than the muscles. Physical or massage therapists with training in these special techniques can often reduce lymphedema symptoms dramatically.

Diuretics (water pills) do not work with lymphedema because the lymph fluid is too "thick." However, many people with lymphedema are seeing slow but encouraging results from various drugs in the benzo-pyrone family. These pills, taken over several months, help dissolve the protein plaques in lymphedema; they are used along with other treatments. While they have not yet been approved for lymphedema by the FDA, the benzo-pyrones are inexpensive and appear to be quite safe and free of side effects. They can be ordered from Europe, or lower-strength derivatives (rutin and bio-flavenoids, three grams a day) can be purchased in healthfood stores in the U.S.

Unfortunately, many doctors are not yet aware of new advances in lymphedema treatment. And some ignore or undertreat lymphedema because of their personal—and very human —difficulty coping with the fact that the therapy they gave is partially responsible for a difficult problem. The National Lymphedema Network (2211 Post Street, Suite 404, San Francisco, CA 94115; 1-800-541-3259) provides information, support, and a newsletter for people with lymphedema and their doctors.

Menopause—
Without Hormone Replacement

Menopause occurs when the ovaries stop their production of the sex hormones estrogen and progesterone. The major physical concerns are immediate problems such as hot flashes, night sweats, and vaginal changes, and potential long-range problems such as osteoporosis ("thinning" bones) and heart disease.

Normally, menopause is a gradual process, occurring over several years as the body adjusts to these natural changes. Some kinds of cancer therapy, however, can send a woman into an abrupt, all-at-once menopause. Her ovaries may be removed surgically or become nonfunctional after radiation or certain kinds of chemotherapy.

Many women in the U.S. now rely on **hormone replacement therapy (HRT)** to counter the effects of decreased hormones after menopause. HRT may be prescribed as estrogen and/or progesterone pills, patches, or creams.

HRT is an option for many women with a cancer history. But most doctors currently consider it too risky to use when the woman has been treated for a cancer that can "feed" on hormones. If there are any stray cancer cells anywhere in the body, the doctors want to starve them, not nourish them. While HRT may sound dangerous in theory, however, more research needs to be done about whether it is dangerous in practice.

Any woman who picks up a popular magazine today and reads the ads can be forgiven for fearing that, without HRT, she will have nonstop hot flashes, no sex life, brittle bones, and a faltering heart. It is hard to remember that, not many years ago, *all* women went through menopause without the option of HRT—and billions of them survived and even thrived!

With an abrupt menopause, a woman's symptoms may come on more dramatically than those of other women, but menopause is an absolutely individual experience. Some women experience minimal symptoms, while others suffer significantly. Any woman with concerns deserves to get from her doctor clear factual information and help with symptom relief.

No one knows yet exactly how the drop in hormones

triggers the sudden expansions and contractions in the blood vessels that can leave a woman suddenly dripping with sweat. Simple strategies for warding off hot flashes and night sweats include dressing lightly so that the woman does not get too hot, layering clothing, and keeping a paper fan handy.

"Keeping cool" emotionally can help but is not usually a cure. Yoga or slow deep breathing works for some. Some women find symptom relief through such complementary health therapies as herbal medicine and acupuncture or acupressure. Also, engaging in stimulating activity can distract a woman from hot flashes and may actually make them occur less often.

For severe hot flashes, doctors may prescribe a patch of clonidine, a blood pressure medication. Diphenhydramine (Benadryl), an antihistamine that also makes people drowsy, is a mild sleeping aid that lets some women sleep through the night. More potent sleep medications tend to lose their effectiveness and cause drug dependence if they are taken for more than a few days.

Dryness and thinning of the vagina walls can make sexual penetration uncomfortable. It can also make the woman more prone to infections because of tiny breaks in the vaginal lining. Drug stores offer several over-the-counter, water-based lubricants that can be applied to the vagina or penis during intercourse. (Vaseline works poorly, does not clean off well, and is a haven for the organisms that cause yeast infections.) Some doctors recommend a vaginal moisture-replenishing product to use a few times a week to keep the vagina comfortable. An estrogen vaginal suppository, developed in Denmark and being tested in the U.S., supposedly releases estrogen so slowly that it can help the vagina without getting into the bloodstream. This may become available soon in the U.S.

Many of my friends swear by regular use of prescription vaginal creams made from the male hormone testosterone, which actually decreases vaginal thinning and atrophy. One of these, 1% testosterone enanthate in a Velvachol base, was developed several years ago by William Goodson III, M.D., faculty surgeon and chief of the Breast Screening Clinic at the University of California in San Francisco, working with UCSF pharmacologist Phil Hoffman. Since testosterone is not a female hormone, it does not appear to promote growth of cancer cells. Used as directed, it does not cause masculine changes in a woman. (The only side effect Dr. Goodson has seen in over twelve years was acne in one patient; this disappeared promptly when she stopped taking the drug.)

The cream must be prescribed by a doctor and compounded by a pharmacist; it is somewhat difficult to mix, but the woman must insist on a Velvachol base which absorbs easily from the vagina. Then, using the kind of standard vaginal applicator used for inserting antiyeast infection creams, the woman inserts two grams (one inch in the applicator) of cream every day for a week, and then uses one inch every ten to fourteen days for maintenance. The idea is to use the minimum amount necessary as seldom as possible. (If the medicine comes in a jar, women can transfer the contents to the kind of open-end tube that campers fill with peanut butter; these are available where camping/hiking supplies are sold.)

Some women find that tamoxifen, used as anti-estrogen therapy for breast cancer, makes hot flashes and night sweats worse—but acts as a mild estrogen in the reproductive tract and may relieve vaginal thinning slightly. Other women have not found it effective for vaginal changes. Regular sexual activity (including masturbation) helps keep the vagina open and healthy.

For the woman experiencing problems with menopause, there may be a specific menopause group in her area, since this is a problem for many women with no cancer history. Several books on menopause offer hints on solving both physical and emotional concerns. The woman who should not use HRT needs to choose a book that does not focus entirely on the benefits and joys of hormone replacement. Pamphlets published by drug companies naturally tend to stress the hormone replacement medications from which they make their profit.

Women begin to lose bone mass during young adulthood, but the process accelerates dramatically as estrogen decreases at menopause. Estrogen protects a woman's bones somewhat, and if bones become too porous, they break easily. To maintain as much bone density as possible, women who do not take HRT can exercise regularly, especially by doing weight-bearing exercise such as walking, jogging, jumping, and dancing, which builds bone in legs, hips, and spine.

A well-balanced diet can help prevent osteoporosis. It includes generous servings of food rich in calcium and vitamin D, which the body needs to absorb calcium. There are many calcium-rich foods besides the obvious dairy products, but women who like and can digest dairy products can make tasty blender drinks from nonfat (or low-fat) milk and yogurt, one or more kinds of fruit, and perhaps a bit of sweetener; these give plenty of calcium but few calories and minimal fat. Calcium from pills can supplement calcium from food.

Yo-yo dieting, in which a woman frequently loses weight and then regains it, changes the body's metabolism and draws calcium out of the bones. Smoking, too, decreases the effectiveness with which the body processes calcium.

Researchers are currently studying several drugs that may help women maintain bone density and even reverse bone loss. One class of these drugs is called the bisphosphanates (etidronate is one). Tamoxifen appears to have some protective effects against both osteoporosis and heart disease.

Many of the anti-osteoporosis strategies, such as exercise and not smoking, work as well to keep the heart healthy. Many researchers believe that diets low in saturated fats build up less "sludge" in the body's blood vessels so that the blood moves freely; that means less work for the heart and less chance of a clot forming in the heart. Other researchers are convinced that a diet low in all fats decreases the risk for breast cancer and some other cancers.

Menopause is a normal, natural process. But because menopause means that a woman can no longer bear a child, she may equate this stage of life with growing old or with losing her femininity and worth. A cancer diagnosis can make those feelings more acute.

Many women, however, happily bid adieu to menstrual periods. Because she no longer has monthly blood loss, a woman may feel more energetic than she has felt for years. *Post-menopausal zest*, a phrase coined by anthropologist Margaret

Mead, says it accurately for many women. Freed from the possibility of pregnancy, they are eager to dream new dreams, step out in new directions.

EMPLOYMENT AND INSURANCE

Some women with a job never break step after a cancer diagnosis. They may take sick leave for treatment, but they have secure jobs they like and can continue to do, and never face an employment problem.

For others, employment after cancer is a major concern. Some have lost jobs during a period of disability (or for any other reason), and fear their health history will make it more difficult to find a new job. Some women can no longer meet the physical demands of a particular job (such as heavy lifting) or find that the job makes them feel so stressed and unhappy that it probably is not healthy for them. And some women just want to spread their wings . . . .

Whenever a woman looks for a new job, there are basic tips she can follow appropriate for all job-seekers, such as arriving on time, dressing appropriately for any interview, and applying for only those jobs for which she is qualified. The woman who can no longer perform her former job because of cancer or its treatment may get the state department of rehabilitation to finance job retraining.

Liking oneself and communicating that good self-image to a potential employer make a difference. The woman can give herself positive "self-talk," and possibly role-play with a mentor or support group. It helps to practice beforehand answering questions that the personnel department might ask so that she can appear confident rather than defensive. The library or bookstore, state department of employment, and private employment agencies all offer information about basic job-seeking skills.

Specifics tips include downplaying any cancer-related gaps in employment history by organizing a resume by skills and achievements rather than chronological dates of employment. In any job application or interview, the woman must answer honestly any direct questions about her health history, but is not obliged or advised to volunteer any information. She can make honest positive statements about her health. If her health history comes into question, her doctor can write a letter to the employer.

In the U.S, the employment rights of the person with a cancer history are protected somewhat by the *Rehabilitation Act of 1973* and the *Americans with Disabilities Act of 1990*. Many U.S. employers can no longer base hiring decisions on what are *perceived* to be disabilities. State laws may also apply. Federal and state agencies give information about these laws and enforce them.

The National Coalition for Cancer Survivorship offers packets of current information about both employment and insurance issues—and fights to make the situation better. "Facing Forward: A Guide for Cancer Survivors," a pamphlet that is a joint venture of the National Coalition for Cancer Survivorship and NCI, is available free from NCI's Cancer Information Service, and gives tips about these practical problems as well as about emotional and physical survival. Another free booklet, "Cancer: Your Job, Insurance, and the Law" is available from the American Cancer Society Hotline at 1-800-ACS-2345. Local chapters of the American Cancer Society can provide information about current laws, and how to fight apparent discrimination.

Insurance

To remain profitable, most health insurance companies prefer to insure people who will not cost them much money. This often means that the people who need health insurance most have the most trouble getting and keeping it. After treatment, a cancer patient may cost no more than anyone else—in fact, may cost less because she takes better care of her health—but insurance companies look at actuarial tables of averages rather than at individuals.

If a woman is insured through work, she may cling to a job she does not like in order to keep her health insurance ("job trap") or may have trouble finding a new job that covers her. Since insurance companies may pass on their potential future costs to employers or a group of employees, an employer may be leery of hiring a woman who might cost more. Other potential problems include obtaining new insurance that covers her preexisting condition, getting the insurance company to pay for procedures (especially ones it sees as "experimental," such as autologous bone marrow transplants for breast cancer), and affording premiums and copayments.

These are not concerns in countries with national health insurance, such as Canada. In the U.S., federal or state governments offer basic health care for some groups of people: most people 65 or older and the permanently disabled (Medicare); armed service veterans (VA); and some people who are in low-income brackets (Medicaid, or Medi-Cal in California).

Any kind of large-group insurance plan in which the risks and costs are spread out among many people is apt to be easier to obtain and pay for than individual or small-group policies. Besides a regular company plan for the employed woman with a cancer history, options include: dependent coverage under a spouse's insurance plan; a health maintenance organization (HMO) with an open enrollment period in which a person must be accepted regardless of health history; and group insurance through a professional or other organization to which the woman belongs.

The woman who is insured under a group health plan through an employer and leaves her work for any reason can continue her same coverage for eighteen months under the federally-mandated COBRA program (Consolidated Omnibus Budget Reconciliation Act of 1985). She pays the full cost of the policy, including what her employer used to pay, but because it is a group-rate policy, the cost is much less than for individual coverage. After eighteen months, she may be able to "convert" to an individual policy with the same company, which will cost more and often cover less but will insure her despite her preexisting condition.

Some states offer "high risk" health insurance pools for people who cannot get insurance any other way. Blue Cross and

Blue Shield have open enrollment periods in some states. A phone call to the National Coalition for Cancer Survivorship will bring information. Some independent insurance brokers can match up a woman with some kind of insurance, although the coverage may have high premiums and deductibles and limited coverage.

Occasionally, legal action about insurance becomes appropriate, especially in cases where the insurance company refuses to pay for a procedure it considers experimental but which the medical community contends is state-of-the-art. Currently, however, the federal "ERISA" provisions mean that most cases involving insurance through an employer must be tried in federal court. Since federal courts do not allow damages for emotional distress or punitive damages, this reduces incentives both for attorneys to take on the woman's case, and for insurance companies to settle (since it costs them little to stall).

More and more people consider health insurance in the U.S. an expensive scandal. Whether this will translate into concrete action remains to be seen, but several groups are formulating plans to give more people better coverage at less cost. Part of this process means asking how limited health dollars should be allocated in order to serve both individuals and society best. Balancing the needs of the individual woman for health insurance, of all insured people for coverage at reasonable rates, and of the insurance company and/or the employer to remain profitable enough to stay in business can call for the wisdom of Solomon—and probably the charity of Mother Teresa.

Kerry McGinn

Chapter 23

❖

Cancer *Is* a Political Issue

One of every four Americans now living will get cancer, and half of these people are women. Breast cancer claims the lives of at least 46,000 women each year—more American lives lost *each year* than during the entire Vietnam War. This year alone, some 180,000 American women will learn that they have breast cancer. Lung cancer kills another 53,000 women annually and is the single leading cause of cancer deaths for women in this country. Even though lung cancer is not just a "women's cancer," lung cancer is definitely a women's issue. Twenty-one thousand woman will be told this year that they have ovarian cancer and 12,000 women will die of this disease. Close to 4,500 women die annually from cervical cancer *despite* the fact that a simple, relatively cheap method of finding cervical cancer at a curable stage has been around for over thirty years.

Over $20 billion has been spent on America's "War on Cancer" since 1971. The combined cure rate for all cancers is now about 50%. Some kinds of cancers offer fair odds for survival, others, much less. And some kinds of cancer are more common now than they were in 1971. Certainly cancers affecting women occur in more women now than was true in the past. Breast cancer now affects 1 of every 9 American women, while just a few short years ago, that incidence was 1 in 15. Cancers of the cervix occur more in younger women now than in years before, and these cancers seem to be more deadly. For many Americans, especially those who are poor, black, or Hispanic, victories in the "War on Cancer" have been watched from the sidelines. Lack of insurance and/or access to screening and early treatment is reflected in their higher death rates. While the search for "the magic bullet"—a cure for cancer—goes on, little has been done to search for the reasons cancer happens in the first place. Many people believe we do not have enough to show for our dollars.

One woman described a clinic nurse's attempt to help her understand chemotherapy. The nurse tried to reassure her by explaining that the anticancer drug she was going to get had been used for over 20 years. The woman, who is a newspaper writer, did not find this encouraging: why, in a world where computer programs are outdated every two or three months and cars are redesigned nearly as often, must women depend on 20-year-old technology? Good question!

Many issues complicate healthcare policy and politics. For example, the so-called abortion pill developed in France, RU-486, may be able to shrink tumors in breast cancer. But because of the pro-choice versus pro-life argument, RU-486 is banned in the United States. Our scientists cannot even study the tumor effects of this drug. Many women's groups and many women became especially outraged when, in August 1992, newspapers reported that a man was to be treated with RU-486 for a brain tumor. A representative from Oregon stated "this is a real step forward." Is it a step forward when one man with a rare tumor can be treated with this drug, and at the same time, 180,000 women diagnosed with breast cancer are not afforded the same chance?

In 1990 less than 14% of the National Institutes of Health (NIH) research dollars were spent on women's health issues. There is evidence that most medical research is so slanted toward men that many women are misdiagnosed and inadequately treated. NIH's 1992 appropriation includes $133 million earmarked for breast cancer research ($169 million is directed for AIDS research). The approval of this budget hinged on President George Bush's reservations about amendments related to fetal tissue research. In October 1991, breast cancer activists hand-delivered petitions with 600,000 signatures to Congress demanding more breast cancer research; unfortunately, the event was overshadowed by the Clarence Thomas Supreme Court confirmation hearings and did not receive the attention it deserved.

Seventeen of our fifty states do not have state reimbursement for mammography screening for breast cancer, and most healthcare insurance plans do not cover expenses related to screening tests such as Pap smears, mammography, and breast exams, but these are *vital* to women's health.

Each year, lung cancer kills nearly 150,000 Americans. Most experts estimate that at least 85%—127,500 people— are killed by cigarettes. There is scientific evidence that women may be more susceptible to lung tissue damage caused by tobacco smoke. So why are we not up in arms about cigarette brands and advertising schemes targeted (like a loaded gun) right at women? This advertising also targets our kids. Studies show that slick ads work to recruit new smokers, and women's magazines, even magazines with a feminist message, are largely supported by tobacco advertising. The tobacco industry, seeing its tobacco revenues decrease as more Americans stop smoking and veteran smokers die off, seeks export of tobacco products to Third World countries. Why does the federal government issue studies that document the health hazards of tobacco use and at the same time continue to allow tax breaks to tobacco companies and subsidize tobacco farming? You can enter a Virginia congressman's Capitol Hill office and see the prominent position given to a framed collection of cigarettes manufactured in his state to find the answer to that question. But, the Marlboro Man himself just died of lung cancer; he was 51.

Most cancer research is funded through the United States' National Institutes of Health and the National Cancer Institute. Like all Federal agencies, NIH and NCI are subject to the whims of the Federal budget process, where the squeaky wheel syndrome prevails. The most pressing need, usually defined as the loudest voice, gets funding priority. AIDS activists have successfully put the squeaky wheel concept to use. So where are cancer activists? Why are not we out on the streets or the halls of Congress demanding long-overdue attention to women's health and women's cancer issues?

I think a major reason people affected by cancer are not as

politically active as people affected by AIDS is related to the way the two diseases act. People infected with the AIDS virus often know they are infected long before they actually get AIDS. They have months and even years to get really angry—and active—about their almost certain death from AIDS. Most significant may be the fact that so many people with AIDS, at least in the United States, are young.

On the other hand, people with cancer discover they have the disease and go into a treatment phase almost immediately. Treatment is a drawn-out process that zaps people of strength and energy. Most people with cancer are older: 57% of all cancers occur in people over 65 years old. Many older people take the cards life deals them and do not—or cannot—fight the system. Some people with cancer try to keep a low profile: they don't want anyone to know they have cancer because they fear loss of a job, loss of friends, loss of a spouse, loss of life. Lastly, the activist tendencies of women as a group have diminished since Margaret Sanger. Women like Betty Friedan and Gloria Steinem are relatively quiet about women's cancers, even though Gloria is a breast cancer survivor. Women, particularly the group of women most likely to have cancer, are still fairly passive and apolitical. But women with cancer are often victims of the highly patriarchal healthcare system.

Some critics believe that the politics of cancer are extensive and even sinister. In his book *The Politics of Cancer*, Samuel Epstein tells us that the lack of advances in the "War on Cancer" is related to a conspiracy involving the Establishment—the government, NCI researchers, and drug companies—who are more interested in treatment than prevention. Epstein is not a flake: he is professor of occupational and environmental medicine at Illinois University. In a May 5, 1992, presentation to the National Cancer Advisory Board (NCAB), Epstein charged that two former chairmen of NCAB had serious conflicts of interest. He said that the first chair, Benno Schmidt, had ties with drug industries, and the other, the late Armand Hammer, was chairman of Occidental Petroleum, one of America's leading producers of chemicals that cause cancer (carcinogens). Epstein asserts that executives from agricultural, drug, oil, chemical and tobacco industries sit on boards of major cancer research institutions that make more money *treating* cancer than they could by *preventing* cancer.

1 in 3: Women with Cancer Confront an Epidemic, edited by Judy Brady, is a testimony to the politics of cancer in women's lives. The essays in *1 in 3* describe women's reactions to the cancers that changed their lives, and their anger at pollution, chemicals, radiation, and the politics that they believe caused their cancers. Brady suggests that government "will not be a willing ally in any battle against cancer."

"Politics" is much more than people who work on Capitol Hill or offices in state capitols. It can be finding ways to meet the needs of a community health center or a prevention and screening clinic. It can be letting elected officials know what you think about issues. Letters to these people *do have meaning*. Federal and state legislators or city council members respond to constituents. But they are not mindreaders. And silence usually gets interpreted as approval.

Politics can mean challenging the male-dominated practice of gynecology. Eighty percent of all gynecologists are men—men who act and think like men. Could this relate to the fact that nearly a million hysterectomies are performed each year? There are only a few real reasons to have a hysterectomy, but over 1,000 women die each year as a result of this operation. The political and policy consequences of this gender imbalance is not even being discussed, let alone addressed.

Things are changing for the better, but change is slow in coming. The Women's Health Equity Act of 1991 (WHEA) is a package of legislation devoted to the healthcare needs of women, introduced by Representatives Patricia Schroeder (D-Colorado) and Olympia Snowe (R-Maine). It is the creation of women legislators who have banded together to form the Congressional Caucus for Women's Issues. Various bills in the package deal with women's health research, informed consent, adolescent pregnancy, prenatal care and infant mortality, breast cancer screening, equality in clinical trials, ovarian cancer, AIDS, and other issues. For more information about the Women's Health Equity Act, contact the Congressional Caucus for

Women's Issues, 2471 Rayburn Building, Washington, D.C. 20515 or call (202) 225-6740. The office provides updates on WHEA as well as information on other women's issues being addressed through the legislative process.

The National Institute of Health created the Office on Women's Health Research and appointed Vivian Pinn, M.D., as director. Dr. Pinn is known for her work on educating minority women on the need for breast and cervical cancer screening. This office is charged with strengthening NIH's efforts to improve and increase research on the prevention, diagnosis, and treatment of illnesses that affect women.

There is a hopeful beginning of cancer activism. In 1986, the National Coalition for Cancer Survivorship (NCCS) was founded by Dr. Fitzhugh Mullan, a survivor of testicular cancer. This organization exists to be a voice for people affected—or disaffected—by cancer. NCCS promotes everyone's right to healthcare insurance despite a history of cancer. At one time, employers could exclude people who had had cancer from certain jobs. Today, that is illegal—but one-fourth of workers who survive cancer are still fired from their jobs. NCCS supports the right of people to work without this discrimination. Other new groups centered around a specific cancer are growing. Most numerous are organizations for women who have had breast cancer. The organizations Y-ME, Breast Cancer Action, and the Breast Cancer Network are part of the larger National Coalition of Breast Cancer Organizations (NABCO). Us Too is a group for men who have had prostate cancer. The Candlelighters Foundation provides support for parents and families of children and young people with cancer.

A grassroots movement of cancer activism is out there, and it grows every time someone new has to hear "You have cancer."

WHAT YOU CAN DO

The ability to influence our healthcare system on the local, state, or national level is related to events that occur long before we call or write a city council member or senator. The most important step in the process is determining who is nominated and elected. Women can participate in campaigns to help elect officials who are sensitive to our views. Political party activity provides a vehicle for developing relationships with elected officials and is essential to building a politically active network. Even very simple things, like helping on a telephone bank or volunteering time in an elected official's office can begin to give a woman an "inside track" to the political process.

The power of numbers is very great. That is why working with groups that reflect your own views is important. For example, it helps support my opinion to say that it is shared by 20,000 other cancer nurses in this country, or that my idea is endorsed by a professional organization. The power of numbers is an important reason for organizations like the National Coalition for Cancer Survivorship and Y-ME to exist.

I recently learned a very important political principle. I went to a congressman's Washington, D.C. office to ask for a copy of a bill he was going to introduce. The bill, I believe, will add another obstacle to people's ability to get narcotic analgesics for the treatment of cancer pain. I ended up talking to his legislative aide, who it turned out, was the major author of the bill. The aide expressed total shock that I was at all interested in this legislation. Despite the fact that several drafts of the bill had been circulating for months and were reviewed by medical and pharmaceutical groups, not one nurse had uttered (or written) a word of concern about it.

The fact that the nurses had not voiced concerns was interpreted as approval. That was my big revelation. Since then, I have become a sort of "pen-pal" to my elected officials. I write to them about legislation I think might curb the tobacco industry's efforts to addict more people (like selling cigarettes to Third World countries). I wrote to express my objections to the so-called "gag rule." I write when pending legislation might affect women's health—particularly when the issues involve cancer prevention, early detection, and care. And I write about funding for nursing education and nursing research. Recently, an estimated 200 California cancer nurses wrote or called the

Governor to encourage his support for a bill that mandates insurance companies' reimbursement for certain drugs used in cancer and AIDS treatment. The governor did sign the bill.

So, let your elected officials know who you are, what you think, and what you'd like to see them do. The addresses and telephone numbers of all officials are in the phone book. If you are not sure who your representative is, call the local League of Women Voters; they can give you this information. Western Union offers a public opinion message service; call them at 800-325-6000 and ask to send a public opinion message to the representative you need to reach. It doesn't matter how you do it. In most instances, handwritten letters are more likely to get attention; it is obvious that they are not mass-produced and that the writer went to some trouble to write them.

Tips on writing to an elected official:

1. Be concise, informed, and polite

2. Stick to one typewritten or hand-written page; if writing longhand, make it legible

3. If you are writing about a bill, cite it by name and number

4. Be factual and support your position with factual information about how the bill might affect you

5. If you believe that legislation or a proposal is wrong— say so; state the likely adverse effects and suggest a better approach

6. Ask for the official's views, but do not demand support

7. Be sure your name and return address are legible

Most important, be visible. Express your opinions and ideas. After all, elected officials will not know your opinion until you tell them.

"Politics" also goes beyond what we think of as the traditional political arena. The media, for example, is a powerful, political tool. Women can write "letters to the editor" in newspapers and magazines to present pertinent ideas or respond to issues of the day. Television and radio offer public service announcements or other free, public opinion forums. Boycotts of products (including magazines and TV shows) accompanied by written and publicized messages of protest can send a potent message. Silence is approval. Visibility creates reality.

Judith Brady's words in her essay "The Goose and the Golden Egg" summarize the need for women in cancer-related politics:

> Our ultimate salvation from the ravages of cancer lies not in the doctor's office nor the pharmaceutical laboratory, but in the political arena. *1 in 3*

Pamela Haylock

Afterword

I can check them off on my fingers, my "sisters" from the Monday night cancer support group alumnae:

Margaret is enjoying her husband and rambunctious seven-year-old son, her part-time work, and (more or less) their extensive home remodeling project.

Jenny quit the job she detested, pulled up stakes, and is gloriously happy now with a new career as a park ranger.

Jill has taken off for another state with her new boyfriend, but keeps in touch periodically by phone.

Elizabeth is putting her amazing organizational skills into starting a breast cancer foundation.

And Linda . . . Linda died of her cancer. We will never forget Linda, with her keen artistic eye, her spunk, or that crazy sense of humor. She was the one who coined the term "CRS syndrome" ("can't remember shit") for the memory glitches we all complained about during chemotherapy. We honor her memory and will always mourn her loss.

But then there's Marty, who is involved in . . .

That's what cancer is. Both sadness and joy. Both dreams put on hold—and bright new beginnings.

And that is why I treasure, and wear with pride, the bold yellow button given to me by one of my "sisters":

Enjoy life. This is not a dress rehearsal.

Kerry McGinn

Resources

❖

Books and Publications

General Cancer Information

Coping Magazine (4 times/year) 2019 North Carothers, Franklin, TN 37064

Dollinger, M., Rosenbaum, E., and Cable, G. *Everyone's Guide to Cancer Therapy.* Andrews and McMeel, 1991.

Morra, Marion, and Eve Potts. *Choices: Realistic Alternatives in Cancer Treatment.* Avon, 1987.

Renneker, Mark. *Understanding Cancer.* (3rd ed.) Bull Publishing, 1988.

Cancer Therapies

Bruning, Nancy. *Coping with Chemotherapy.* The Dial Press, 1985.

Chemotherapy and You: A Guide to Self-Help During Treatment. (booklet) NIH Publication No. 83-1136, National Cancer Institute. (Available free from Cancer Information Service [CIS])

Eating Hints: Recipes and Tips for Better Nutrition during Cancer Treatment. (booklet) NIH Publication No. 87-2079. National Cancer Institute. (Available free from CIS)

Graham and Lomer, *Something's Got to Taste Good.*

Lerner, Michael. *Choices in Cancer.* Bolinas, CA: Commonweal.

Ramstack, J., Rosenbaum, E., and Carter, B. *Nutrition for Chemotherapy Patients.* Bull Publishing, 1990.

 Radiation Therapy and You: A Guide to Self-Help During Treatment. (booklet) NIH Publication No. 84-659, National Cancer Institute. (Available free from CIS)

What are Clinical Trials All About? (pamphlet) NIH Publication No. 85-2706. National Cancer Institute. (Available free from CIS)

Feelings and Relationships

Benjamin, Harold. *From Victim to Victor.* Jeremy Tarcher, 1987.

Brack, Pat and Ben. *Moms Don't Get Sick.* Melius Publishing, 1990.

Fiore, Neil A. *The Road Back to Health: Coping with the Emotional Side of Cancer.* Bantam, 1984.

Kushner, Harold S. *When Bad Things Happen to Good People.* Schocken Books, 1981.

Noyes, Diane and Mellody, Peggy. *Beauty and Cancer.* AC Press, 1988.

Sontag, Susan. *Illness as Metaphor.* Farrar, Straus and Giroux, 1978.

Surviving!: A Cancer Patient Newsletter. (6 times/year) c/o Stanford University Hospital, Department of Radiation Oncology, Division of Radiation Therapy, Room A035, 300 Pasteur Drive, Stanford, CA 94305.

Unconventional Cancer Therapies. Washington, D.C.: U.S. Government.

Taking Time: Support Groups for People With Cancer and the People Who Care About Them. (booklet) NIH Publication No. 88-2059, National Cancer Institute.

When Someone in Your Family Has Cancer. NIH Publication No.90-2685. National Cancer Institute. (For children; available free from CIS)

Breast Disease and Treatment

The Breast Cancer Digest: A Guide to Medical Care, Emotional Support, Educational Programs and Resources. 1984. NIH Publication No. 84-1691, National Cancer Institute.

Brinker, N. and Harris, C. E. *The Race is Run One Step at a Time.* Simon and Schuster, 1990.

Bruning, Nancy. *Breast Implants: Everything You Need To Know.* Hunter House, 1992.

Dackman, Linda. *Up Front: Sex and the Post-Mastectomy Woman.* Viking, 1990.

Kahane, Deborah. *No Less A Woman: Ten Women Shatter the Myths About Breast Cancer.* Prentice Hall, 1990.

Kaye, Ronnie. *Spinning Straw into Gold: Your Emotional Recovery from Breast Cancer.* Simon & Schuster, 1991.

Kelly, Patricia. *Understanding Breast Cancer Risk.* Temple, 1991.

Love, Susan and Lindsey, Karen. *Dr. Susan Love's Breast Book.* Addison-Wesley, 1991.

McGinn, Kerry. *The Informed Woman's Guide to Breast Health: Breast Changes That Are Not Cancer.* Bull Publishing, 1992.

Murcia, Andy and Stewart, Bob. *Man to Man: When the Woman You Love Has Breast Cancer.* St. Martin's, 1989.

Radiation Therapy: A Treatment for Early Stage Breast Cancer, NIH Publication No. 84-659. 1987. National Cancer Institute. (Available free from CIS)

Rollin, Betty. *First, You Cry.* New American Library, 1986.

Seltzer, Vicki. *Every Woman's Guide to Breast Cancer.* Viking Books, 1987.

Survivorship and Practical Issues

Acute Pain Management: Operative or Medical Procedures and Trauma, and *Pain Control After Surgery: A Patient's Guide.* U.S. Health and Human Services Agency for Health Care Policy and Research Publications Clearinghouse, P.O. Box 8547, Silver Spring, MD 20907, 800-358-9292 or 301-495-3453.

Cancer Treatments Your Insurance Should Cover. (pamphlet) Available free from the Association of Community Cancer Centers, 301-984-9496.

Cancer: Your Job, Insurance and the Law. (pamphlet) Available free from American Cancer Society.

Facing Forward: A Guide for Cancer Survivors. (booklet) NIH Publication No. 90-2424. 1990. National Cancer Institute. (Available free from CIS)

Larschan, Edward and Richard. *The Diagnosis is Cancer: A Psychological and Legal Resource Handbook for Cancer Patients, Their Families and Helping Professionals.* Bull Publishing, 1986.

National Coalition for Cancer Survivorship. *An Almanac of Practical Resources for Cancer Survivors: Charting the Journey.* (Mullan, Fitzhugh and Hoffman, Barbara, ed.). Consumer Reports Books, 1990.

Nessim, Susan and Ellis, Judith. *Cancervive: The Challenge of Life After Cancer.* Houghton Mifflin, 1991.

Ojeda, Linda. *Menopause Without Medicine.* Hunter House, 1992.

INFORMATION & SUPPORT ORGANIZATIONS

American Cancer Society   (800) ACS-2345
1599 Clifton Road NE, Atlanta GA 30329
(local chapters; Reach to Recovery; I Can Cope; Look Good, Feel
Better, etc.)

The Boston Women's Health Book Collective   (617) 924-0271
47 Nichols Avenue, Watertown MA 02172
(information on several women's health issues)

Breast Cancer Action   (415) 922-8279
P.O. Box 460185, San Francisco CA 94146
(political action, newsletter)

Breast Cancer Advisory Center   (301) 984-1020
11426 Rockville Pike, Suite 406, Rockville MD 20859
(information)

Cancer Information Service (CIS)   (800) 4-CANCER
(service of the National Cancer Institute)
(information over the phone or in a mailed packet)

Cancer Pain Hotline   (800) 422-6237

The Cancer Support and Education Center   (415) 327-6166
1035 Pine Street, Menlo Park CA 94025
(support, counseling, seminars)

Cancervive   (213) 203-9232
6500 Wilshire Boulevard, Suite 500, Los Angeles CA 90048
(support groups for people who have finished cancer treatment)

Congressional Caucus for Women's Issues   (202) 225-6740
2471 Rayburn Building, Washington D.C. 20515
(information on women's issues being addressed by the legislature)

The Commonweal Cancer Help Program   (415) 868-0970
P.O. Box 316, Bolinas CA 94924
(family consulting, children's training, other projects)

DES Action   (510) 465-4011
1615 Broadway, Suite 510, Oakland CA 94612
(information and support for DES-caused cancers or related concerns)

DES Cancer Network   (716) 473-6119
Box 10185, Rochester NY 14610
(meetings, telephone counseling, newsletter)

Encore (YWCA) (212) 614-2827
726 Broadway, 5th Floor, New York NY 10003
(local groups, exercise, and discussion for women with breast cancer)

The Komen Alliance (800) I'M AWARE
(Susan B. Komen Foundation)
(breast cancer information; sponsors "Race for the Cure")

National Alliance of Breast Cancer Organizations (212) 719-0154
1180 Avenue of the Americas, 2nd Floor
New York, NY 10036
(fact sheets and newsletter)

National Coalition for Cancer Survivorship (301) 585-2616
1010 Wayne Avenue, 5th Floor, Silver Spring MD 20910
(newsletter, insurance and employment information)

National Lymphedema Network (800) 541-3259
2211 Post Street, Suite 404, San Francisco CA 94115
(clearinghouse for information, newsletter)

National Women's Health Network
1325 G Street NW, Washington DC 20005
(information packets and booklets about women's health topics)

Planetree Health Resource Center (415) 923-3680
2040 Webster Street, San Francisco CA 94115
(will conduct literature searches of conventional and complementary
therapies for fee)

Physicians Data Query (PDQ) fax: (301) 402-5874
(service of the National Cancer Institute)
(information on the latest cancer treatments and research)

United Ostomy Association (800) 826-0826
36 Executive Park, Suite 120, Irvine CA 92714-6744
(self-help groups and information for people with colostomies and/or
urostomies)

Wellness Community (213) 393-1415
1235 Fifth Street, Santa Monica CA 90401
(support and education for emotional recovery, some local chapters)

Y-ME Breast Cancer Support Program (708) 799-8228 (24 hrs.)
18220 Harwood Avenue (800) 221-2141(9 A.M.-5 P.M. CST)
Homewood, IL 60430
(support, education, political action, newsletter, some local chapters)

Glossary

adjuvant chemotherapy—anticancer drugs used after all the known cancer has been removed with surgery/radiation, when there is a high risk of hidden cancer cells in the body

alopecia—partial or complete hair loss

aneuploid—cancer cells that do not contain the standard number of chromosomes

angiogenesis—the process by which cancerous tumors are able to induce the production of new blood vessels

atypia—cells that look abnormal under the microscope

autologous bone marrow transplant—the planned infusion of a patient's own tissue, previously withdrawn from the body and stored, as a rescue after very high-dose chemotherapy has destroyed the bone marrow in the body

axilla—armpit

axillary lymph nodes—the lymph nodes (bean-shaped filters) in the armpit

axillary node dissection—removal of the lymph nodes from the armpit during breast cancer surgery

barium enema—special X-ray of the colon and rectum after liquid barium has been given in an enema

benign—not cancerous

benign breast changes—collective term for any breast lump, lumpiness, nipple discharge, or pain that is not caused by cancer

bimanual pelvic examination—examination of the internal reproductive organs with both hands, two fingers of one hand in the vagina and the other hand on the abdomen

biological response modifier—a naturally-occuring substance, often grown in the laboratory, that changes the body's defenses

biological therapy—use of biological response modifiers to fight cancer *biopsy*—removal of a piece of body tissue so that it can be examined under a microscope

brachytherapy—radiation therapy given from a sealed radioactive source placed in the body

breast reconstruction—surgery to restore the breast mound (and sometimes areola and nipple) after a mastectomy

BSE (breast self-examination)—inspection and palpation of the breast tissue by the woman herself

CA 15-3—a breast cancer tumor marker measured with a specific laboratory blood test

CA-125—an ovarian cancer tumor marker measured with a specific laboratory blood test

calcifications—see *microcalcifications*

cancer—a condition in which highly abnormal cells, with the capacity to invade nearby body tissues and spread to other organs in the body, are growing abnormally

cancer risk counseling—advice given by medical geneticist or other health professional based on an individual's family history and other risk factors for cancer

capsular contracture—the formation of a fibrous shell around a breast implant

carcinogens—substances that can cause cell changes leading to cancer

carcinoma—cancer that develops in the covering or lining tissues of body organs

carcinoma in situ—presence of highly abnormal cells confined within a local area, without evidence of any invasion of nearby tissues. Some people consider this the earliest stage of cancer, while others believe it may be the most abnormal form of benign breast changes.

cathepsin-D—an enzyme that can be measured in breast cancer tissue, a high value of which is associated with a more aggressive cancer

CEA (carcinoembryonic antigen)—a tumor marker in some breast cancers and other kinds of cancers, measured with a specific laboratory blood test

chemotherapy—treatment of cancer with drugs to kill cancer cells

CIN (Cervical Intraepithelial Neoplasia)—premalignant changes in the cervical cells

clinical trial—a study that tests the safety and effectiveness of a new treatment in humans

colonoscopy—passage of a flexible lighted tube from the anus through the entire large intestine to inspect the colon and remove biopsy specimens if needed

colony stimulating factor (G-CSF or GM-CSF)—a substance that increases the blood cell production of the bone marrow

colposcopy—inspection of the cervix, vagina, and vulva through special lighted "binoculars" on a stand with wheels

Community Clinical Oncology Program (CCOP)—one of the local community programs that participates in clinical trials under the direction of the National Cancer Institute

complementary therapy—a treatment from a source other than traditional Western medicine that a patient uses along with traditional therapy

complete remission—disappearance of all signs of a cancer

Comprehensive Cancer Center—a specialized cancer hospital/research center that meets criteria set by the National Cancer Institute

cone biopsy (conization)—removal of a cone of tissue around the opening of the cervix to check for the presence of cancer cells

consent form—a piece of paper a patient signs before surgery or other procedures to indicate that she or he has been informed about the procedure and agrees to it

CT scan (CAT scan, computerized tomography)—a special X-ray study that gives cross-sectional views of the body organs

culdoscopy—inspection of the area behind the uterus and between the uterus and the rectum through a tube inserted through a tiny incision in the vagina

cyst—a benign fluid-filled sac

cystoscopy—inspection of the bladder (and removal of tissue specimens as needed) through a lighted tube inserted through the bladder opening

cytology—examination of cells under a microscope for the presence of cancer (as with a Pap smear)

D&C (dilation and curettage)—a gynecological procedure in which the cervix is enlarged (dilated) with a special instrument and the lining of the uterus in scraped out for diagnosis and/or treatment

DES (diethylstibesterol)—a synthetic estrogen given at one time to prevent miscarriages, now known to initiate rare gynecologic cancers in offspring; still used as treatment for some metastatic cancers

DNA (deoxyribonucleic acid)—genetic material in cells which determine inherited cell characteristics

detection—finding a body change that could be either benign or malignant

diagnosis—the process (or the doctor's conclusion) when the pathologist examines body tissues under the microscope to discover what a change means

diaphanography—a technique for imaging the breasts by directing an infrared light through the breast, photographing the transmitted light, and reading the film

diploid—cells having the normal number of chromosomes (46)

disease-free interval—the period of time after initial cancer therapy during which the person has no signs or symptoms of cancer

distant metastasis—spread of cancer cells through the blood or lymph system to a body organ away from the organ where it started

dominant breast lump—in breast examination, a three-dimensional lump that stands out from the surrounding tissue

Doppler study—a technique that images the blood vessels by transmitting sound waves through them

doubling time—the time it takes for a group of cells to double

duct carcinoma in situ (DCIS, intraductal carcinoma, noninvasive carcinoma, noninfiltrating carcinoma)—highly abnormal cells confined within the duct(s) of the breast

dysplasia—abnormal cells, often used to refer to atypical cells of the surface layer of the cervix

early detection—finding cancerous changes during their silent period or soon after, before they cause symptoms

endometrial biopsy—removal of a small piece of tissue from the lining of the uterus for examination by a pathologist

endoscopy—examination of a hollow organ or body cavity with a tubular instrument

estrogen—the female hormone that acts on the reproductive tract and the breasts

estrogen receptor—protein on some cells that attaches to the female hormone estrogen. A cancer tumor that is estrogen receptor positive has this protein on its cells and responds to the hormone.

excisional biopsy—removal of the entire lump during an open surgical biopsy

external radiation—radiation therapy delivered from a machine outside the body

false negative—an imaging study or biopsy that does not show cancer although cancer is present

false positive—an imaging study that shows suspicious changes that do not prove to be cancer

fibroadenoma—a kind of benign solid breast lump

"fibrocystic breast disease"—inaccurate and outdated term used for any breast change that is not cancer

flow cytometry—a test that analyzes the DNA content of a cancer to see if the cells have the normal number of chromosomes

FNA (fine needle aspiration)—withdrawal of fluid or a few cells from a breast lump through a needle into a syringe for diagnosis

frozen section—the freezing and slicing of biopsy tissue to make a slide for immediate diagnosis

grading—a way of judging how aggressive a cancer is likely to be by its appearance under a microscope

hematoma—a "pocket" of blood, usually as a complication of surgery

Her-2/neu oncogene—a specific rapid-growth gene found in about 30% of breast cancers

hormone receptor assay—test to check whether breast cancer cells contain specific proteins sensitive to the female hormone(s) estrogen and/or progesterone

hormone therapy—use of female or male hormones or antihormones to influence cancer growth

HPV—human papillomavirus or "genital warts"

HRT—hormone replacement therapy

HSV—herpes simplex virus type II, or "genital herpes"

hyperplasia—too much cell growth

hysterectomy—surgical removal of the uterus

hysteroscope—lighted tube that can be inserted through the cervix to see inside of the uterus *imaging technique*—any one of several techniques to picture the inside of the body without direct visualization (e.g., X-rays)

incisional biopsy—removal of a piece of a suspicious lump during an open surgical biopsy

infiltrating cancer—see *invasive cancer*

informed consent—a legal standard of minimum information a patient must receive before agreeing to surgery or other invasive procedure

initiators—substances/factors that cause direct cell damage leading to cancer

internal radiation—radiation therapy using a source of radiation inside the body, such as ovoids

intra-arterial chemotherapy—a way to deliver chemotherapy agents directly to a body organ by infusing them into the artery leading to that organ

intraperitoneal chemotherapy—delivery of chemotherapy through a special catheter into the space around the abdominal organs to "bathe" the tissues there

intravenous pyelogram—a special X-ray of the urinary tract after a contrast fluid has been injected into the patient's vein

invasive cancer (infiltrating cancer)—cancer cells that have penetrated and taken over surrounding normal tissue

laparoscopy—use of a narrow lighted tube inserted through a small skin incision to see inside the body

LATS flap (latissimus dorsi flap)—a breast reconstruction procedure in which skin and a piece of muscle from below the shoulder blade area are tunneled under the skin to help form a new breast covering

linear accelerator—a type of machine that delivers external radiation therapy

local therapy—a treatment for cancer in the organ where it originated

lumpectomy (tylectomy, quandrantectomy, wide excision, partial mastectomy)—removal of a cancerous breast lump with a margin of normal tissue as treatment (with radiation) of some breast cancers

lymphatic system—the system of lymph vessels and lymph nodes

lymphedema—swelling of an arm or leg because of blocked drainage of lymph fluid in the armpit or groin

lymph nodes—bean-sized filters along the lymph system which contain special white blood cells and which sometimes trap cancer cells

magnification views—special mammogram views that show breast tissue in more detail

malignant—cancerous

malignant transformation—the process by which a healthy cell becomes a cancer cell

mammograms—X-rays of the breasts

margin—the strip of apparently normal surrounding tissue removed with a cancer or a biopsy specimen

mastalgia—breast pain

metastasis—the spread of a cancer from one organ to another via the bloodstream or lymph system

microcalcification (calcification)—tiny calcified specks seen on a mammogram that can be associated with either benign or cancerous breast changes

microscopic nodal invasion—spread of cancer cells to nearby lymph nodes in numbers that can be seen only with a microscope

mitosis—the process of cell division

modified radical mastectomy—removal of island of breast skin with nipple and areola, all the breast tissue, and some or all of the armpit lymph nodes, but no chest muscle

MRI (magnetic resonance imaging)—method of imaging body by using magnetic field and radiowaves

multiple hits—a theory that an individual cancer requires several changes or "hits" to the normal cell

mutagen—anything that can cause a cell to change (mutate)

mutation—the process by which a cell changes

nadir—after a chemotherapy drug is given, the point at which the white blood cells and platelets reach their lowest level

needle biopsy—withdrawal of a core of tissue from a suspicious area through a special, wide "tru-cut" needle

needle localization biopsy—see *wire localization biopsy*

neoplasia—abnormal new growth that can be either benign or malignant

neutropenia—the condition of having too few of the white blood cells that protect against infection

noninfiltrating carcinoma—see *carcinoma in situ*

noninvasive carcinoma—see *carcinoma in situ*

nonproliferative change—a benign increase in body cells because the old cells are not being disposed of as fast as they should be

nuclear grade—a way of estimating the aggressiveness of a cancer by its appearance under the microscope

nuclear scan (bone scan, brain scan, etc.)—an imaging study done after an injection of a small amount of radioactive tracer into the vein

oncogenes—specific pieces of DNA in the cell that can be activated and cause uncontrolled cell division

oncologist (medical oncologist, radiation oncologist)—a doctor who specializes in cancer treatment

open biopsy—surgery to obtain a specimen of tissue that can be examined under the microscope

ostomy (colostomy, urostomy, etc.)—rerouting the healthy end of digestive or urinary tract to a new opening on the abdomen

palliation—the giving of treatment to relieve symptoms

palpation—examination of body tissue by feeling with the fingers

Pap smear—process of scraping a few cells from the cervix, placing them on a slide, staining them, and examining the slide under a microscope for presence of abnormal cells. Similar experimental process for fluid suctioned from nipple of breast.

partial remission—decrease in size of tumor by at least 50%

pathologist—doctor who specializes in examining tissue under a microscope for diagnosis

PCA (patient-controlled analgesia)—use of a preprogrammed intra-venous pump that delivers a set dose of pain medicine when the patient pushes a button

PDQ (Physicians Data Query)—computer information service run by the National Cancer Institute to make current cancer treatment information available, primarily to physicians

permanent section—lengthy process by which the pathologist slices and prepares biopsy tissue for definitive diagnosis

poorly-differentiated—cancer cells that look very different from normal cells in the same organ, associated with poorer prognosis

positive lymph node—a lymph node with cancer cells in it

proctosigmoidoscope (sigmoidoscope)—a lighted instrument inserted through the anus to look directly at the last twelve inches of the large intestine and take biopsy specimens if needed

P.R.N.—"as needed or requested," usually referring to when medication is given

progesterone—female hormone associated with producing breast milk and reproductive function

progesterone receptors—proteins that some cells have which are sensitive to the female hormone progesterone

prognosis—the statistically likely outcome of a disease

proliferative change with atypia—benign buildup of cells because abnormal cells are dividing more often than normal

proliferative change without atypia—benign buildup of cells that appear normal themselves but are dividing more often then normal

promoters—factors that encourage the development of cancer, but do not initiate the process

prophylactic mastectomy—surgical removal of a breast when there is no known cancer in it as a preventive measure

psychoneuroimmunology—the study of the influence of the brain on the immune system and the development of disease

radiation oncologist (radiation therapist)—doctor who specializes in treating cancer with radiation

radiation therapy (radiation oncology)—treatment of cancer with energy from atoms in transition

radiologist—doctor who specializes in imaging studies such as X-rays and CT scans

Reach to Recovery—American Cancer Society volunteer organization that pairs the woman undergoing breast cancer treatment with another woman who is a veteran of that treatment

recurrence—return of cancer after a period when it was thought to be gone (used by some people to mean only the return of cancer in the same organ)

regional extension—spread of cancer cells directly to an adjoining organ (not through bloodstream or lymph system)

RNA (ribonucleic acid)—material associated with the control of cell level chemical activities and DNA replication

sarcoma—a cancer that begins in the connective or supporting tissue of the body (bones, muscle, etc.)

sclerosing adenosis—a benign breast change, sometimes marked by microcalcifications on mammograms

screening tests—physical examinations, imaging studies, and/or laboratory tests used to check for the presence of disease in apparently healthy people

second opinion—therapy recommendation from a doctor other than the treating physician

seroma—collection of tissue fluid under the skin, usually after surgery

silent period—the time between when a cancer begins growing and when it begins causing signs or symptoms

simulation—"mockup" of radiation therapy from machine done before the treatment begins

sonography (ultrasound)—a kind of imaging study that records the echoes of soundwaves passing through the body

specimen radiography—technique for examining by X-ray a biopsy specimen of a breast change that cannot be palpated but shows on mammograms

staging—process for classifying a cancer by how extensive it is

stereotactic guided needle biopsy—a procedure for using a needle placed by computer to obtain a biopsy specimen of a breast change that shows only on mammography

stomatitis—inflammation of the lining of the mouth, often as a side effect of chemotherapy

systemic therapy—cancer therapy that treats the whole body

tamoxifen—a hormone medication used commonly in breast cancer treatment

tamoxifen chemoprevention trial—clinical trial of tamoxifen in 16,000 apparently healthy women to test whether it is safe and effective in preventing or postponing breast cancer

thermography—a breast imaging technique that measures body heat at skin level to identify hot spots due to inflammation or cancer

thrombocytopenia—the condition of having a serious deficiency of platelets in the blood

tissue expander—a kind of breast implant used in breast reconstruction, consisting of an expandable chamber connected to a port; the chamber is slowly expanded with weekly injections of salt water through the skin into the port

TNM classification—a system to classify cancers by the size of the tumor (T), lymph node involvement (N), and distant metastasis (M)

TRAM flap (transverse rectus abdominus myocutaneous flap)—a technique for reconstructing the breast by tunneling abdominal muscle, skin, and fat under the skin to make a new breast mound

transvaginal sonography—an imaging technique for the ovaries that measures the echoes of soundwaves transmitted by a probe placed in the vagina

tumor—a swelling or lump that can be either benign or malignant

tumor board—a group of cancer doctors from different specialties who meet periodically to pool their expertise and recommend therapy for individual cancer patients

tumor marker—a physical change that is not itself cancer but often occurs in connection with a cancer (e.g., elevated CEA or CA-125 in blood tests)

tylectomy—see *lumpectomy*

ultrasound—see *sonography*

upper GI series—X-rays taken of the upper digestive tract after patient swallows barium

VAIN (vaginal intraepithelial neoplasia)—carcinoma in situ of the vaginal canal

VIN (vulvar intraepithelial neoplasia)—or carcinoma in situ of the vulva

well-differentiated—cancer cells that still look somewhat similar to normal cells from the same organ, usually associated with a less aggressive cancer

wide excision—see *lumpectomy*

wire localization biopsy (needle localization biopsy)—special technique for surgical biopsy of the breast when the abnormality appears only on mammogram. The radiologist marks the area first with wires (or needles) and often dye, and then the surgeon cuts out the marked area.

xeromammograms—breast mammograms done using blueprint-type paper and white lines rather than film

Bibliography

Chapter 2

American Cancer Society. *Cancer Facts & Figures–1992*. American Cancer Society, Atlanta, 1992.

Boring, C. C., Squires, T. S., Heath, C. W. Cancer Statistics for African Americans. *Ca: A Cancer Journal for Clinicians*. 42(1):7-17, 1992.

Cohen, R. F., Frank-Stromberg, M. Cancer Risk and Assessment. In Groenwald, S. L., Frogg, M. H., Goodman, M., Yarbro, C. H. *Cancer Nursing Principles and Practice*. Second edition, Boston: Jones and Bartlett, 1990, 103-118.

Hay, L. L. *Heal Your Body*. Carson, CA: Hay House, Inc., 1988.

Johnson, E. Y., Lookingbill, D. P. Sunscreen Use and Sun Exposure: Trends in a White Population. *Archives of Dermatology*. 120:727-731, 1984.

LeShan, L. An Emotional Life-history Pattern Associated with Neoplastic Disease. *Annals of the New York Academy of Sciences*. 125:780-793, 1966.

Rowe, W. Identification of Risk. In *Risk and Reasons: Risk Assessment in Relation to Environmental Mutagens and Carcinogens*. New York: Alan R. Liss, 1986, 3-22.

Samet, J. M., Nero, A. V. Indoor Radon and Lung Cancer. *New England Journal of Medicine*. 320(9):591-593, 1989.

Selye, H. *The Stress of Life*. New York: McGraw-Hill, 1956.

Siegel, B. S. *Love, Medicine and Miracles*. New York: Harper & Row, 1986.

United States Department of Health & Human Services, Public Health Service. *Healthy People 2000: National Health Promotion and Disease Prevention Objectives*. 1990. (Publication #017-001-00474-0)

Chapter 9

American College of Sports Medicine Preventive and Rehabilitative

Exercise Committee. *Guidelines for exercise testing and prescription.* Fourth edition. Philadelphia: Lea & Febiger, 1991, 178-180.

The Cancer Letter. 18(23). NCI Plans Trials of Burzynski's 'Antineoplaston.' June 5, 1992.

The Cancer Letter. 18(26). Unorthodox Panel Considers NIH Madated Role in Study of Unconventional Medical Practices. June 26, 1992.

The Cancer Letter. 18(37). Politics, Short Tempers, Grievances Dominate NIH Panel on Unconventional Medical Practices. September 25, 1992.

Carlson, R. and Shield, B. *Healers on Healing.* Los Angeles: Jeremy P. Tarcher, Inc., 1989.

Coping. Radical Treatments in Mexico. Spring 1992, 30-31.

Cousins, N. *Head First: The Biology of Hope.* New York: E. P. Dutton, 1989.

Dehart, O. W. Quackery: The Modern Highwayman. (Editorial) *Southern Medical Journal.* 85(8):793-794, 1992.

Gorman, J. Take a Little Deadly Shade and You'll Feel Better. *The New York Times Magazine.* August 30, 1992.

Harner, M. The Hidden Universe of the Healer. In Carlson, R. and Shield, B. *Healers on Healing.* Los Angeles: Jeremy P. Tarcher, Inc., 1989.

Hay, L. L. *Heal Your Body.* Carson, CA: Hay House, Inc., 1988.

Issues. Special report prepared for the Technical Committee on Spiritual Well-Being. White House Conference on Aging. Washington, D.C.: Government Printing Office, 1971. Government Document No. 14369.

Krieger, D. The Timeless Concept of Healing. In Carlson, R. and Shield, B. *Healers on Healing.* Los Angeles: Jeremy P. Tarcher, Inc., 1989.

Lane, D. Music Therapy: A Gift Beyond Measure. *Oncology Nursing Forum.* 19(6):863-867, 1992.

Lane, I. W. and Comac, L. *Sharks Don't Get Cancer.* Avery Books, 1992.

Lerman, C., Rimer, B., Blumberg, B., Cristinzio, S., et al. Effects of Coping Style and Relaxation on Cancer Chemotherapy Side Effects and Emotional Responses. *Cancer Nursing,* 13(5):308-315, 1990.

Lerner, I. J. and Kennedy, B. J. The Prevalence of Questionable Methods of Cancer Treatment in the United States. *Ca: A Cancer Journal for Clinicians.* 42(3):181-191, 1992

Lerner, M. *Choice In Cancer: Integrating the Best of Conventional and Alternative Approaches to Cancer Treatment and Care.* Bolinas, CA: Commonweal, 1992.

McGinnis, L. S. Alternative Therapies, 1990: An Overview. *Cancer.* 67(6):1788-1792, 1991.

O'Connor, A. P., Wicker, C. A., and Germino, B. B. Understanding the Cancer Patient's Search for Meaning. *Cancer Nursing.* 13(3):167-175, 1990.

Pasquali, E. A. Learning to laugh: humor as therapy. *Journal of Psychosocial Nursing and Mental Health Services.* 28:31-5, 1990.

Payer, L. *Medicine and Culture: Varieties in Treatment in the United States, England, West Germany, France.* New York: Holt, 1988.

Radziewicz, R. M., and Schneider, S. M. Using Diversional Activity to Enhance Coping. *Cancer Nursing.* 15(4):293-298, 1992.

Siegel, B. S. *Love, Medicine & Miracles.* New York: Harper & Row, 1986.

Siegel, B. S. *Peace, Love and Healing.* New York: Harper & Row, 1989.

Simonton, O., Simonton, S. M., and Creighton, J. *Getting Well Again.* Los Angeles: Jeremy P. Tarcher, Inc., 1978.

Stein, D. *All Women are Healers: A Comprehensive Guide to Natural Healing.* Freedom, CA: The Crossing Press, 1990.

U.S. Congress, Office of Technology Assessment. *Unconventional Cancer Treatments.* OTA-H-405 Washington, DC: U.S. Government Printing Office, September 1990.

U.S. Congress, Office of Technology Assessment. *Unconventional Cancer Treatments.* OTA-H-406. Washington, DC: U.S. Government Printing Office, September 1990.

U.S. Department of Helth and Human Services. *Quackery: The Billion Dollar Miracle Business.* HHS Publication No. 85-4200.

Vines, S. W. The Therapeutics of Guided Imagery. *Holistic Nursing Practice.* 2(3):34-44, 1988.

Waitzkin, H. Information Giving in Medical Care. *Journal of Health Social Behaviors.* 26:81-101, 1985.

White, J. A. Touching With Intent: Therapeutic Massage. *Holistic Nursing Practice.* 2(3):63-67, 1988.

Winningham, M. L. Walking Program for People With Cancer: Getting Started. *Cancer Nursing.* 14(5):270-276, 1991.

Winningham, M. L. and MacVicar, M. G. The Effect of Aerobic Exercise on Patient Reports of Nausea. *Oncology Nursing Forum.* 15(4):447-450, 1988.

Young, J. H. *The Medical Messiahs*. Princeton: Princeton University Press, 1975 (expanded printing 1992).

Young, J. H. *American Health Quackery*. Princeton: Princeton University Press, 1992.

Chapter 16

American Cancer Society. *Cancer Facts and Figures—1992*. Atlanta, 1992.

DiSaia, P. J. and Creasman, W. T. *Clinical Gynecologic Oncology*. Third edition. St. Louis: C. V. Mosby, 1989.

Hubbard, J. L. and Holcombe, J. K. Cancer of the Endometrium. *Seminars in Oncology Nursing*. 6(3):206-213, 1990.

Sutton, G. P. The Significance of Positive Peritoneal Cytology in Endometrial Cancer. *Oncology*. 4(6):21-26, 1990.

U.S. Department of Health and Human Services, National Cancer Institute. *Cancer of the Uterus: Endometrial Cancer*. Research Report. NIH Publication No. 91-171, 1991.

U.S. Department of Health and Human Services, Public Health Service, National Institute of Health. *What You Need to Know About Cancer of the Uterus*. NIH Publication 88-1562, 1988.

Chapter 17

Andersen, B. L. How Cancer Affects Sexual Functioning. *Oncology*. 4(6):81-93, 1990.

DiSaia, P. J. and Creasman, W. T. *Clinical Gynecologic Oncology*. Third Edition, St. Louis: C. V. Mosby, 1989.

Gross, A. and Ito, D. *Women Talk About Gynecological Surgery*. New York: HarperCollins, 1991.

Jenkins, B. Patients' Reports of Sexual Changes After Treatment for Gynecologic Cancer. *Oncology Nursing Forum*. 15(3):349-354, 1988.

Nolte, S. and Hanjani, P. Intraepithelial Neoplasia of the Lower Genital Tract. *Seminars in Oncology Nursing*. 6(3):181-189, 1990.

Smith, J. M. *Women and Doctors*. New York: The Atlantic Monthly Press, 1992.

Thompson, L. J. Cancer of the Cervix. *Seminars in Oncology Nursing*. 6(3):190-197, 1990.

Chapter 18

Braun, M. L. *Still With Us: Research Needs of the DES-Exposed*. Presented to the National Institutes of Health Office of Research on Women's' Health. Bethesda, MD, June 12, 1991.

Chamorro, T. Cancer of the Vulva and Vagina. *Seminars in Oncology Nursing*. 6(3):198-205, 1990.

DiSaia, P. J. and Creasman, W. T. *Clinical Gynecologic Oncology* Third edition. St. Louis: C. V. Mosby, 1989.

DiSaia, P. J. and Creasman, W. T. *Clinical Gynecologic Oncology*. (Third Edition) Management of the female exposed to diethylstilbestrol. (Ch. 2, 49-66) St. Louis: C.V. Mosby, 1989.

Greenberg, E. R., Barnes, A. B., Resseguie, L., Barrett, J. A., et al. Breast Cancer in Mothers Given Diethylstilbestrol in Pregnancy. *New England Journal of Medicine*. 311(22):1393-1398, 1984.

Journal of the National Cancer Institute, NEWS. DES-Related Cancers Under Renewed Scrutiny. 84(8):565-6, April 15, 1992.

Journal of the National Cancer Institute, NEWS. DES Consensus Conference. 84(12):925-926, June 17, 1992.

Melnick S., Cole, P., Anderson, D. et al. Rates and Risks of Diethylstilbestrol-related Clear Cell Adenocarcinoma of the Vagina and Cervix: An Update. *New England Journal of Medicine*. 316(514):, 1987.

Nolte, S. and Hanjani, P. Intraepithelial Neoplasia of the Lower Genital Tract. *Seminars in Oncology Nursing*. 6(3):181-189, 1990.

Otte, D. M. Gynecologic Cancers. In Groenwald S. L., Frogge, M. H., Goodman, M. Yarbro, C. H. *Cancer Nursing: Principles and Practice* Second edition. Boston: Jones and Bartlett, 1990, 873-875.

PDQ. Vaginal Cancer: Information for Patients. National Cancer Institute, September, 1992.

PDQ. Vaginal Cancer: Information for Physicians. National Cancer Institute, September, 1992.

Robboy, S. J., Noller, K. L., O'Brien, P., Kaufman, R. H., et al. Increased Incidence of Cervical and Vaginal Dysplasia in 3,980 Diethylstilbestrol-Exposed Young Women. *Journal of the American Medical Association*. 252(21):2979-2983, 1984.

Seaman, B., and Seaman, G. *Women and the Crisis in Sex Hormones*. New York: Rawson Associates, 1977.

Smith, O. W. and Smith, G. V. S. Diethylstilbestrol and Treatment of

Complications of Pregnancy. *American Journal of Obstetrics and Gynecology*. 58: 821-834, 1948.

Chapter 19

Andersen, B. L., Hacker, N. F. Psychosexual Adjustment After Vulvar Surgery. *Obstetrics and Gynecology*. 62:459, 1983.

Chamorro, T. Cancer of the Vulva and Vagina. *Seminars in Oncology Nursing*. 6(3):198-205, 1990.

DiSaia, P. J. Current Treatment of Small Vulvar Cancers. The Article Reviewed. *Oncology*. 4(8):26-28, 1990.

DiSaia, P. J. and Creasman, W. T. *Clinical Gynecologic Oncology*. St. Louis: C. V. Mosby, 1989.

Hacker, N. F. Current Treatment of Small Vulvar Cancers. *Oncology*. 4(8):21-25, 1990.

Homesley, H. D. Current Treatment of Small Vulvar Cancers. The Article Reviewed. *Oncology*. 4(8):33, 1990.

Lamb, M. Vulvar Cancer: Patient Information Booklet. *Oncology Nursing Forum*. 31(6):79-82, 186.

Nolte, S. and Hanjani, P. Intraepithelial Neoplasia of the Lower Genital Tract. *Seminars in Oncology Nursing*. 6(3):181-189, 1990.

Phillips, G. L. Current Management of Vulvar Melanoma. *Oncology*. 4(9):61-64, 1990.

Sandella, J. Vulvar Self-Examination. *Oncology Nursing Forum*. 14(6):71-73, 1987.

Thiadens, S. R. J. *Lymphedema: An Information Booklet*. San Francisco, National Lymphedema Network.

Chapter 22

Brady, J. *1 in 3: Women with Cancer Confront an Epidemic*. Pittsburgh: Cleis Press, 1991.

Stocker, M. (ed.) *Cancer As a Woman's Issue*. Chicago: Third Side Press, 1991.

Epstein, S. S. *The Politics of Cancer*. San Francisco: Sierra Club Books, 1978.

Moss, R. W. *The Cancer Industry*. New York: Paragon House, 1991.

White, L. C. *Merchants of Death: The American Tobacco Industry*. New York: Beech Tree Books, 1988.

Index

ORDER FORM

10% DISCOUNT on orders of $20 or more —
20% DISCOUNT on orders of $50 or more —
30% DISCOUNT on orders of $250 or more —
On cost of books for fully prepaid orders

NAME

ADDRESS

CITY/STATE   ZIP

COUNTRY [outside USA]   POSTAL CODE

TITLE	QTY	PRICE	TOTAL
Breast Implants	@	$7.95	
Menopause Without Medicine	@	$12.95	
The New A-to-Z of Women's Health	@	$16.95	
The A-to-Z of Women's Sexuality	@	$14.95	
Once A Month	@	$9.95	
Getting Pregnant and Staying Pregnant	@	$12.95	
The Fertility Awareness Handbook	@	$11.95	
Running on Empty (paperback)	@	$13.95	
Running on Empty (hardcover)	@	$21.95	
Women's Cancers (paperback)	@	$14.95	
Women's Cancers (hardcover)	@	$24.95	

Shipping costs:
*First book: $2.50
($3.50 for Canada)
Each additional book:
$.75 ($1.00 for
Canada)
For UPS rates and
bulk orders call us at
(510) 865-5282*

TOTAL		
Less discount @_____%		( )
TOTAL COST OF BOOKS		
Calif. residents add sales tax		
Shipping & handling		
TOTAL ENCLOSED		
Please pay in U.S. funds only		

❑ Check   ❑ Money Order   ❑ Visa   ❑ M/C

Card # _____ Exp date _____

Signature _____

3602

Complete and mail to
Hunter House Inc., Publishers
PO Box 2914, Alameda CA 94501-2914
Phone (510) 865-5282 Fax (510) 865-4295
❑ Check here to receive our book catalog

OAM-R2 8/93